Aromatherapy for Health Professionals

For Churchill Livingstone

Commissioning Editor: Inta Ozols
Project Editor: Dinah Thom
Copy Editor: Michael Dean
Indexer: Nina Boyd
Project Manager: Valerie Burgess
Design Direction: Judith Wright
Pre-press Project Manager: Neil Dickson
Pre-press Desktop Operator: Kate Walshaw
Sales Promotion Executive: Maria O'Connor

Aromatherapy for Health Professionals

Shirley Price FISPA MIFA
Practitioner and Lecturer in Aromatherapy, Hinckley, Leicestershire

Len Price MIT FISPA
Lecturer in Aromatherapy, Hinckley, Leicestershire

Foreword by

Dr Daniel Pénoël
International Consultant and Lecturer in Clinical Aromatology, Aouste-sur-Sye, Drôme, France

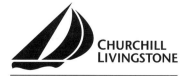
CHURCHILL
LIVINGSTONE

EDINBURGH HONG KONG LONDON MADRID MELBOURNE NEW YORK AND TOKYO 1995

CHURCHILL LIVINGSTONE
Medical Division of Pearson Professional Limited

Distributed in the United States of America by Churchill
Livingstone Inc., 650 Avenue of the Americas, New York,
N.Y. 10011, and by associated companies, branches and
representatives throughout the world.

First published 1995
    Reprinted 1995
    Reprinted 1996

ISBN 0 443 04975 0

British Library Cataloguing in Publication Data
A catalogue record for this book is available from
the British Library.

Library of Congress Cataloging in Publication Data
A catalog record for this book is available from
the Library of Congress.

The
publisher's
policy is to use
**paper manufactured
from sustainable forests**

Produced through Longman Malaysia, GPS

Contents

Foreword

It is an honour and a joy to write the foreword for the first work on aromatherapy published in English specifically covering the use of aromatherapy in hospital settings.

Aromatic plants have been used for thousands of years in every part of the world by numerous civilizations which, driven by their intuition and their sense of observation, were able to find answers to their health problems in the plant environment. The lack of understanding of the biochemical mechanism of action of a substance has never been an obstacle to its effective use!

Fortunately, the progress of analytical chemistry enables us to begin to understand the extraordinary laboratory which exists inside the aromatic plant cell; we can only be spellbound by realizing the fantastic complexity of this biochemical manufacture, and the harmonious and powerful result represented by the aromatic substance inside the plant called the essence.

Essential oils, made out of natural aromatic molecules, are endowed with so many physiological and pharmacological properties that they find applications in almost every field of medicine, not only curatively but also from a preventive medicine point of view.

Len and Shirley Price rightly insist upon the importance of using whole essential oils from the highest quality aromatic plants. Having created strong links with growers and distillers, in particular in the Drôme area, which is the foremost county in France for the production of aromatic and medicinal plants, they know that excellent therapeutic results can only be obtained by the use of top quality products and that poor quality or adulteration will lead to disappointment and eventually to discarding the whole method.

Provided that the practitioner has the relevant information and has undergone the appropriate training, and that the aromatic extracts used conform to medical quality criteria, aromatherapy and aromatology can bring real complementary help to many patients, far beyond the anti-stress massage approach.

I am convinced that this book paves the way for a massive development of the use of essential oils medically and pharmaceutically in the UK. I congratulate Shirley and Len Price wholeheartedly for their dedication and their continuous efforts to promote true aromatherapy, and I wish this book the great success it deserves.

D.P.

Acknowledgements

The authors are grateful to the following people for supplying information about the practice of aromatherapy in different countries that appears in Chapter 15:

- Dr D. Pénoël, aromatologist and medical doctor—France
- Mary Killeen SRN RCT and Catherine Pepper SRN SCM PHN, both aromatherapists—Republic of Ireland
- Marlene Cadwallader BAppSci (Nursing) and Margaret Meyer SRN and midwife, both aromatherapists, and Margaret Tozer, aromatherapy tutor and practitioner—Australia
- Laraine Kyle MSN RN CMT, aromatherapist and nurse tutor, and Eli Muller, research associate and licensed massage therapist at the Touch Research Institute, University of Miami Medical School—USA
- Lucile Bischoff, aromatherapy tutor and practitioner, and Karen Ten Velden, aromatherapist—South Africa
- Margaret Demleiter, occupational therapist and naturopath, and Ulrike Rädlein, State Registered Nurse, both aromatologists—Germany

- Gian Furrer, Rosemary Mathys, Ueli Morgenthaler and Jan Straub; the last three are all aromatologists and nurses—Switzerland.

The authors would also like to thank the following people, whose understanding and help has been much appreciated: Alan Barker, for the tremendous interest and support he has given us over the last months; Daniel Pénoël, for his notable interest in the book and for writing the foreword and the text on aromatherapy in France; Dinah Thom and Michael Dean (who checked our work so thoroughly) for their editorial advice; Katya Svoboda, Jane Buckle, Susan Lundie, Maureen Farrell, for reading relevant parts of the text at manuscript stage; David Witty, for his specialist advice on essential oil research; Marie Hélène Grandvoinnet, Doreen Bishop and Harry Thomte for their patient willingness to be photographed for the massage section; the secretarial staff of Shirley Price Aromatherapy Limited, Justine Finney, Julie Dillabough and Suzanne Jordan, for their prompt attention to requests (even when otherwise occupied) and last but not least our five grandchildren, for not minding too much the infrequency of their overnight visits.

S.P.

Preface

Many books have been written on aromatherapy aimed at the general public, and although they can be of interest to the health professional, they are of limited use. This book directly addresses health professionals and their need for properly targeted information on aromatherapy.

Since the 1980s standards of training in aromatherapy have been much improved, guided by leading schools and the professional associations. This prompted the writing of my *Aromatherapy Workbook* (1993) aimed at helping student aromatherapists acquire in-depth knowledge of the physiological and psychological effects of essential oils. Amongst other things it stresses the importance of specifying accurately the essential oils employed, for example by using botanical names in preference to the common ones.

In addition, because professionals such as physiotherapists, occupational therapists and nurses have become increasingly aware of the possibilities of using essential oils in hospices, hospitals, clinics and community care work, my husband, Len, and I felt the time was ripe for a book aimed specifically at health professionals. This feeling was confirmed at the lectures and workshops we gave at hospitals throughout the UK in the period 1992 to 1994. It became clear that many nurses were introducing essential oils into their hospitals without attending an accredited training course. This may be because much aromatherapy course time is concerned with full-body-massage—something which professionals in healthcare situations rarely have the time to carry out. In response to this, we have introduced aromatology (aromatic medicine) courses (without full-body-massage) into our college. We also feel that a book which emphasizes the need to obtain extensive knowledge of essential oils before using them on sick people will discourage the incorrect application of these powerful agents—which in several unfortunate cases has led hospitals to forbid their use.

This book also contains guidelines on the preparation of a professionally based policy and protocol to present to hospital management when applying for permission to use essential oils in a healthcare setting. In those hospitals where the use of essential oils has already been introduced on a correct footing, many trials and projects have been carried out. Although not constituting research in the accepted scientific sense of the word, such studies are extremely valuable to the future acceptance of aromatic medicine. It is hoped that, by publicizing some of them here, more health professionals will be encouraged to continue the good work. It is not possible to do double blind tests with an aromatic substance—the presence or absence of an aroma being immediately obvious to the participants—so many more trials, projects and single-case studies are needed to demonstrate unequivocally the efficacy of these holistic medicines.

We trust that this book will be of value to you and your colleagues.

Hinckley, 1995   S.P.

Botanical abbreviations

The following Latin botanical terms and abbreviations are used in this book:

Latin	Abbreviation	English
caulis	caul.	stem
cortex	cort.	bark
flos	not abbreviated	flower
folium	fol.	leaf
fructus	fruct.	fruit
herba	herb.	herb
lignum	lig.	wood
pericarpium	per.	peel
radix	rad.	root
ramunculus	ram.	twig
resina distillata	res. dist.	distilled resin
rhizoma	rhiz.	rhizome
semen	sem.	seed
strobilus	strob.	cone

Introduction

Historical use of essential oils

Plants and their extracts have been used since time immemorial to relieve pain, aid healing, kill bacteria and thus revitalize and maintain good health. Many books have now been written on aromatherapy, its history usually being included in more or less detail. Suffice it to say here that although the word itself was not coined until this century, the distilled extracts from plants—the essential oils—have been employed by mankind for countless years in religious rites, perfumery and hygiene. Cedarwood oil, known to have been used by the Egyptians for embalming and for hygienic purposes 5000 years ago, was probably the first 'distilled' oil to have been produced although the process used is open to speculation (Ch. 2). Both the plant and the essential oil of lavender were used by the abbess Hildegard of Bingen as early as the 12th century and by the 15th century it is thought that essential oils of turpentine, cinnamon, frankincense, juniper, rose and sage were also known and used (Pignatelli 1991). About 60 oils were known and used in perfumes and medicines by the beginning of the 17th century (Valnet 1980 p. 28).

Modern evidence for the antiseptic powers of essential oils

Towards the end of the 19th century, the first acknowledged research to prove the antiseptic properties of essential oils was by Chamberland (Chamberland 1887). This was followed early in

1

the 20th century by Cavel's research into the individual effects of 35 essential oils on microbial cultures in sewage. The most effective oil required to render inactive 1000 cc of culture was found to be thyme (0.7 cc). Two other well-known oils showing high efficacy were sweet orange (1.2 cc, 3rd) and peppermint (2.5 cc, 9th) (Cavel 1918). The antiseptic power of several oils has now been proved to be many times greater than that of phenol. Certain essential oils have also been shown to be effective against different bacteria, e.g. lemon, which is one of the best in its antiseptic and bactericidal properties, neutralizing both the typhus bacillus and *Staphylococcus aureus* in a matter of minutes. Cinnamon kills the typhus bacillus when diluted 1 part in 300 (Valnet 1980 p. 36).

Professor Griffon, a member of the French Academy of Pharmacy, made up a blend of seven essential oils (cinnamon, clove, lavender, peppermint, pine, rosemary and thyme), to study their antiseptic effect on the surrounding air when sprayed from an aerosol; all the staphylococci and moulds present were destroyed after 30 minutes (Valnet 1980 p. 37). See Chapter 6 for more recent studies on the antiseptic properties of essential oils.

The bacteriological approach of aromatherapy is an extremely complex field of the utmost interest, opening the way to the ecological understanding and management of the different colonies and floras that live in cohabitations—or at war—within us. Allopathic medicine begins to realize that the misuse of antibiotics leads to numerous side-effects and sometimes results in chronic disastrous conditions (i.e. systemic candidosis) that could have been avoided if medical aromatherapy had been implemented in due time (Pénoël 1993 personal communication).

Today, the properties of herb volatile oils are researched in many centres throughout the world. A typical case is the excellent work carried out in Scotland since the early 1980s by Deans and Svoboda at the Scottish Agricultural College, Auchincruive (Ch. 4), assessing antibacterial and antifungal properties of essential oils and their constituents.

Wide-ranging application

Essential oils can be put to a multitude of uses both in general practice and in hospitals, as this quote from Dr J Valnet illustrates:

The doctor who is familiar with essential oils can use them to treat a whole range of infections—pulmonary, hepatic, intestinal, urinary, uterine, rhinopharyngeal and cutaneous (infected wounds and suppurating dermatoses). The use of these oils usually produces satisfactory results, provided they have been prescribed wisely and that, in the case of certain long-standing complaints, the treatment is followed for a long enough period. Aromatic therapy can neutralise enteritis, colitis and putrid fermentations, and can relieve chronic bronchitis and pulmonary tuberculosis. The colon bacillus cannot resist essential oils.

(Valnet 1980 p. 41)

Orthodox medicine currently uses plant material to help cure diseases which previously had a high death rate. 20 years ago, four out of every five children with leukaemia lost their lives; now, four out of five are returned to health with the aid of vincristine and vinblastine, derivatives of the rosy periwinkle—a plant used for hundreds of years by tribal healers as a medicine (Craker 1990). The snakeroot plant from India is now used in the western world to treat hypertension; digitalis, for heart conditions, is produced from the humble foxglove and the well-known rhododendron is used in the treatment of fatigue. 'Plants are an intrinsic part of natural medicine, and not even the most orthodox doctor can get by without them; indeed they represent the link between the natural and the orthodox, the traditional and the ultra-new' (Pahlow 1980).

Phytotherapy is the name increasingly given to the use of the whole, or part, of the plant for medicinal purposes. Aromatherapy and aromatology (similar to aromatherapy but without massage) are branches of this, utilizing only the essential oils produced by distillation and citrus oils produced by expression. These are simple to use and administer, yet can compete with the steroids and antibiotics used in allopathic medicine today without the body's defence mechanism becoming exhausted or tolerance developing to them.

The basic reason which accounts for the diversity of conception and application of aromatherapy lies in the very nature of the aromatic substance. Lending itself to easy cutaneous penetration, being endowed with the capacity to influence the mind through its powerful impact upon the olfactive sense, and owing multiple and strong pharmacological properties to its highly active molecular components, it was natural for the aromatic substance to find developments in so many areas.

(Pénoël 1993 personal communication)

Powerful healing agents

Many plant extracts used in the production of conventional medicines are, like the foxglove, poisonous and therefore exceptionally low doses are employed. Some essential oils are also toxic when used incorrectly and the most powerful of these are not normally available to aromatherapists (Chs 3 and 4). Essential oils are concentrated and intensely energetic in their effects, so very little is needed (even of those in general use) for successful treatment—dilutions generally being in the range 0.05-3%, depending on the oil used. Apart from the difference in the intensity of the aroma, no apparent benefit is gained from higher concentrations, particularly where the problem is an emotional one, although they are used in certain medical conditions and aromatology.

Their mode of action

It cannot yet be proved exactly *how* they work, but research and extensive anecdotal evidence exists to prove that they *do* work. In the distant past, essences have been used to heal wounds, inhibit the decay of flesh (as in mummification) and reduce the spread of infection (as in the time of the Black Death)—all without anyone knowing how they worked, just as the humble aspirin was in use for many years before anyone knew its mode of action.

Bios is the Greek word for life and essential oils may be classed as probiotic (for life), as opposed to antibiotic (against life). To illustrate this point, antibiotics kill not only harmful bacteria, but also the beneficial flora that we need to keep us healthy, leaving the body in a weakened state.

Carefully selected essential oils kill only the bacteria inimical to the successful functioning of the body (Valnet 1980 p. 45). Some essential oils also possess antiviral and fungicidal qualities. 'A serious condition obviously authorises the use of antibiotics, and in high doses; but one should be aware that the price of a cure may be a permanent disability' (Valnet 1980 p. 54).

User-friendly

Natural, whole essential oils can be used on living tissue with minimal unwanted effects (unlike some synthetic drugs, however successful these may be against their intended targets). Also, the human body accustoms itself to the effects of chemical synthetics, leading to escalating doses. This has not been found to be the case with essential oils, which retain their effectiveness in repeated applications and can in fact strengthen the living tissue while killing off the unwanted bacteria (Valnet 1980 p. 48).

Quantities of essential oils used

Tens of thousands of tonnes of essential oils are used by the food and perfume industries (Verlet 1993). It is important to realize that the total amount of essential oil used by the aromatherapy profession is extremely small compared with these industries, and this contributes to the difficulties of obtaining high quality, pure, natural oils (Ch. 2). Some oils which could be beneficial when used in aromatherapy are not generally supplied by distillers because they are not required by the giant users. Fortunately, however, a small number of independent distillers produce essential oils solely for aromatherapy use, although such products tend to be more expensive.

Economy of use

Compared with the very high price of drugs (perhaps due to the tremendous research and development costs) essential oils are extremely inexpensive—a factor which should interest those in charge of public health funds. Not only that, they are pleasant to use for both patient and carer.

In many hospitals and hospices they are used not only to improve the quality of a patient's life but in waiting rooms to relieve the anxiety of relatives and friends. More specifically, they can be used in place of secondary drugs, which might be prescribed to counteract iatrogenic effects of the primary drugs being taken. They have been found to aid relaxation effectively, both pre- and post-operatively, to regenerate tissue in cases of severe burns and inflammation, and to relieve pain in cases of rheumatoid arthritis. They have helped to improve the quality of life for the terminally ill, and they have also found important uses in maternity care.

Areas of use

Essential oils are used extensively by aroma-therapists and aromatologists to improve or uplift a patient's state of mind. The effect of the attitude of mind on a person's health is being recognized more and more and essential oils can play an important part here. Florence Nightingale said 'what nursing has to do ... is to put the patient in the best condition for nature to act upon him', reinforcing the ancient tag *medicus cura, natura sanat*—the doctor treats, nature cures.

By far the majority of essential oil users are outside the medical profession, some people using them merely on instruction from one of the many books written for the general public on the subject. They are simple to use and it should come as a relief to GPs that minor everyday ailments such as a sore throat or a winter cold, and even some more serious problems like bronchitis, sinusitis and rheumatism can be treated in the home easily and successfully, leaving the doctor's time free for the cases requiring expert knowledge.

All this is achievable by anyone, without professional medical skills. However, in France (where aromatherapy came to the UK from) doctors prescribe essential oils for internal use in capsules or in drops diluted in alcohol, or in suppositories and pessaries (Ch. 15). They are used externally in dressings, fumigations, inhalations, ointments and in foot, hand or complete baths. The original concept of aromatherapy in England, as introduced by Mme Maury was to use the essential oils in massage only—suitably diluted in a fixed vegetable oil. This unfortunately led to the belief that that is all there is to aromatherapy, and the authors are actively trying to correct this image. It needs the medical profession not only to take an interest but also to use its professional skills to utilize these precious commodities to their fullest capabilities in order to bring the benefits of this aromatic therapy to the hospitals of the world in the 21st century.

The subject of aromatherapy involves pharmacy and farming, botany and bodies, medicine and chemistry, toxicity and safety, all so intertwined and interconnected that it is scarcely possible to disentangle the ramifications for the purpose of setting them down without some repetition and much cross-referral.

REFERENCES

Cavel L 1918 Sur la valeur antiseptique de quelques huiles essentielles. Comptes Rendus (Académie des Sciences) 166: 827

Chamberland M 1887 Les essences au point du vue de leurs propriétés antiseptiques. Annales Institut Pasteur 1: 153–154

Craker L E 1990 News and commentary. The Herb, Spice and Medicinal Plant Digest 8(4): 5

Pahlow M 1980 Living medicine. Thorsons, Wellingborough, p. 9

Pignatelli M F 1991 Viaggio nel mondo della essenze. Muzzio, Padora

Valnet J 1980 The practice of aromatherapy. Daniel, Saffron Walden

Verlet N 1993 Commercial aspects. In: Hay, Waterman (eds) Volatile oil crops. Longman, Harlow, ch. 8

Essential oil science

SECTION CONTENTS

1

The genesis of essential oils

Introduction

Aromatherapy involves the use of essential oils, all of which are derived from plants. Anyone wishing to practise aromatherapy must gain as full an understanding of the plants concerned as possible, so that the oils can be used knowledgeably to their best effect. This chapter enables the practitioner to do this, looking beyond the oil in the little glass bottle to the plant from which it was extracted, its growing environment and the family to which it belongs.

BOTANY FOR AROMATHERAPISTS
Taxonomy

The precise identification of plants was made possible by the Swedish naturalist Carl von Linné or Linnaeus (1707–1778) who developed the system of classifying organisms in groups according to their similarities. Over the years the Linnaean method of classification has been subject to modification but is still at the core of the international taxonomical system used today. Each plant belongs to a family and is given a generic name based on structural characteristics (written in italics with an initial capital), and a specific name (lower-case italics). For example, lavender is classified in the following way:

Kingdom	Plantae
Division	Tracheophyta
Subdivision	Spermatophytina
Class	Dicotyledons
Subclass	Asterdae
Order	Lamiales
Family	Lamiaceae (syn. Labiatae)
Genus	*Lavandula*
Species	*angustifolia*

To identify a plant accurately it is necessary to give at least the generic and the specific name: lavender is therefore referred to as *Lavandula angustifolia*. However, there are further divisions below this level, such as subspecies (often denoting a geographic variation of a species), variety (see below), forma (denoting trivial differences), cultivar, chemotype and hybrid (see below). Therapists prescribing essential oils must take care to identify precisely the plants from which they are derived, and this means giving not only the generic and specific names but also specifying, where necessary, the chemotype, variety, cultivar etc., as well.

Variety: indicates a rank between subspecies and forma. They are named by adding var. and the italicized variety name, e.g. *Citrus aurantium* var. *amara*. It used to indicate a major sub-division of a species, or a variant of horticultural origin or importance (although these are now labelled cultivar), and many names of horticultural origin reflect the historical use of the variety rank.

Cultivar: cultivated variety, and a rank known only in horticultural cultivation. These names are nonlatinized and in living languages (usually the name of, or chosen by, the originator). They are not italicized, and appear within quotation marks, e.g. *Lavandula angustifolia* 'Maillette'.

Chemotype: visually identical plants with significantly different chemical components, resulting in different therapeutic properties. Chemotypes occur naturally in plants grown in the wild, and some species throw up many chemical variations. Named by the abbreviation ct. followed by the constituent, e.g. *Thymus vulgaris* ct. alcohol, *Thymus vulgaris* ct. geraniol etc.

Hybrid: natural or manmade crosses between species. Represented by ×: e.g., *Mentha × piperita*, a cross between *M. aquatica* and *M. spicata*.

Metabolism

Each plant is a vibrant chemical factory capable of transforming the electromagnetic rays from the sun into energetic substances which are then available for the plant's use. The plant takes up water and minerals from the soil through its roots and carbon dioxide from the air through its leaves. These supplies are then converted by the energy absorbed from the sun into a simple 6-carbon sugar, glucose, which provides food for the plant's growth. The waste product of this chemical change is oxygen. The whole process is called photosynthesis, and because it is essential to the life of the plant it is termed primary metabolism. Secondary metabolism products include alkaloids, bitters, glycosides, gums, mucilages, saponins, steroids, tannins and essential oils, which are not necessary for the vital functions of the plant. Of these secondary metabolites the essential oils have the greatest commercial significance, being used in many industries (Verlet 1993).

The metabolic changes in plants are made possible by the action of protein catalysts known as enzymes. Enzymes are highly specific and assist in only one particular reaction (as they do in humans). To function they need manganese or iron combined with a tiny amount of energy which is to be found stored in phosphate bonds in the plant chemicals. The secondary metabolites vary widely in chemical structure and their purpose and function in the plant is little understood. Whatever else they may do, they give the plant its aroma and flavour and often have a significant physiological effect on people.

Why does a plant contain essential oil?

Before seeing how an essential oil comes into being, it is worth reflecting on what value essential oils have for plants. This has been debated for many years and there is as yet no definitive answer. Perhaps there never will be, given that science is much better at answering the question 'how?' than the question 'why?', and that there is no obvious commercial advantage in this knowledge. Most research effort is put into investigating the properties and effects of the oils themselves, and it is left to disinterested investigators at universities to look into what possible use the essential oils may be to the plant. However, conjecture on the subject has thrown up many possible reasons:

- To prevent attack by herbivores: both mono- and sesquiterpenes are involved in various ways, such as acting as insect hormones to interfere with the development of the feeding insects, or a straightforward repellent action.
- To prevent attack from insects: it has been shown that the number of oil glands in a plant increases when it is under attack by insects (Carlton 1990, Carlton et al 1992).
- To prevent attack by bacteria, fungi and other microorganisms: there is ample in vitro proof available of the antifungal and bactericidal properties of herb volatile oils (see section on aromatograms in Ch. 6).
- To aid pollination by attracting bees and other insects such as moths and bats (Harborne 1988).
- To help in the healing of wounds inflicted on the plant itself, and to act as an energy reserve.
- To help survival in difficult growth conditions: for instance by the production of allelopathic compounds, such as 1,8-cineole and camphor, which are freely given off from the plant and find their way to the soil where they prevent other plants from growing (Deans & Waterman 1993).
- To prevent dehydration and afford some degree of protection in hot dry climates by surrounding the plant with a haze of volatile oil, thus helping to prevent water loss from its foliage. One of the oldest plants in the world whose leaves can be 10% oil by weight, is the eucalyptus. Living root stock of this plant has been found dating back thousands of years to the Ice Age (Dr Mike Crisp 1986 Australian National Botanic Gardens). The free oil vapour emanating from other ancient plants, e.g. the pine trees, can be smelt easily when walking in pine forests on a sunny day.

The genesis of essential oils

Plants produce a tremendous variety of chemicals, including a major group of compounds, the terpenes. According to Harborne (1988) there are more than 1000 monoterpenes and possibly 3000 sesquiterpenes presently identified. The phenylpropanoids constitute another much smaller but significant group. In essential oils most of the components belong either to the terpene group, based on the mevalonic acid pathway, or to the phenylpropene group which is based on shikimic acid.

Terpenic structures

The starting point for the terpenes is acetyl coenzyme A (mentioned also in Ch. 6), which leads to the 6-carbon mevalonic acid. This is then modified to the 5-carbon skeleton known as the isoprene unit (Fig. 1.1) which occurs in two forms: IPP (isopenteny1 pyrophosphate) and DMAPP (dimethylallylpyrophosphate).

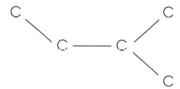

Fig. 1.1 isoprene carbon skeleton

Monoterpenes are hydrocarbons (consisting only of carbon and hydrogen atoms) and are formed from two isoprene units; sesquiterpenes are formed from three isoprene units and diterpenes from four isoprene units. Molecules larger than this do not occur in essential oils because their molecular weight exceeds the limit imposed by the distillation process. Monoterpenes constitute the most commonly occurring kind of terpene in plant volatile oils and exist in acyclic (open ended chain) and cyclic (closed circle chain) forms. The latter can be either monocyclic or bicyclic. Further complexity arises when double bonds are added (oxidation) or subtracted (reduction), and also by the addition of various oxygen-containing active groups. Numerous alcohols, ketones, aldehydes and esters are formed by this process.

Phenylpropanoid structures

Precursors (phenylalanine, tyrosine, cinnamic acid) of these molecules act to form compounds which have a 6-carbon benzene ring attached to a

Fig. 1.2a anethole

Fig. 1.2b apiole

short (3-carbon) chain to form a phenylpropene. Even though phenylpropenes occur much less frequently in essential oils than terpenes, they can have a great impact on the aroma, flavour and therapeutic effect. Examples of phenylpropenes in essential oils are estragole in tarragon oil, cinnamaldehyde in cinnamon bark oil, apiole (Fig. 1.2b) in fennel seed oil and anethole (Fig. 1.2a) in aniseed oil.

The chemistry of essential oils is discussed further in Chapter 2.

Secretory structures

There are different sites in which the essential oils are synthesized and stored, broadly dependent on the plant family. Oils may be found in various parts of plants, e.g. leaves, seeds, petals, roots, bark etc. Sometimes different oils occur in more than one site in a plant, for example two oils are produced by the cinnamon tree (bark, leaf), and three different oils by the orange tree (leaf, blossom, peel).

Essential oils and their mixtures with resins and gums are commonly found in special secretory structures. The type of structure is one of the characteristics of a family, as is shown below.

- Oil cells and resin cells
  —Lauraceae (e.g. cinnamon)
  —Zingiberaceae (e.g. cardamom, ginger, turmeric)
  —Piperaceae (e.g. black pepper)
  —Myristicaceae (e.g. nutmeg)
- Cavities, sacs, oil reservoirs (schizolysigenous)
  —Rutaceae (e.g. orange)
  —Myrtaceae (e.g. clove, eucalyptus)
- Oil or resin canals
  —Apiaceae or Umbelliferae (e.g. dill)
  —Pinaceae (e.g. pine, cedarwood)
  —Burseraceae (e.g. myrrh)
- Oil ducts
  —Compositae or Askraceae (e.g. tarragon)
- Glandular hairs
  —Labiateae or Lamiaceae (e.g. lavender, rosemary)
- Internal hairs
  —Orchidaceae (e.g. vanilla).

Stereochemistry

The word stereo comes from the Greek meaning solid, and here refers to the spatial arrangement of atoms within the molecule. A different relative position of the same atoms in a molecule has an influence on the chemical activity, and this influence may be slight or very great. In the phenylpropenes the short carbon chain may be attached to the benzene ring at three different locations, known as ortho, meta and para. A molecule may adopt a different shape with side chains differently orientated. These isomers are known as cis and trans forms.

Some molecules are dextrorotatory (+) and others laevorotatory (-) which indicates their capability to rotate light. The stereochemical form of the molecules will determine the odour and flavour attributes of the oil (Craker 1990). For example, carvone is present as as (+)-carvone in spearmint, where it has the aroma of spearmint, and as (-)-carvone in caraway, where it has the aroma of caraway. Clearly, a small change in shape can have a significant effect.

Fig. 1.3a   l-carvone

Fig. 1.3b   d-carvone

CHEMICAL VARIATION WITHIN SPECIES

Chemotype is a term applied to plants of the same genus and species, which have the same external appearance but differ, sometimes considerably, in their internal chemical composition. These chemotypes usually occur naturally in plants growing in the wild, and can be due in part to cross-pollination. The place and manner of growing will also promote internal changes and many essential-oil-bearing plants, e.g. rosemary and thyme, are prone to this kind of change due to genetic and environmental factors. They become resistant to local pests and diseases and have adapted to make the best use of the soil and other surrounding conditions. Such plants are termed landrace, and strains which yield specified chemical constituents are sought and selected for propagation by cloning. Cuttings are then cultivated which will produce the specific oils required. Included in this category are the thymes and lavenders flourishing wild on the sunny dry hills of Provence.

Thyme chemotypes

The thyme plant is particularly prolific in spontaneously producing strains bearing essential oils of different composition. Some of these are described below:

- *Thymus vulgaris* ct. thymol. The thymol-bearing thyme is strongly antiseptic and aggressive to the skin due to the presence of this phenol. Cut in the spring the essential oil contains 30% thymol plus paracymene (a monoterpene hydrocarbon). When the same plant is cut in the autumn the essential oil may be found on analysis to have 60–70% thymol and less paracymene.

- *Thymus vulgaris* ct. carvacrol. This variant behaves in the same way as the thymol chemotype of thyme, but the phenol involved is carvacrol. In the spring the essential oil contains 30% carvacrol which increases to 60-80% in the autumn.

Fig. 1.4   thymol

Fig. 1.5   carvacrol

The thymol and the carvacrol chemotypes do not flourish at high altitudes but are cultivated in the valleys. Both of these chemotypes are often referred to as red thymes, and they are major antiinfective agents with a wide range of action (Belaiche 1979). The alcohol-containing chemotypes below are referred to as yellow or sweet thymes.

• *Thymus vulgaris* ct. linalool. The linalool-bearing thyme has a herbaceous smell and (like the thujanol and terpineol thymes) is grown at high altitudes. It contains the alcohol linalool and the ester linalyl acetate, therefore the essential oil from the linalool thyme is gentle in action. This chemotype is antibacterial, fungicidal (e.g. against *Candida albicans*),

Fig. 1.6   linalool

viricidal, parasiticidal and vermifugal, and neurotonic and uterotonic (Franchomme & Pénoël 1990 p. 403).

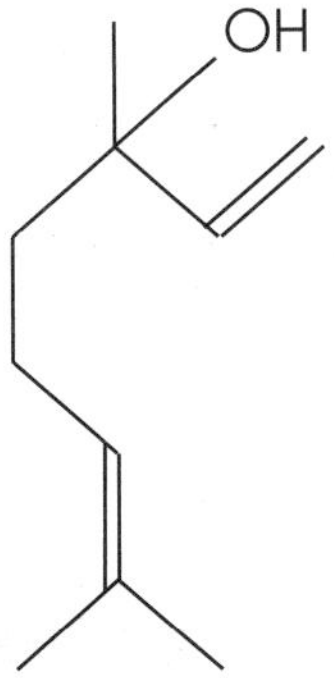

• *Thymus vulgaris* ct. thujanol-4. In contrast to all the other chemotypes of thyme, the thujanol-4 type does not show seasonal variation in the constitution of the essential oil, but is the same all year round with a content of 50% of the alcohol trans-thujanol-4, 15% approximately of terpinen-4-ol and 15% approximately of cis-myrcenol-8. It is found only in the wild because it has resisted all attempts to cultivate it— cloning has not yet been successful. It has a floral smell. The oil is antiinfective, bactericidal (against chlamydia), and a powerful viricide. It stimulates the immune system (by augmenting IgA) and the circulation. It is described as a neurotonic, balancing to the nervous system, hormonelike and antidiabetic (Franchomme & Pénoël 1990 p. 403). According to Roulier (1990 p. 305) this oil is a notable hepatic regenerant, and is non-irritant.

• *Thymus vulgaris* ct. α-terpineol. The oil from this chemotype contains the ester terpenyl acetate (more so in the spring) and the alcohol α-terpineol (80–90% free and esterified). The smell is slightly peppery. This chemotype, like that of geraniol and linalool, does not possess the aggressive effects of the red thymes (thymol and carvacrol) and can be used safely on children, sensitive skins and mucous surfaces (Roulier 1990 p. 305).

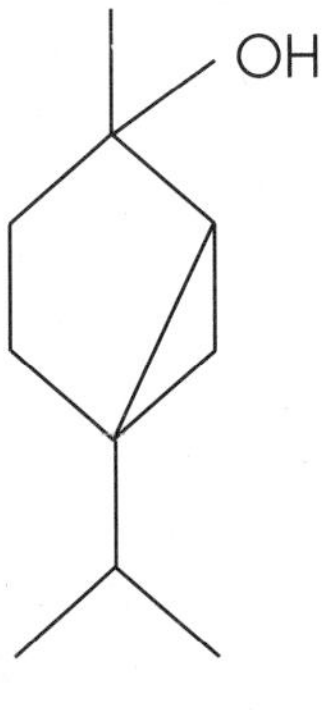

Fig. 1.7   thujanol-4

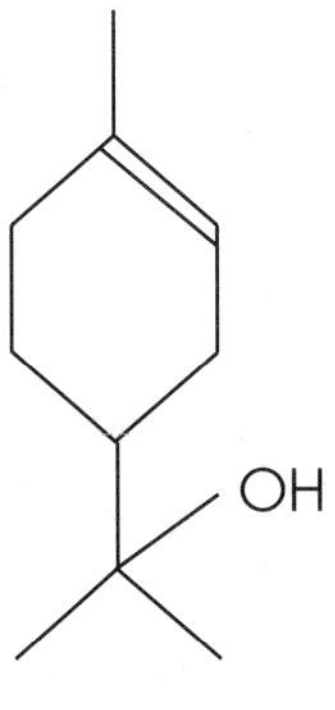

Fig. 1.8   α-terpineol

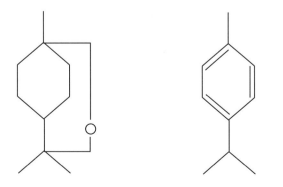

Fig. 1.9 geraniol

Other *Thymus vulgaris* chemotypes also exist. The cineole-bearing plant has 80–90% 1,8-cineole. According to Franchomme and Pénoël (1990 p. 403), the paracymene chemotype is analgesic when applied to the skin, a notable antiinfective agent and useful for rheumatism and arthritis.

Altitude and light

The following effects on the essential oil are more pronounced the lower down the thyme plant is grown:

- the essential oil becomes more aggressive—more phenolic, antiseptic
- the colour of the essential oil changes also, from a light straw to a more reddish hue
- the structure of the main component molecule goes from open chain to cyclic chain to benzene ring base.

These effects are due in part to the quality of light available to the plant. At high altitude (1000 m) there is a relatively high amount of free ultraviolet, and at low altitude there is less ultraviolet but a proportional increase in the more penetrating infrared frequencies. The plant responds to the quality of light falling on it (and to other growing conditions) and will produce different chemicals accordingly. Another influencing factor is the latitude of the country of origin. The further north, the more phenols are produced—for instance *Thymus vulgaris* grown in Finland produces up to 89% phenol (von Schantz et al 1987).

More changes may be expected in oil bearing plants in the future due to chlorofluorocarbon damage to the ozone layer. Higher levels of ultraviolet radiation are expected to reach the surface of the earth, and research carried out to test the possible effects of this on plant growth suggests that alpine species will be least affected by increased ultraviolet radiation. The tests involved *Aquilegia canadensis* and *Aquilegia caerulea*. The first normally grows at low altitude, and showed less growth during the test, but the second, Alpine, plant was not affected in this way: it even grew extra leaves (Gates 1991).

- *Thymus vulgaris* ct. geraniol. The geraniol thyme is grown at high altitude and the oil contains the ester geranyl acetate and the alcohol geraniol (80–90% in free and esterified forms); again there is a seasonal variation. This thyme is very assertive and when grown in a field of mixed thymes it gradually predominates. It has a lemony smell. It is interesting to note that the creeping wild thyme (*Thymus serpyllum*) which is found everywhere in the hills also has a somewhat lemony smell because the geraniol chemotype is dominant and is gradually taking over. The properties are antiviral, antifungal and antibacterial, and uterotonic, neurotonic and cardiotonic (Franchomme & Pénoël 1990 p. 402).

Fig. 1.10a 1,8-cineole   **Fig. 1.10b** *p*-cymene

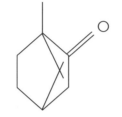

Fig. 1.11a verbenone   **Fig. 1.11b** camphor

Rosemary chemotypes

Rosemary has three chemotypes, all of which are used in aromatherapy.

- *Rosmarinus officinalis* ct. camphor (camphor 30%) with the properties: mucolytic, cholagogic, diuretic, circulatory decongestant/stimulant (vein), emmenagogic (non-hormonal), muscle relaxant.
- *Rosmarinus officinalis* ct. cineole (1,8-cineole 40–55%) whose properties are anticatarrhal, mucolytic, expectorant, fungicidal (e.g. *Candida albicans*), bactericidal (*Staphylococcus aureus, Staph. alba*).
- *Rosmarinus officinalis* ct. verbenone (verbenone 15–40%, alpha pinene 15–35%). It is anti-catarrhal, expectorant, mucolytic (Roulier 1990 p. 298); and antispasmodic (which Roulier attributes to the cineole and camphor chemotypes—this has been our experience also), cicatrizant and an endocrine system regulator (Franchomme & Pénoël 1990 p. 393).

Roulier (1990) classes the camphor and cineole chemotypes together as being similar in effect.

Other chemotypes

Some further examples of plants with different chemotype forms are:

- *Artemisia dracunculus* [TARRAGON] ct. estragole, ct. sabinene (Tucker & Maciarello 1987)
- *Ocimum basilicum* [BASIL] ct. linalool, ct. estragole, ct. eugenol (Sobti et al 1978)
- *Salvia officinalis* [SAGE] ct. thujone, ct. cineole (there is also a thujone-free chemotype) (Tucker & Maciarello 1990, Tegel 1984)

- *Valeriana officinalis* [VALERIAN] ct. valeranone, ct. valeranal, ct. cryptofouranol (Bos et al 1986).

There are also two chemotypes of melissa: *Melissa officinalis* ct. citral, *M. officinalis* ct. citronellal (Lawrence 1989).

Clones of lavender and lavandin

True lavender grown from seed is properly called *Lavandula angustifolia* Miller (syn. *L. officinalis, L. vera*). However, many cultivated lavender plants are cloned (i.e. grown from cuttings taken from the hardiest, healthiest and biggest plants with a high yield of good quality oil), the name of the most popular clone being *L. angustifolia* 'Maillette'. In contrast, all cultivated lavandin plants are grown from cuttings—they are all clones.

Three lavenders are described below:

- *Lavandula angustifolia* contains mainly alcohols and esters. It is a calming oil recommended to induce sleep. However, an overdose has the opposite effect—another pointer to the importance of using these potent oils correctly. It has been recommended for respiratory ailments, asthma, spasmodic cough (whooping cough), influenza, bronchitis, tuberculosis and pneumonia (Valnet 1980) on account of its antiinflammatory properties.
- *Lavandula latifolia* [SPIKE LAVENDER] (syn. *L. spica*) is a much bigger plant, with larger florets than true lavender. It contains very few esters and is slightly lower in alcohol content also, containing instead about 30% of the oxide 1,8-cineole and about 15% of the ketone, camphor. It is an efficient expectorant and is also indicated for severe burns (Franchomme & Pénoël 1990 p. 365) because it is well tolerated on all parts of the skin surface. It is especially useful in chest and throat infections, whether for children or adults (Roulier 1990 p. 276).
- *Lavandula stoechas* contains about 75% ketones, of which almost two thirds is fenchone. It shares some properties with the previous two, being anticatarrhal, antiinflammatory and cicatrizant. This plant has never been cultivated

commercially (Meunier 1985) and is not easily available, which is perhaps fortunate because it is sometimes confused with true lavender, which is almost free of ketones. Its effects can be found in many other, safer oils.

Lavandins

Lavandin is the natural hybrid between *Lavandula angustifolia* Miller and *Lavandula latifolia* Medicus and the resulting plant has been given many taxonomical classifications, such as *Lavandula × burnatii* 'Briq.', *Lavandula spica-latifolia* 'Albert', *Lavandula × hortensis* 'Hy', *Lavandula × leptostachya* 'Pau', etc. All these are in common use along with other names—Duraffourd (1982 p. 77) calls it *Lavandula fragrans*. This confused state of affairs prompted Tucker (1981) to research the situation and he reported that the correct name for lavandin is *Lavandula × intermedia* 'Emeric' ex 'Loiseleur', which covers all the lavandin cultivars, and is the name used in this book.

The × in the names above indicates that the plant is a hybrid or cross-pollinated plant and should not be mistaken for a variety of true lavender. Lavandin plants occur naturally, but cultivators have attempted for many years to find a plant that combines the oil yield of *L. latifolia* with the aromatic quality of *L. angustifolia*. As a result there are many cultivars which are currently grown, including *L. × intermedia* 'Abrialis', *L. × intermedia* 'Super', *L. × intermedia* 'Grosso' and *L. × intermedia* 'Reydovan'. Although the Abrialis clone is deteriorating after long use, other cultivars are now producing large quantities of lavandin oil.

When lavandin is used, especially in clinical trials, it is necessary to specify the particular clone. The two clones of lavandin most used in aromatherapy are:

- *Lavandula × intermedia* 'Reydovan'. Principally antibacterial, antifungal and antiviral, it is also a nerve tonic and expectorant.
- *Lavandula × intermedia* 'Super' (as can be seen from the above, sometimes known under other names, e.g. *L. × burnatii* 'Super') is, on the other hand, calming and sedative and antiinflammatory. In fact, it seems to have most of the

properties of its mother plant true lavender (Franchomme & Pénoël 1990 p. 364), and its production is on the increase. It was this oil which was used by Buckle (1993) along with true lavender in tests on cardiac patients and the oil from this cultivar of lavandin was found to be more effective than oil of lavender in this instance.

Other factors in plant change

Not only nature brings about changes in the chemicals produced in the plant: farmers have an influence too. The use of chemicals in the form of artificial fertilizers influences some of the plant's secondary metabolites, but has little effect on the essential oils. These are composed in the main of carbon, hydrogen and oxygen, whereas fertilizers are made up of nitrogen, phosphates and potassium. However, as fertilizers cause an increase in plant growth, there may be an overall gain in the yield of essential oil.

Herbicides, pesticides, and heavy metals are absorbed by the plant, and the more pesticides absorbed, the more there are as residue. A safe level of residue may be regarded as 2 mg (per) 1 kg of dry material. Some safe herbicides are decomposed in the plant, but still add to the residue levels. In Europe, toxic pesticides are prohibited, but unfortunately they are still manufactured and sent to third-world countries (Wabner 1993). Heavy metals do not pass over in the steam distillation process.

Toxic residues are easily transferred to expressed essential oils, absolutes and vegetable oils, which makes it imperative to know the source and the manner of growing of such oils before using them therapeutically. Although many pesticides contain volatile molecules, it is not clear how many of these are taken into a distilled oil. Wabner (1993) also concludes that 'aromatherapy is much safer than eating' because 'no clear cut correlation has been established between pesticide residues in oils and detrimental effects on the human organism' and 'essential oils are used in much smaller quantities and much less frequently than food products'. This article emphasizes the fact that health professionals should purchase their oils for therapeutic use from a trusted supplier, who knows where to buy high quality pesticide-free and unadulterated essential oils and fixed vegetable oils, especially as the latter normally make up 97% or more of any oil prepared for application to the skin.

Yield of essential oils

Many factors affect the yield regarding both quantity and quality of an essential oil. Some are under the control of the farmer, e.g. time of harvest, chemicals used and plant selection, and others are more or less beyond control, e.g. available light, altitude, temperature and rain (although drought can be remedied by use of a watering system).

Essential oils are not spread equally throughout all parts of the plant, and the quantity of essential oil varies throughout the growing season to such a degree that the time of harvesting, even to the time of day, can have a critical effect on the quantity and quality of essential oil derived (see Fig 1.12).

The farmer may have to face the fact that the time of maximum yield of essential oil may not coincide with the quality required. This is especially so when the oils are intended for therapeutic use, when compromise on quantity against quality cannot be accepted.

SOME ESSENTIAL-OIL-PRODUCING FAMILIES

Plants are divided into families, and it is generally recognized that familial therapeutic characteristics may be ascribed to many of the individual plants in a particular family, e.g. the beneficial influence on the digestive system of the citrus oils or the warming action of oils from the ginger family. There can also be toxic familial effects as with the solanaceae and umbelliferae.

Several hundred essential oils of plant origin have been identified worldwide. Many are not commercially available, either because the yield of distilled oil is so small that the cost is prohi-

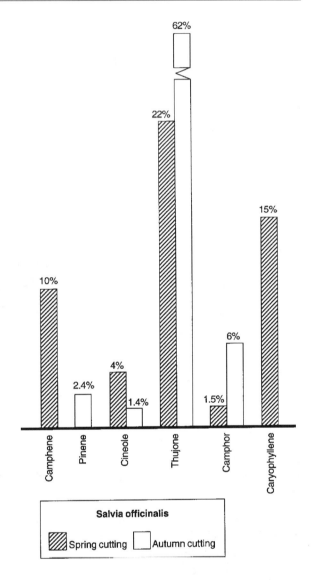

Fig. 1.12 Variation in sage oil constituents between spring and autumn cuttings (Lamy 1985, 1988)

bitive (as in the case of lime blossom oil) or because there is no commercial demand for them. Between 40–60 essential oils are normally used by the professional aromatherapist, and most of their suppliers offer in the region of 70–80 oils. These oils generally belong to just a few of the many plant families, and the families dealt with below include the majority of plants utilized in the production of essential oils.

In the text below, the common names have been used, since to name each species or variety is not necessary when giving general familial characteristics. The botanical name will be used when talking about a specific essential oil. Where only one oil from a family is used in aromatherapy, no family characteristics will be given, only the therapeutic properties of that individual oil. Where there are several oils in a family, only the family properties will be given. Individual properties of selected individual oils can be found in Appendix A. The lists are not comprehensive, since reference can be made to the many books written on the properties of essential oils for details of oils not mentioned here. Neither will every essential oil appear on the lists—the main purpose of this book is to make health professionals aware of the principal beneficial essential oils.

Reference sources for the properties and effects of the essential oils below are as follows: Bardeau (1976), Bernadet (1983), Duraffourd (1982), Franchomme & Pénoël (1990), Lautié & Passebecq (1984), Mailhebiau (1989), Roulier (1990). Other references will be mentioned individually.

Angiospermae

Because they bear seeds, all the plants used to obtain essential oils belong to the spermatophytina subdivision. The vast majority also belong to the class angiospermae, or flowering plants.

Annonaceae

This family consists of only one species, *Cananga odorata*, with two varieties, of which ylang ylang is one (*C. odorata* forma *genuina*). Distillation of *Cananga* forma *odorata* is carried out in several stages, and the resulting oils (superior, extra and grades 1, 2, and 3) each have a slightly different aroma. It is not easy to procure the complete oil, which would be preferable for the holistic aspect of aromatherapy (Price 1993). *Cananga odorata* is antiinflammatory, antispasmodic, hypotensive, sedative and a tonic to the pancreas.

Apiaceae (or Umbelliferae)

Examples include aniseed, caraway, coriander, dill, fennel. In this family the oils are usually extracted from the seeds, which are renowned for their digestive properties, having been used in digestive and aperitif drinks and consumed for centuries with bread, and as an accompaniment with cheeses such as Munster. Umbellifer therapeutic qualities are aromatic, carminative, stimulating, tonic and warming when they are grown naturally in dry regions. It should be noted that this family is also known as the hemlocks. If grown in the shade or humid regions a narcotic principle can develop (particularly so for green anise), and many of the oils in this family are neurotoxic due to the presence of particular ketones or phenolic ethers.

Asteraceae (or Compositae)

Examples include calendula (only available in a fixed oil), chamomiles, tagetes and tarragon. The essential oils from plants in the asteraceae are taken from the flowerheads. In the case of calendula they are macerated in a fixed oil—not distilled, so the fixed oil also contains larger nonvolatile plant molecules, e.g. some colour molecules. Two of the main characteristics of essential oils in this family are their anti-inflammatory and antiseptic action on the skin and digestive tract. Many toxic oils come from this family, e.g. the artemisias, which contain a high percentage of ketones or phenolic ethers. *Tagetes glandulifera* also contains a ketone (tagetone) at 50% and should be used with caution.

Burseraceae

Examples include frankincense (olibanum) and myrrh. These two are available as distilled oils and as resinoids, but the distilled oils are required for therapeutic use. The family has cicatrizant properties, indicating their use for scar tissue, ulcers and wounds. They are also expectorant, and useful in catarrhal conditions. *Boswellia carteri* is also indicated in the treatment of depression, immune system deficiency and perhaps cancer (Franchomme & Pénoël 1990 p. 328).

Geranaceae

The oil utilized from this small family comes from one or two species belonging to the *Pelargonium* genus. The essential oil of *Pelargonium graveolens* has antiinflammatory, astringent, cicatrizant, haemostatic properties and is antidiabetic (Valnet 1980 p. 133).

Lamiaceae (or Labiatae)

Examples include basil, clary, hyssop, lavandin, lavender, marjoram, melissa, origanum, patchouli, peppermint, rosemary, sage, savory and thyme. Of all the families in the plant kingdom none offers a greater array of healing aromatic plants than the labiatae. These plants are strongly aromatic due to the volatile essence stored in special glandular trichomes, which are found principally on the leaves. In general the labiatae family produce aromatic and stimulating essential oils, which bring vigour and energy to the whole body (or sometimes to just one system in particular, e.g. the respiratory system). They have remarkable antiseptic and antispasmodic properties and are also emmenagogic and sudorific. Oils derived from the lamiaceae are generally safe, with one or two exceptions. These include *Salvia officinalis* and *Hyssopus officinalis* [HYSSOP], both of which contain ketones (thujone and pinocamphone respectively) which could be neurotoxic in overdose. Ingestion of large quantities of these oils can lead to serious disorders, as pointed out by the Centre anti-poisons de Marseille (Rouvière & Meyer 1983 p. 6).

Many of the plants in this family have been in constant culinary use for thousands of years, not only to add flavour but for their preservative and health giving properties as well. The use and ingestion of herbs and their essential oils in small doses over such a long period of time proves their fundamental safety.

Lauraceae

Examples include cinnamon and camphor. Members of this family generally have a pleasant aroma, sometimes strong and penetrating, a warm pungency, sometimes bitter. All the oils are considered to be uplifting in their effects (Rouvière & Meyer 1983 p. 7). However, the majority of the family are highly toxic (e.g. cassia, laurel and sassafras), and they will not be recommended in this book because similar therapeutic properties can be found in other safer oils. Even when they are not actually dangerous, these oils still need extra care in use.

Myrtaceae

Examples include cajuput, eucalyptus, niaouli, clove and tea tree. The essential oils from this family are contained in cells in the body of the leaf. They are powerful antiseptics (especially to the respiratory system) as well as being antiviral (see Table 4.6), astringent, stimulant and tonic. It is advisable to use them with caution as they can be irritant. This is particularly so of the oils of clove and adulterated niaouli. It is worth mentioning that the latter oil is adulterated more often than not and will not have the desired therapeutic effect. Care should be taken to obtain the genuine oil. Rectified *Eucalyptus globulus* [TASMANIAN BLUE GUM] is irritant because the natural balance has been destroyed. It can be identified because the rectification process renders it clear, but unfortunately very little of the eucalyptus oil harvest escapes this fate.

Oleaceae

Jasminum officinale is a well-loved oil, but a steam-distilled essential oil does not exist and the absolute is subject to the most deplorable adulteration. 'A large number of synthetic materials, some of them chemically related to the jasmones ... are of great help ... to reproduce the much wanted jasmine effect at a much lower cost. ... Jasmine absolute is frequently adulterated. Its high cost seems to tempt certain suppliers and producers beyond their moral resistance' (Arctander 1960 pp. 310–311). If it is to be used therapeutically at all, only the finest quality should be sought and purchased. On account of its aroma it is often used as a relaxant.

Piperaceae

Examples include black pepper and cubeb. *Piper nigrum* is the most used of the two oils and possesses analgesic, anticatarrhal, expectorant, stimulant and tonic properties.

Poaceae or Gramineae

Examples include citronella, lemongrass, palmarosa, vetiver. Most of this family have antiinflammatory and tonic properties, *Vetivera zizanioides* [VETIVER] also being stimulating to the immune system (Franchomme & Pénoël 1990 p. 405). Oils from this family, together with lemon and/or grapefruit oil are used to make a cheap 'melissa' oil.

Rosaceae

The only essential oil utilized from this family is rose otto, whose aroma is less sweet than the absolute oil obtained by solvent extraction. Strictly speaking, only the distilled oil should be used by health professionals (see *Jasminum officinale*). Rose otto has astringent, antihaemorrhagic, cicatrizant, hormonal and neurotonic properties.

Rutaceae

As mentioned above, citrus oils are derived from three different sites in the plant. Examples are:

- peel: bergamot, grapefruit, lemon, mandarin and orange
- leaf: petitgrain oils, mainly from the bitter orange, but occasionally from other citrus trees
- flower: neroli.

To obtain citrus peel oils for aromatherapy the rinds are not distilled, but mechanically squeezed by a method called expression. They are therefore not strictly essential oils and contain many large molecules which would not come over in distillation. These include colour and waxes, and the latter can precipitate if the oils are stored incorrectly or kept for a long time. In storage these oils are especially susceptible to oxidation and the precious active aldehydes may degrade into acids. To help prevent this, nitrogen gas is used to displace the air as the oil is decanted. For small bottles, the air can be displaced with tiny glass beads (see Useful Addresses) as the level of the oil goes down with use.

Expressed oils from the citrus family have a refreshing aroma and are antiseptic, stimulating and tonic, having significant effects on the whole of the digestive tract. This is especially true of bergamot and bitter orange, which are stomach anti-spasmodics. These two are also sedative to the nervous system.

Both leaf and flower oils from *Citrus aurantium* [ORANGE] are obtained by distillation and their aroma is sweeter and more floral than the peel oils. The best leaf and flower oils are obtained from the bitter orange, *C. aurantium* var. *amara*: both of these oils are effective on the nervous system, relieving irritability and promoting sleep (Mailhebiau 1989 pp. 269–270). Petitgrain bigarade from the bitter orange tree (bigarade means bitter) is indicated for infected acne, whereas neroli bigarade is indicated for varicose veins and haemorrhoids, and is also a hypotensor.

Styraceae

The only extracts from this family which are of interest to aromatherapists are the resinoids from *Styrax tonkinensis* and *S. benzoin* (both have the common name benzoin). This resinoid is anticatarrhal and expectorant. It is also cicatrizant, promoting healing on cracked and dry skin. Care should be taken when purchasing this oil: some sources abroad still use benzene as a solvent (forbidden in Europe), and a high proportion of benzene may remain in the final product.

Valerianaceae

Examples include valerian and spikenard. The general family effects are calming and sedative, and are helpful in the reduction of varicose veins and haemorrhoids. Valerian provided the blueprint for the drug valium, and the true oil is very difficult to obtain.

Verbenaceae

Lippia citriodora [TRUE VERBENA] is rarely obtainable; like jasmine it is frequently grossly adulterated and *Thymus hiemalis* is often sold in its place as Spanish verbena (Arctander 1960 pp. 648–649).

Coniferae

The conifer class display their seeds directly, rather than hiding them within a structure of petals.

Cupressaceae and pinaceae

Examples include cypress, juniper (cupressaceae), and pine, cedar (pinaceae). The chief common characteristics of essential oils derived from plants in these two families of the conifer class are their good general hygienic qualities, particularly in the air and on the skin. Cedar, cypress and juniper also have specific individual properties for urinary tract infections, the circulatory system and scalp maladies (Rouvière & Meyer 1983 p. 7). Thuja belongs to the pinaceae, but is not used in aromatherapy because of its high ketone content.

Summary

Traditionally, plants have been the main source of materials to maintain health and prevent ill-health, and it is only comparatively recently that they have been replaced by synthetics. The study of plant structure and function should not be regarded as an interesting but inessential requirement for aromatherapy. The more knowledgeable the therapist is about the exact botanical derivation of the oils used, the more effective he or she can be in practice.

REFERENCES

Arctander S 1960 Perfume and flavor materials of natural origin. Published by the author, Elizabeth, New Jersey

Bardeau F 1976 La médecine aromatique. Laffont, Paris

Belaiche P 1979 Traité de phytothérapie et d'aromathérapie. Maloine, Paris, vol. 1: 93

Bernadet M 1983 La phyto-aromathérapie pratique. Dangles, St-Jean-de-Braye

Bos R, van Putten F M S, Hendriks H 1986 Variations in the essential oil content and composition in individual plants obtained after breeding experiments with a *Valeriana officinalis* strain. In: Brunke E J (ed) Progress in essential oil research. W de Gruyter, Hamburg, pp. 223–230

Buckle J 1993 Does it matter which lavender essential oil is used? Nursing Times 89 (20): 32–35

Carlton R R 1990 An investigation into the rapidly induced responses of *Myrica gale* to insect herbivory. Unpublished PhD Thesis, University of Strathclyde

Carlton R R, Gray A I & Waterman P G 1992 The antifungal activity of the leaf gland oil of sweet gale (*Myrica gale*). Chemecology 3: 55–59

Craker L E 1990 Herbs and volatile oils. Herb, Spice and Medicinal Plant Digest 8(4): 1–5

Deans S G, Waterman P G 1993 Biological activity of volatile oils. In: Hay R K M, Waterman P G (eds) Volatile oil crops. Longman, Harlow pp 100–101

Duraffourd P 1982 En forme tous les jours. La Vie Claire, Périgny

Franchomme P, Pénoël D 1990 L'aromathérapie exactement. Jollois, Limoges

Gates P 1991 Gardening in tomorrow's world. Gardener's World July: 4

Harborne J B 1988 Introduction to ecological biochemistry. Academic Press, London

Lamy J 1985 De la culture à la distillerie. Quelques facteurs influant sur la composition des huiles essentielles. Chambre d'Agriculture de la Drôme, Valence

Lamy J 1988 Présentation de 30 huiles essentielles typées produites dans la Drôme. Congress des Parfumeurs Allemandes: 23–25

Lautié R, Passebecq A 1984 Aromatherapy. Thorsons, Wellingborough

Lawrence B M 1989 Progress in essential oils. Perfumer & Flavorist 14(3): 71

Mailhebiau P 1989 La nouvelle aromathérapie. Vie Nouvelle, Toulouse

Meunier C 1985 Lavandes et lavandins. Edisud, Aix-en-Provence

Price S 1993 The aromatherapy workbook. Thorsons, London, p. 192

Roulier G 1990 Les huiles essentielles pour votre santé. Dangles, St-Jean-de-Braye

Rouvière A, Meyer M C 1983 La santé par les huiles essentielles. M A Editions, Paris

Sobti S N, Pushpangadan P, Thapa R K, Aggarwal S G, Vashist V N, Atal C K 1978 Chemical and genetic investigations in essential oils of some *Ocimum* species, their F1 hybrids and synthesised allopolyploids. Lloydia 41: 50–55

Tegel C 1984 Morphologische und chemische Variabilität sowie Anbau und Verwendung von *Salvia sp* (Salbei). Unpublished MSc Thesis, Technical University of Munich

Tucker A O 1981 The correct name of lavandin and its cultivars (Labiatae). Baileya 21: 131–133

Tucker A O, Maciarello M J 1987 Plant identification. In: Simon J E, Grant L (eds) Proceedings of the first national herb growing and marketing conference. Purdue University Press, West Lafayette

Tucker A O, Maciarello M J 1990 Essential oils of cultivars of Dalmation sage (*Salvia officinalis* L). Journal of Essential Oil Research 2: 139–144

Valnet J 1980 The practice of aromatherapy. Daniel, Saffron Walden

Verlet N 1993 Commercial aspects. In: Hay R K M, Waterman P G (eds) Volatile oil crops. Longman, Harlow, ch. 8

von Schantz M, Holm Y, Hiltunen R, Galambosi B 1987 Arznei- und Gewürzpflanzenversuche zum Anbau in Finnland. Deutsche Apotheke Zeitung 127: 2543–2548

Wabner D 1993 Purity and pesticides. International Journal of Aromatherapy 5(2): 27–29

2

Chemistry and quality

Introduction

The highest possible quality of medicament is always required in therapy. This chapter shows that aromatherapy is no exception to the rule. The main chemical groups found in essential oils are outlined, along with an account of methods of testing for quality.

GENUINE ESSENTIAL OILS

In medicine the quality and wholeness of any essential oils used is of paramount importance irrespective of the cost, whereas when used in flavours and fragrances the taste and the aroma respectively are the most important considerations. For the food and perfume industries essential oils may be adjusted or changed to suit the particular need of the purchaser or the vendor.

In these commercial enterprises the price is an important consideration, and standardized essential oils are necessary to ensure repeatability and consistent quality. It is tacitly accepted that traders in essential oils add other cheaper oils or synthetics to the genuine oils, in order to maintain the same standard taste, aroma and price for successive repeat deliveries to the same customer.

Natural and commercial variations

Wine is a commodity which is expected to have a different taste and character from year to year although harvested, processed and bottled at the same vineyard and from the same vines. The differences are even welcomed and certainly make for conversational one-upmanship! Plants, whether grown to make wine or essential oils, are subject to varying amounts of sunshine, frost, rain, heat or cold each year and it is these factors, plus the composition of the soil, which are responsible for the quality variations in the plant extracts, and the bouquet in the case of essential oils, which occur naturally from year to year. However, in the essential oil world of perfumery and flavouring, this natural variation cannot be tolerated. Haarmann & Reimer (1984) outline some contributory factors that lead essential oil merchants to modify the natural product: 'bad harvests, political conflicts, exhaustion of the soil or transportation difficulties are imponderables which make it impossible for the perfumer to rely entirely on Nature's raw materials. Against that background, synthetic fragrance substances appear as *economically indispensable substitutes for Nature's originals*' (authors' italics).

Most aromatherapy suppliers purchase their essential oils from importers who mainly supply the perfume and food industries, but this is not always a good and reliable source for unadulterated oils for therapeutic use. As Steffen Arctander explains in his book:

The author has nothing in principle against the addition of foreign or 'unnatural' materials to essential oils etc. as long as the intention *and the result* is an indisputable improvement in respect to perfumery performance and effect. … However, the above philosophy should not indicate that the author approves of adulteration of natural perfume materials. On the contrary. But the meaning of the term adulteration should be taken literally: with the intention of acquiring the business (order) through a devaluation of the oil in relation to the labelling of its container. The consumers of perfume oils are buying odor, not physico-chemical data. If the odor and the perfumery (or flavor-) effect is in agreement with the customer's standards, there is no reason to talk about adulteration: the oil is then worth the full price of a true, natural oil and the 'adulteration', if any, has not been a means of direct economical gains.

(Arctander 1960)

In contradistinction to the above, the aromatherapist is buying not merely an odour, but wishes above all to acquire the physicochemical characteristics; however they may vary from harvest to harvest.

Essential oils are made up of distinct natural chemicals, many of which are found in more than one oil. It is a fairly simple matter for the chemist to remove a desired constituent from a cheap oil and add it to an expensive oil in order to lower the price for a customer, or to sell a modified 'pure' oil to an unsuspecting customer for a high price. Adulteration also takes place when a synthetic isolate is added, especially to one of the costly oils such as rose otto, when synthetic phenyl ethyl alcohol (occurring naturally in rose otto) is used as the adulterant. Alcohol, and occasionally a small amount of vegetable oil, both good solvents for essential oils, are also used to adulterate, stretch, or cut Nature's gifts, and many descriptive words are used to justify the standardization sometimes necessary in the fragrance and food industries. 'Certain suppliers with highly developed imagination will even use the term "ennobling" for the disfiguration of an essential oil' (Arctander 1960).

The need for genuine oils

The following case cited by Valnet illustrates perfectly the need to use genuine essential oils in therapeutic treatments:

A patient being treated for a fistula of the anus by the instillation of *pure and natural* drops of lavender and who was beginning to recover, had to go on a journey. Having forgotten his essential oil, he purchased a further supply from a chemist. Unfortunately, this essence was neither pure nor natural; one single instillation resulted in such severe inflammation that the patient was unable to sit down for over two weeks.'

(Valnet 1980 p. 27)

Essential oils used in the fragrance industry often have their terpenes partly or wholly removed on account of their insolubility in alcohol, which would result in cloudiness—a distinct commercial and aesthetic disadvantage in a perfume! To the therapist however, a deterpenated oil is incomplete. It then contains a higher percentage of the remaining constituents of the oil. For example, the deterpenation of peppermint increases the content of the possibly hazardous ketone, menthone. 'In perfumery, certain essential oils are deterpenised, because too high a degree of terpenes reduces their solubility in alcohol. In aromatherapy, there is no necessity for this, and … it is preferable to avoid interfering with the natural balance of the essence' (Lautié & Passebecq 1984 p. 15).

Some therapists purchase bergapten-free bergamot oil, as this constituent (a furocoumarin) is responsible for phototoxicity of the skin in sunlight. It is understandable that the cosmetic industry was restrained from using the complete oil of bergamot in suntanning creams and lotions, but for therapists to use an incomplete oil for therapeutic purposes, not related to tanning, is baffling to say the least. All that is needed in this instance is proper labelling, to the effect that a person should not go out into the sun for at least an hour after using oil of bergamot. The IFRA (International Fragrance Research Association) recommendation is 0.4% maximum in the consumer product, which is equivalent to 8 drops of bergamot in 100 ml.

Natural wholeness and synergy

It is important also to preserve the wholeness of an essential oil in order to guard its natural synergy (Greek, *syn* = together, *ergon* = work). The components making up an essential oil cooperate to produce their healing effect and, if these are altered in any way, the natural synergy is upset. When a single active component is removed, not only is the synergy of the remaining constituents diminished, but the isolated component generally needs much greater care when used alone. It may produce side-effects with continued use. However, when present in the whole oil, the other constituents seem to act as 'quenchers' of these unwanted effects, enabling the oil to be used without harm (see Synergy and Quenching in Ch. 3).

It is extremely difficult to judge the probable effects of an essential oil solely by knowing its principal chemical constituent(s), important though this knowledge is. The whole oil has to be considered in all its complexity, the mixture of possibly hundreds of different types of molecules, their molecular energy and the overall synergy.

There is no simple direct relationship between any one of the chemical constituents and the therapeutic effect—or even the hazard—of the whole essential oil (Price 1990).

Ambiguous BP standards

Some essential oils listed in the British Pharmacopoeia are stocked in hospital pharmacies, but oils prepared to BP standards may not be suitable for use in aromatherapy. One reason for this is that many plants, for example thyme, *Thymus vulgaris*, exist in the wild as many different chemotypes, some of which are propagated and grown from cuttings, each chemotype producing quite a different essential oil in make-up and therapeutic action (see Ch. 1), but these differences are not reflected in the pharmacopoeia. Another reason is imprecise specification. For instance, a request for lavender may produce *Lavandula angustifolia*, *L. × intermedia* or perhaps *L. spica* all of which have different properties and indications. According to the British Pharmacopoeia (1993) eucalyptus essential oil may be any one of four different species, which when unrectified may have different properties and indications, even though the principal constituent in each case is the oxide 1,8-cineole. The same source states that it is not always the whole oil which is used therapeutically—it may be an incomplete oil (e.g. terpeneless), an active constituent, or even prepared synthetically.

CHEMISTRY OF ESSENTIAL OILS

For the safe practice of aromatherapy it is essential to have at least a basic understanding of the chemistry of the essential oils before being able to use them in a meaningful, caring and effective way—not at random, or indiscriminately. Such understanding makes it evident that certain chemicals may have certain effects—'may', because, as stated above, there is no direct link between even the major components of an essential oil and the effects of the complete oil. These complex relationships are little understood at present because hundreds of different chemicals are involved, and many of them are unknown. Suffice it to say that knowledge of the basic composition of each oil contributes to the overall background knowledge of aromatherapy, thus promoting confidence and aiding selection of the oils to be used, until such time as more is discovered about the interaction of the plant chemicals within the human body.

The list of the physiological and pharmacological properties of aromatic molecules encompasses almost all the organs and all the functions of the organism, from skin conditions to psychological disturbances. Chemists have identified more than 3000 different aromatic molecules, and new ones are being discovered. Fortunately, these molecules are gathered in main groups or families, with a relationship between the chemical function and the pharmacological activities. Although we use whole essential oils and not isolated molecules, it is necessary to undertake the study not only of the classes of molecules but also a few important individual molecules and possible actions.

Fig. 2.1a Carbon skeleton of the isoprene unit

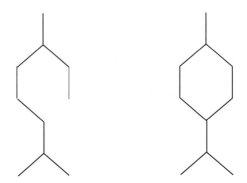

Fig. 2.1b Two isoprene units join to form an acyclic chain

Fig. 2.1c Two isoprene units join to form a cyclic chain

Essential oil components

It is not the intention to give a lesson in organic chemistry in this book, but a brief explanation of the building blocks of essential oils will be helpful. Carbon, hydrogen, oxygen are essential to life itself, and all three are contained in every essential oil. They combine in countless mono- and sesquiterpenic families of hydrocarbons, alcohols, aldehydes, ketones, acids, phenols, esters and coumarins (and furocoumarins).

Hydrocarbons

Terpenic hydrocarbons consist only of hydrogen and carbon atoms, arranged in a chain—which can be either straight or branched. The basic building block for these chains is the isoprene unit—comprising five carbon atoms (Fig. 2.1a). See Chapter 1 and also, for the basic chemistry leading up to the isoprene unit (Price 1993).

Aliphatic chains

Two of these units joined together head to tail form the basis of all monoterpenes (monoterpenic hydrocarbons have 10 carbon atoms) (Figs 2.1b, 2.1c). Three units provide the basic structure for the larger molecules known as sesquiterpenes (sesquiterpenic hydrocarbons have 15 carbon atoms) (Fig. 2.2a). Four isoprene units joined together are diterpenes (diterpenic hydrocarbons have 20 carbon atoms) (Fig. 2.2b), and are not often met with in steam-distilled oils because they are almost too heavy to come over in the distillation process—only a few diterpenes manage it. All these chains are known as aliphatic hydrocarbons.

Terpenic hydrocarbons are generally recognizable from their name: all end in -ene. They are all slightly antiseptic and bactericidal (Franchomme & Pénoël 1990 p. 220, Roulier 1990 p. 51) and may play an important part in the quenching effect mentioned earlier, thus making deterpenated oils unsuitable for aromatherapeutic purposes.

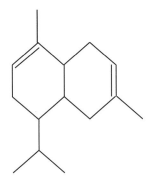

Fig. 2.2a α-cadinene (15C). Three isoprene units join to form a sesquiterpene

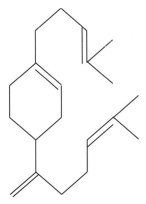

Fig. 2.2b α-camphorene (20C). Four isoprene units join to form a diterpene

In all cases the therapeutic qualities given below are general familial characteristics. Individual molecules may have their own particular properties as well as the general ones quoted.

Explanation of the term cyclic

Sometimes an aliphatic straight chain can, as it were, loop round itself (Fig. 2.1c) and give the *appearance* of an aromatic ring, but it is still a 10-carbon chain. When this looping occurs, the terpene is said to be monocyclic, because one circle has been created, and therefore the complete description is monocyclic monoterpene.

More than one circle can arise in a chain so that it is possible to have a tricyclic sesquiterpenic alcohol. If they do not form a circle at all (i.e. if they form a straight chain) they are said to be acyclic (Fig. 2.1b).

To be precise, these terms describing the chains—or the term 'aromatic' (ring-based—see The aromatic ring below) should be included when describing a particular chemical constituent of an essential oil, e.g:

- geraniol—an acyclic monoterpenic alcohol
- patchoulol—a tricyclic sesquiterpenic alcohol
- citronellal—an acyclic monoterpenic aldehyde
- cinnamic aldehyde—an aromatic aldehyde
- geranic acid—an acyclic monoterpenic acid
- cinnamic acid—an aromatic acid … etc.

Not enough is yet understood about the pharmacological effects of essential oils to know how each type may differ in effect.

Monoterpenes (see Fig. 2.3 for examples) occur in almost all essential oils to varying degrees, and in addition to the antiseptic and bactericidal properties mentioned above they may also be analgesic, expectorant and stimulating (Franchomme & Pénoël 1990 pp. 217–224).

Sesquiterpenes

Additional to the antiseptic and bactericidal properties mentioned above, the sesquiterpenes (Figs 2.2a, 2.4) as a class are antiinflammatory, calming and slight hypotensors; some are analgesic and/or spasmolytic (Franchomme & Pénoël 1990 pp. 217–224).

Diterpenes

Diterpenes (Fig. 2.2b) have the further properties of being expectorant and purgative and some are antifungal and antiviral. Some appear to have a balancing effect on the hormonal system, e.g. the diterpenic alcohol sclareol in *Salvia sclarea* [CLARY] (and also the sesquiterpenic alcohol viridiflorol in *Melaleuca viridiflora* [NIAOULI]) (Pénoël 1993 personal communication).

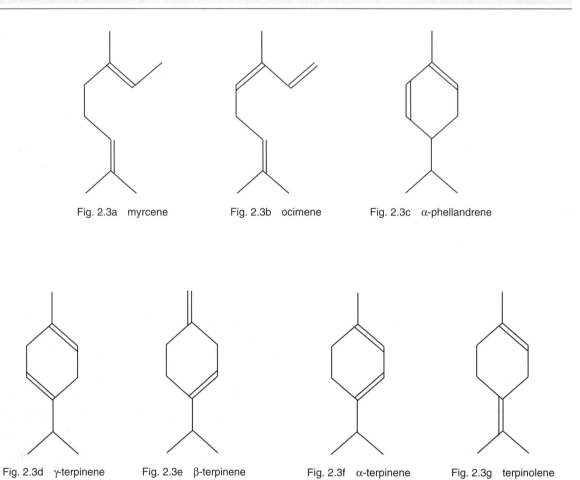

Fig. 2.3a myrcene

Fig. 2.3b ocimene

Fig. 2.3c α-phellandrene

Fig. 2.3d γ-terpinene

Fig. 2.3e β-terpinene

Fig. 2.3f α-terpinene

Fig. 2.3g terpinolene

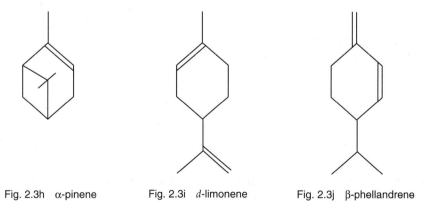

Fig. 2.3h α-pinene

Fig. 2.3i *d*-limonene

Fig. 2.3j β-phellandrene

Fig. 2.3 Examples of monoterpenic hydrocarbons

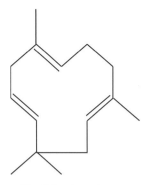

| Fig. 2.4a γ-curcumene | Fig. 2.4b caryophyllene | Fig. 2.4c humulene |

Fig. 2.4 Sequiterpenic hydrocarbons

The aromatic ring

The second building block occurs when six carbon atoms join together in the form of a ring, which has three names in common use:

1. aromatic ring, because many of the substances based on it are aromatic
2. benzene ring, because the substance so formed is benzene
3. phenyl ring, because phenols are formed from this base.

Thus we find both aliphatic and aromatic aldehydes, ketones and organic acids (involving both chain and ring building blocks) occurring naturally in essential oils. However, when the hydroxyl radical -OH is attached to a chain it is an aliphatic alcohol (Fig. 2.5a); when the same radical is attached to a ring it is an aromatic phenol (Fig. 2.5b).

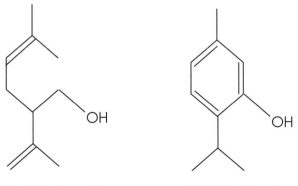

Fig. 2.5a lavandulol
(alcohol)

Fig. 2.5b thymol
(phenol)

Alcohols

When a hydroxyl radical, consisting of one oxygen atom and one hydrogen atom (-OH), joins onto one of the carbons in an aliphatic chain by displacing one of the hydrogen molecules, an alcohol is formed: a monoterpenol, sesquiterpenol or diterpenol, depending on whether the chain to which it attaches itself has two, three or four isoprene units. The name of the alcohol so formed always ends in -ol, e.g. geraniol.

Alcohols are antiinfective, strongly bactericidal, antiviral and stimulating; they are generally nontoxic in use and do not cause skin irritation (Roulier 1990 p. 53, Franchomme & Pénoël 1990 p. 115).

Phenols

When the same hydroxyl group attaches itself to a carbon in the *aromatic* (or phenyl) ring, the resulting molecule is known as a phenol, which, because it is a kind of alcohol, also has strong effects. Phenols, like alcohols, have names which also end in -ol, e.g. carvacrol, and to discriminate between the two it is necessary to learn the most important ones.

Phenols, like alcohols, are antiseptic and bactericidal. Because they stimulate both the nervous system (making them effective against depressive illness) and the immune system, they activate the body's own healing process. However, due to the -OH attachment to a ring rather than a chain molecule, aromatic phenols,

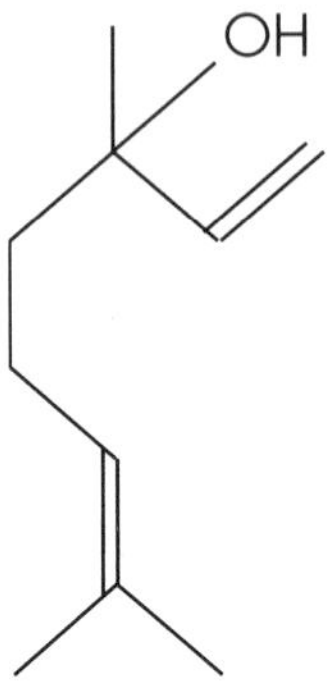

Fig. 2.6a linalool
(aliphatic monoterpenic alcohol)

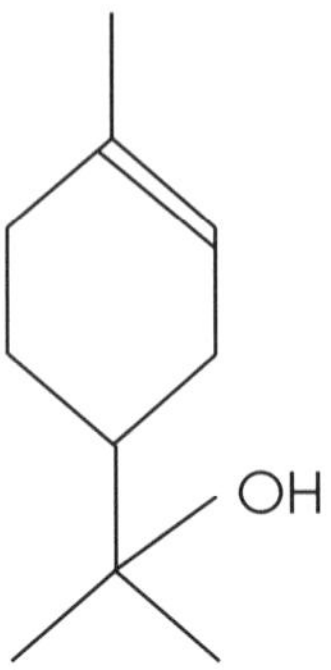

Fig. 2.6b α-terpineol
(monocyclic monoterpenic alcohol)

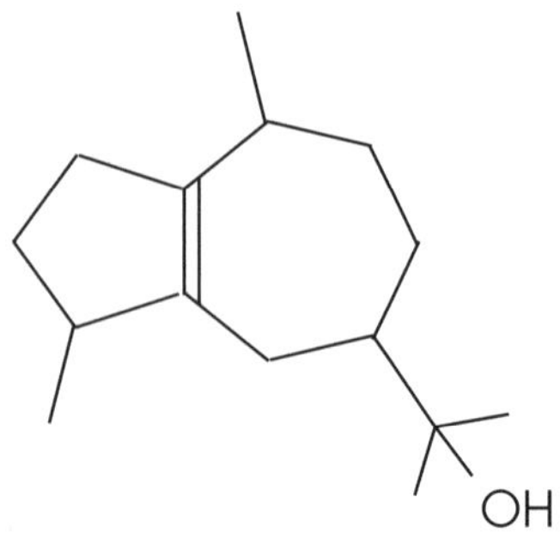

Fig. 2.6c guaiol
(bicyclic sesquiterpenic alcohol)

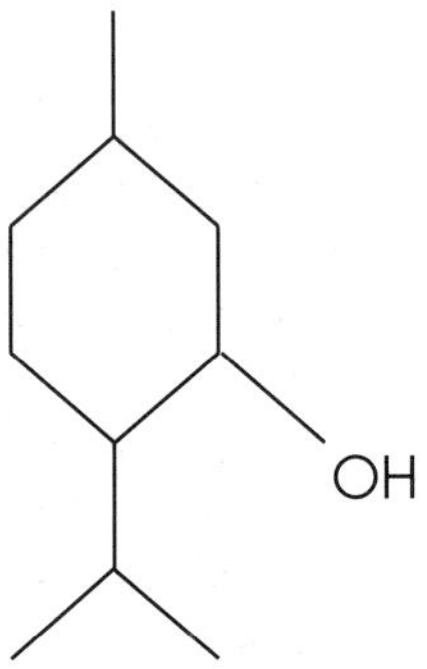

Fig. 2.6d menthol
(monocyclic monoterpenic alcohol)

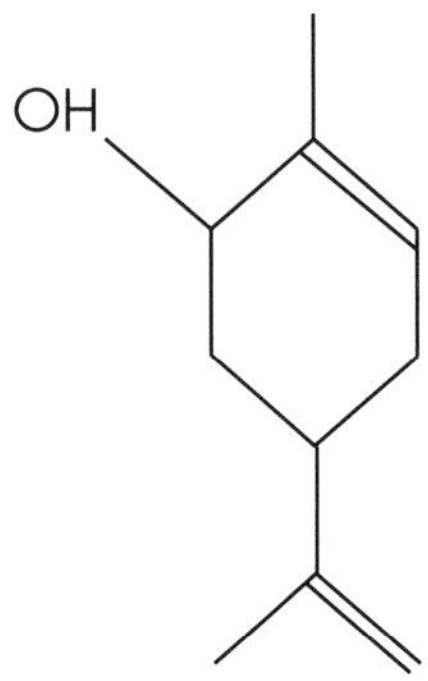

Fig. 2.6e carveol
(monocyclic monoterpenic alcohol)

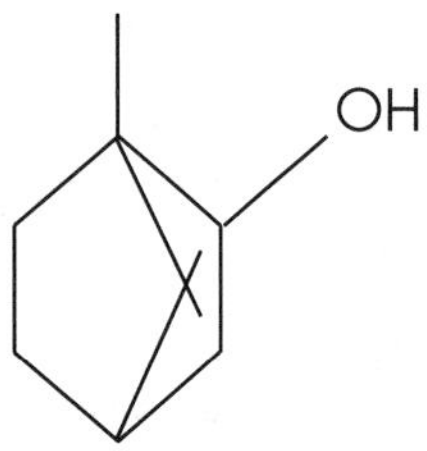

Fig. 2.6f borneol
(bicyclic monoterpenic alcohol)

Fig. 2.6   Alcohols

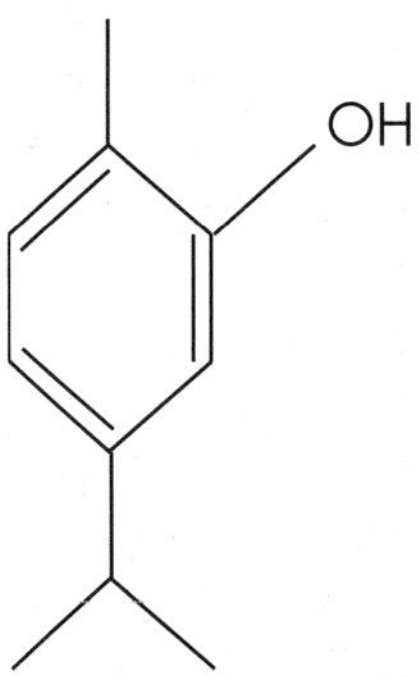

Fig. 2.7a carvacrol (phenol)

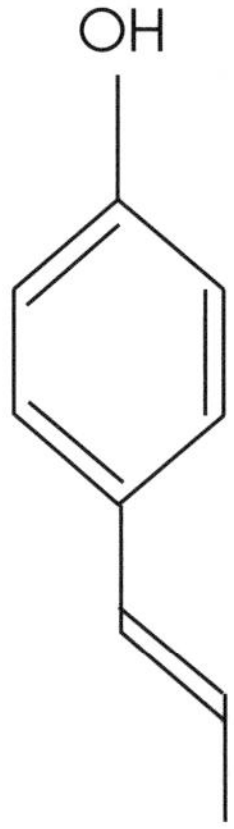

Fig. 2.7b chavicol (phenol)

Fig. 2.7   Phenols

unlike the aliphatic alcohols, can be toxic to the liver and irritant to the skin if used in substantial amounts or for too long a time (Roulier 1990 pp. 51-52). 'Some oils—for example, thyme and origanum—owe their value in the pharmaceutical field almost entirely to the antiseptic and germicidal properties of their phenolic content' (Guenther 1949).

A number of phenols appear in essential oils as phenolic ethers (Fig. 2.8). These are more complicated structures and have various word forms as seen in the following examples: safrole, methyl chavicol, eugenol methyl ether (as distinct from the straight phenol, eugenol) and asarone (confusing because of its similarity to the ketone name ending). Some phenolic ethers occur in two forms, as in trans-anethole and cis-anethole, the latter being the more toxic of the two (Witty 1993 personal communication).

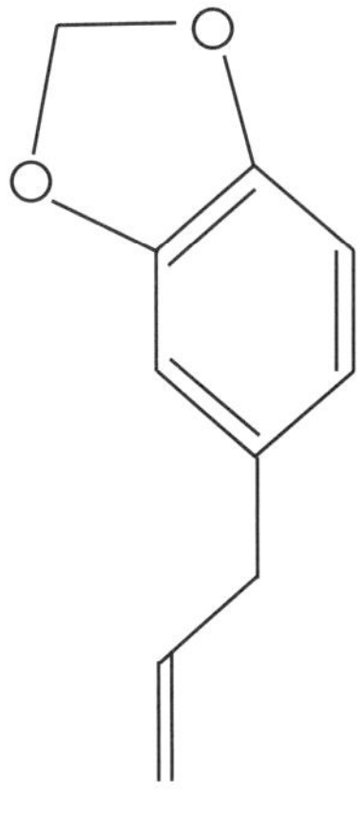

Fig. 2.8a   safrole

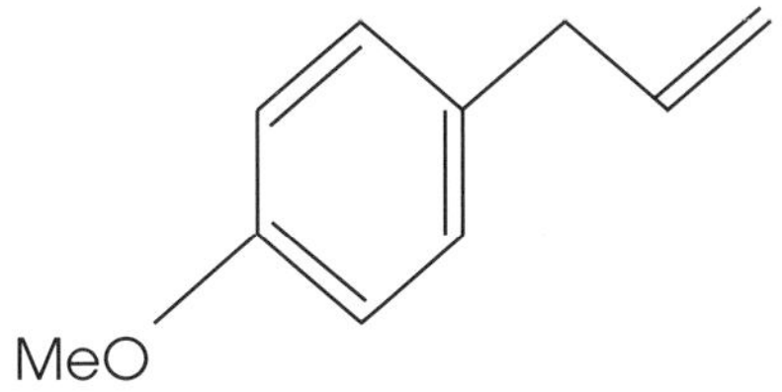

Fig. 2.8b   methyl chavicol

Fig. 2.8   Phenolic ethers

Phenolic ethers have some similar therapeutic effects to phenols, but, being more powerful, several may be neurotoxic if present in large amounts in an essential oil, thus indicating short term use in low concentration.

Ethers rarely, if ever, occur alone in essential oils. The relationship to phenolic ethers is close, their antidepressant, antispasmodic and sedative properties echoing those of the phenolic ethers, as do those of esters (Roulier 1990 p. 53).

Aldehydes

An aldehyde is formed when the carbonyl radical (=O) together with a hydrogen atom (-H) attaches itself to one of the carbon atoms in the basic structure (Fig. 2.9). Recognizing an aldehyde from its name is easy, as aldehydes end either in -al e.g. citral, or the name aldehyde is stated, as in cinnamic aldehyde. They usually have a powerful aroma, making them important to the perfumer, and are very reactive, which means that they must be used with care in aromatherapy.

The beneficial properties of aldehydes are antiviral, antiinflammatory, calming to the nervous system, hypotensors, vasodilators and antipyretic; their negative properties—when used incorrectly or inappropriately—can cause skin irritation and skin sensitivity (Roulier 1990 p. 53, Franchomme & Pénoël pp. 211–214).

Ketones

When the carbonyl group (=O) attaches itself (without a hydrogen atom this time) to a carbon on a chain structure, an aliphatic ketone is formed (aromatic ketones hardly ever occur in essential oils). The ketone names normally end in -one, but look out for false friends like asarone, mentioned above, which is a phenolic ether and not a ketone.

Molecules are not two-dimensional, but occupy space so that changes in molecular spatial shape can take place. Hence differently shaped molecules made up of the same atoms do occur and these seemingly insignificant differences can alter the effect that these molecules have on the body. For example, laevocarvone and dextro-carvone are two examples, one being less toxic than the other. Opdyke suggests α-thujone and

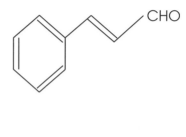

Fig. 2.9a citronellal
(monoterpenic aldehyde)

Fig. 2.9b cinnamic aldehyde
(aromatic aldehyde)

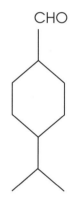

Fig. 2.9c geranial
(monoterpenic aldehyde)

Fig. 2.9d neral
(monoterpenic aldehyde)

Fig. 2.9e cuminal
(monocyclic monoterpenic aldehyde)

Fig. 2.9 Aldehydes

β-thujone may also have differing effects on the body (Opdyke 1973, 1978). Time and research alone will tell.

Generally speaking, ketones (Figs 2.10, 2.11) are cicatrizant, lipolytic, mucolytic and sedative; some are also analgesic, anticoagulant, antiinflammatory, digestant, expectorant or stimulant. They need to be used with care particularly by pregnant women (Roulier 1990 p. 53, Franchomme & Pénoël 1990 p. 193).

Organic acids and esters

Unlike the above there is no active radical whose presence creates an ester. This is formed by the joining together of an organic acid with an alcohol (Fig. 2.12), the formula being:

organic acid + alcohol = ester + water

This chemical reaction is capable of flowing the other way too, which could result in interchanges from acids to esters and back again. Perhaps this is why esters are useful for normalizing some emotional and bodily conditions which are out of balance. There is, however, an acid group (-COOH), which attaches itself to a basic carbon structure and this also plays its part in the formation of an ester. To recognize an ester from its name is not difficult; it usually ends with -ate, e.g. linalyl acetate, or else includes the word ester.

Fig. 2.10a carvone

Fig. 2.10b pulegone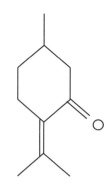

Fig. 2.10c isopulegone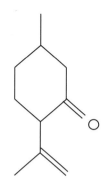

(monocyclic monoterpenic ketones)

Fig. 2.10d menthone

Fig. 2.10e piperitone

Fig. 2.10f germacrone

(monocyclic monoterpenic ketones)

(sesquiterpenic ketone)

Fig. 2.11 thujone
(bicyclic monoterpenic ketone)

Fig. 2.12 benzyl acetate
(ester)

Esters are generally antifungal, antiinflammatory, antispasmodic, cicatrizant and both calming and tonic, especially to the nervous system (Buchbauer et al 1992, 1993) (see Ch. 4). Like alcohols, they are gentle in action, and being free from toxicity they are 'user-friendly'. The exception is methyl salycilate which comprises over 90% of wintergreen and birch oils (neither of which are used in the present British style of aromatherapy).

Oxides

The only oxide known well in aromatherapy is 1,8-cineole, otherwise known as eucalyptol (Fig. 2.13); it may also be regarded as a bicyclic ether (Buchbauer 1993).

Eucalyptol is expectorant and mucolytic, its unwanted effect being skin irritation, especially on young children.

Lactones

Important members of this family occurring in essences are the coumarins and their derivatives (Fig. 2.14). They occur only in the expressed oils and some absolutes, e.g. jasmine, because the molecular weight is too great to allow distillation.

Lactones are reputed to be mucolytic, expectorant and temperature-reducing, their negative aspects being skin-sensitizing and phototoxicity (Franchomme & Pénoël 1990 p. 202). Coumarins

Fig. 2.14a   coumarin

Fig. 2.14b   bergaptene (a furocoumarin)

are anticoagulant hypotensors; they are also uplifting and yet sedative (Franchomme & Pénoël 1990 p. 205, Buchbauer et al 1992). Furocoumarins are known mainly for their phototoxicity, and oils containing these should not be used immediately prior to sunbathing (or sunbeds) due to their ability to increase the sensitivity of the skin to the sun. Some are antiviral and antifungal (Franchomme & Pénoël 1990 p. 206).

There are too many individual essential oil components to name here, but knowledge of the different chemical families will aid recognition of new constituents if they are met with in a listing from a gas chromatograph report (see below).

CHEMICAL VARIABILITY

It is important to recognize that because of the variability of the climate and the soil, no natural chemical will be present in any essential oil in exactly the same proportion at each distillation. Further variations are produced according to the time the plant is harvested. For instance, sage plants cut early in the season contain a much

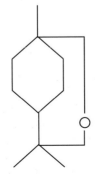

Fig. 2.13   eucalyptol or 1,8-cineole

lower percentage of ketones than those harvested late (Lamy 1985). Constituents can vary sometimes from 20–70% in a genuine oil and suppliers must have obtained an oil from a specific plant grown in the right place and harvested at the right time to ensure the correct proportion of whatever component is required. If this is not the case then the oils may have been adulterated before they reach the buyer, unless he buys it from source. Even a gas liquid chromatograph carried out by an independent authority cannot always be relied upon completely. More than one test is needed when checking the purity of an oil, and not all vendors are able to afford such an expensive procedure as this for each batch. A certificate showing that an oil is of a required standard is no guarantee unless it refers specifically to the batch currently being traded.

Testing oils for quality

Gas–liquid chromatography (GLC)

This apparatus consists of a coiled, temperature-controlled, tubular column into which a minute amount (say 1 microlitre) of essential oil is injected and volatilized. It then passes through the column, which itself may be up to 50 m long and contains a liquid phase and a gas phase. At the other end is a flame ionization detector and a pen recorder which plots a trace (Fig. 2.15) of each component of the essential oil as it exits the column. The smaller, lighter molecules have the shortest retention time and they appear in the shortest time, and so are recorded first on the trace. These are followed by successively larger molecules, the heaviest having the longest retention time and being recorded last. From the resulting trace the percentage of each constituent present in the oil being tested can be calculated. As the reading will always differ for each batch of any one essential oil, a trace for each named essential oil is retained as a standard, to which all future batches are compared. It can be seen that this test is comparative rather than absolute, and although the GLC does not directly identify the constituents present, this can be done by comparing the results obtained with a known standard.

Mass spectrometry

The GLC is a valuable test, but is not the only one. At the forefront of modern technology is the GC-MS, a more expensive process which is capable of analyzing and identifying the individual components of essential oils. The mass spectrometer is interfaced to the gas chromatograph apparatus described above and as the molecules emerge from the GC column they are bombarded with high energy electrons which fragment them. There is a characteristic fragmentation pattern for each molecule, and for identification it is compared by computer to patterns held in a library. Using this technique it is possible to identify each component in a complex mixture such as an essential oil.

Optical rotation

The majority of both mono- and sesquiterpenic compounds are to be found in one stereochemical form in any given essential oil. This results in the oils being what is termed optically active, with the ability to bend plane-polarized light (Table 2.1). The optical activity is measured using a polarimeter and the angle through which the light is rotated is an important physical characteristic by which an essential oil may be recognised.

Refractive index

When light passes through a liquid it is refracted, and this refraction is easily measured to give consistent figures for a particular oil. This refractive index (Table 2.1) is quite consistent for a given oil and is another aid in the authentication of that oil.

Infrared test

When electromagnetic radiation in the infrared region is passed through a sample, the spectrum produced (Fig. 2.16) is a fingerprint from which the level of some of the oil's components can be estimated. Some forms of adulteration can readily be seen by this method, depending to some extent on the skill and knowledge of the person performing the adulteration.

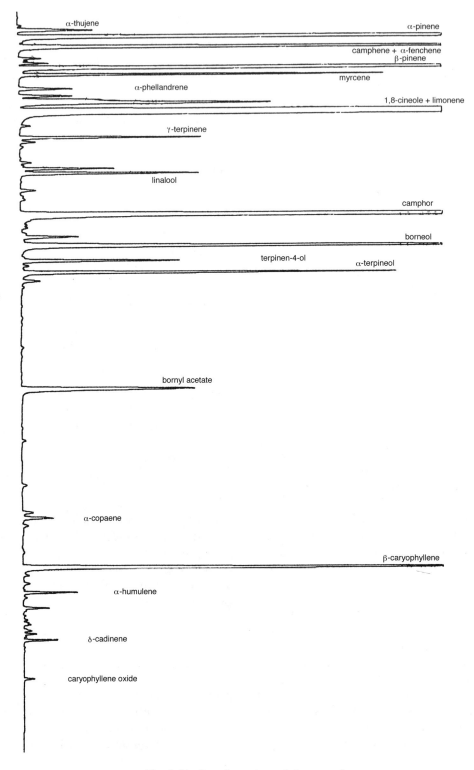

Fig. 2.15 Gas chromatograph (rosemary)

Table 2.1   Physical characteristics of some essential oils

	Family	Optical rotation	Refractive index	Specific gravity
Cananga odorata (flos) [YLANG YLANG]	Annonaceae	−23.44 to −31.45	1.5041–1.5065	0.960–0.986 (20°)
Carum carvi (fruct.) [CARAWAY]	Umbelliferae	+74 to +80	1.485–1.492	0.902–0.912 (20°)
Cedrus atlantica (lig.) [ATLAS CEDARWOOD]	Pinaceae	+34 to +53.8	1.515–1.523	0.953–0.9756 (20°)
Cinnamomum zeylanicum (cort.) [CINNAMON BARK]	Lauraceae	0 to −2	1.573–1.500	1.000–1.040 (20°)
Citrus limon (per.) [LEMON]	Rutaceae	+57 to +65	1.474–1.476	0.849–0.858 (20°)
Citrus bergamia (per.) [BERGAMOT]	Rutaceae	+8 to +24	1.465–1.4675	0.875–0.880 (20°)
Citrus reticulata (per.) [MANDARIN]	Rutaceae	+65 to +75	1.475–1.478	0.854–0.859 (15°)
Citrus aurantium var. *amara* (per.) [ORANGE BIGARADE]	Rutaceae	+94 to +99	1.472–1.476	0.842–0.848 (20°)
Coriandrum sativum (fruct.) [CORIANDER]	Umbelliferae	+8 to +12	1.462–1.472	0.863–0.870 (20°)
Cymbopogon flexuosus (fol.) [LEMONGRASS]	Poaceae	−3 to +1	1.485–1.4899	0.889–0.911 (25°)
Eucalyptus globulus (fol.) [TASMANIAN BLUE GUM]	Myrtaceae	0 to +10	1.458–1.470	0.905–0.925 (20°)
Foeniculum vulgare var. *dulce* (fruct.) [FENNEL]	Umbelliferae	+5 to +16.30	1.5500–1.5519	0.971–0.980 (20°)
Juniperus communis (fruct.) [JUNIPER BERRY]	Cupressaceae	−15 to 0	1.4740–1.4840	0.854–0.871 (20°)
Lavandula angustifolia [LAVENDER]	Labiatae	−5 to −12	1.457–1.464	0.878–0.892 (20°)
Melaleuca leucadendron (fol.) [CAJUPUT]	Myrtaceae	+1 to −4	1.464–1.472	0.910–0.923 (20°)
Melaleuca alternifolia (fol.) [TEA TREE]	Myrtaceae	+6.48 to +9.48	1.4760–1.4810	0.895–0.905 (15°)
Mentha x piperita (fol.) [PEPPERMINT]	Labiatae	−16 to −30	1.460–1.467	0.900–0.912 (20°)
Myristica fragrans (sem.) [NUTMEG EI]*	Myristicaceae	+8 to +25	1.475–1.488	0.883–0.917 (20°)
Myristica fragrans (sem.) [NUTMEG WI]*	Myristicaceae	+25 to +45	1.467–1.477	0.854–0.880 (20°)
Nardostachys jatamansi (rad.) [SPIKENARD]	Valerianaceae	−20	1.5078	0.9649–0.9732 (17°)
Ocimum basilicum (fol.) [BASIL]	Labiatae	−7.24 to −10.36	1.4821–1.4939	0.912–0.935 (20°)
Origanum majorana (fol.) [SWEET MARJORAM]	Labiatae	+14.2 to +19.4	1.4700–1.4750	0.890–0.906 (25°)
Pelargonium graveolens (fol.) [GERANIUM]	Geraniaceae	−7.0 to +13.15	1.461–1.472	0.888–0.896 (20°)
Piper nigrum (fruct.) [BLACK PEPPER]	Piperaceae	−7.2 to +4	1.480–1.492	0.864–0.907 (20°)
Pogostemon patchouli (fol.) [PATCHOULI]	Labiatae	−47 to −70	1.506–1.513	0.955–0.986 (20°)
Santalum album (lig.) [SANDALWOOD]	Santalaceae	−15.58 to −20	1.505–1.510	0.971–0.983 (20°)
Syzygium aromaticum (flos) [CLOVE BUD]	Myrtaceae	−1.5	1.528–1.537	1.041–1.054 (20°)
Vetiveria zizanioides (rad.) [VETIVER]	Poaceae	+19 to +30	1.514–1.519	0.9882–1.0219 (30°)
Zingiber officinale (rad.) [GINGER]	Zingiberacae	−28 to −45	1.4880–1.440	0.871–0.882 (20°)

* EI= East Indies, WI = West Indies

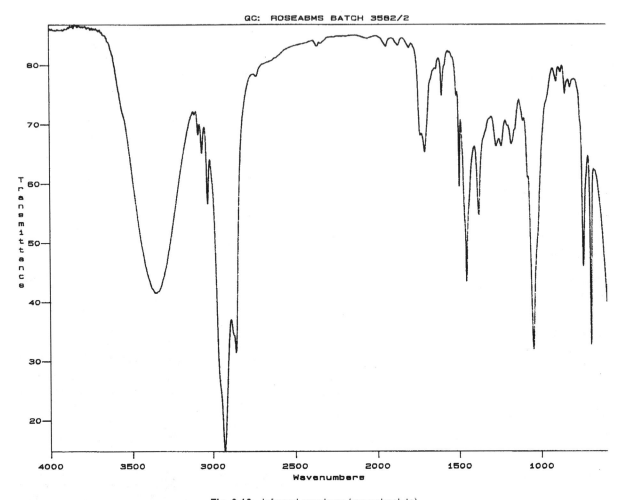

Fig. 2.16 Infrared spectrum (rose absolute)

Essential oils also undergo other checks on their physical characteristics which must be within the accepted tolerances for the given oil. These checks include specific gravity, solubility in alcohol, colour, ester content and so on.

The nose

In addition to all this, possibly the finest tool for some purposes is a well-trained 'nose', who can make an organoleptic assessment of the oil. The trained nose can identify certain molecules at levels that would be impossible low for machines.

The distillation process

Distilling as we know it today can involve efficient cooling systems, electronic control gear to regulate the temperature and pressure of the process, energy-saving steam generators and so on. Some thousands of years ago, to obtain the essential oil, cedarwood pieces would be placed with water in a clay vessel with a lid made of woollen fibres. The vessel would be heated over a wood fire, and as the volatile molecules from the water and the cedarwood escaped they were trapped in the wool. Later they were squeezed out by hand, and the aromatic water and essential oil, being of different densities, would separate and so could be collected.

Over the centuries methods of distillation gradually improved, and 4th century Chinese and 10th century Islamic scientists developed two different methods of obtaining the distillate. Since then, apart from minor improvements, distillation has remained very much the same in principle up to the present day. The availability of modern materials and resources, such as stainless steel and electricity, has permitted much greater control over the whole process and a dramatic increase in the quality of the essential oils produced today. Oils produced in previous centuries, and even at the beginning of this century, cannot be compared with some of the very high quality products we have available for aromatherapy today (assuming they are not adulterated after distillation).

Newer methods have been tried in the 20th century, such as percolation (used on a small scale in France), and new solvents such as supercritical CO_2, which can extract without heat a wider range of molecules from the plant material than is possible by distillation, thus producing a new material which may well be of use to aromatherapists. The oils produced by any of these newer methods have a different molecular mix and until more is known about them, and research carried out on their possibly different therapeutic (and toxic) effects, aromatherapists may be best advised to use only steam-distilled essential oils and expressed essences for the time being. These have been proven by tradition over a long period of time, as well as by the supporting scientific research carried out this century, to be therapeutically effective.

Complexity of essential oils

During the 19th century the first analyses were carried out on essential oils, and attempts made to isolate and identify the various components, some of the terpenes, alcohols and aldehydes being among the first to be named. This was followed by successful attempts to synthesize the individual components; for example, eugenol found naturally in clove bud oil was synthesized in 1822 (Valnet 1980 p. 28).

The complexity of essential oils should be borne in mind when referring to the therapeutic qualities of a given oil, and helps to explain why one oil can be listed at the same time as being 'analgesic, anticonvulsive, antidepressant, antimicrobial, antirheumatic, antiseptic, antispasmodic, antitoxic, carminative, cholagogic, choleretic, cicatrizant, cordial, cytophylactic, deodorant, diuretic, emmenagogic, hypotensive, insecticidal, nervine, parasiticidal, rubefacient, sedative, stimulant, sudorific, tonic, vermifuge, vulnerary'. This staggering array of properties (Lawless 1992) perhaps overstates the case, but demonstrates the 'shotgun' holistic approach in contrast to the 'single bullet' symptomatic approach.

This complexity means that only genuine essential oils should be used therapeutically, even though there is natural variation in the oils. It needs emphasizing that for perfectly valid reasons the fragrance industry requires essential oils which are standardized by one means or another and that many (if not most) essential oils in the general market place may have synthetic or natural additions or fractions removed. As well as these already-mentioned cautions it is also true that some oils are not obtained from plants at all. These laboratory creations are known as reconstructed oils (RCO) and lack many tiny and as yet unidentified components which could well be important to the overall effect of the natural oil.

Summary

The requirements of the food and perfume industries differ dramatically from those of aromatherapy. Essential oils are very complex by nature, and extensive testing is needed to obtain therapeutic quality oils. When altered in any way they will probably not be of a quality suitable for aromatherapy, since the synergy of the natural mix of components in the whole oil will have been destroyed. It goes without saying that they should only be obtained from a reliable and knowledgeable source.

REFERENCES

Arctander S 1960 Perfume and Flavor Materials of Natural Origin. Published by the author, Elizabeth, New Jersey, p. 4

British Pharmacopoeia 1993 HMSO, London, p. 273

Buchbauer G 1993 Biological effects of fragrances and essential oils. Perfumer & Flavorist 18: 22

Buchbauer G, Jirovetz L, Jäger W 1992 Passiflora and lime blossoms: motility effects after inhalation of the essential oils and some of the main constituents in animal experiments. Archiva Pharmaceutica (Weinheim) 325: 247–248

Buchbauer G, Jirovetz L, Jäger W, Plank C, Dietrich H 1993 Fragrance compounds and essential oils with sedative effects upon inhalation. Journal of Pharmaceutical Sciences 82(6): 660–664

Franchomme P, Pénoël D 1990 L'aromathérapie exactement. Jollois, Limoges

Guenther E 1949 The essential oils. Van Nostrand, New York, vol. 2: 499

Lamy J 1985 De la culture à la distillerie: quelques facteurs influant sur la composition des huiles essentielles. Chambre d'Agriculture de la Drôme, Valance, p. 5

Lautié R, Passebecq A 1984 Aromatherapy. Thorsons, Wellingborough

Lawless J 1992 The encyclopaedia of essential oils. Element, Longmead, Shaftesbury, p. 18

Müller J 1984 The H&R book of perfumes. Johnson, London, vol. 1, p. 111

Opdyke D L J 1973 Monographs on fragrance raw materials: laevo-carvone. Food and cosmetics toxicology, vol. 11. Pergamon Press, Oxford, p. 1057

Opdyke D L J 1978 Monographs on fragrance raw materials: dextro-carvone. Food and cosmetics toxicology. Pergamon Press, Oxford, vol. 16: 673

Price L 1990 Lecture notes: theory and philosophy of aromatherapy. Shirley Price International College of Aromatherapy Course, Hinckley

Price S 1993 The aromatherapy workbook. Thorsons, London, ch. 3

Roulier G 1990 Les huiles essentielles pour votre santé. Dangles, St-Jean-de-Braye

Valnet 1980 The practice of aromatherapy. Daniel, Saffron Walden

3

Power and safety

Introduction

The dangers of essential oils have been greatly exaggerated, usually based on insufficient evidence and inappropriate comparisons. This chapter shows that these powerful substances, used knowledgeably and with due caution, pose no threat to health.

SAFETY

It is necessary to begin this chapter on the safe use of essential oils by making three statements. Firstly, there is no doubt that essential oils are powerful mixtures and have physiological, psychological and pharmacological effects when applied to the body. Secondly, in most countries, including the UK, these oils are freely available and there is no restriction on their sale and use. Thirdly, the majority of the people who buy essential oils are members of the general public who cannot be expected to have expert knowledge of their nature and use. It is remarkable then that their safety record is as good as it undoubtedly is. Despite this record, statements are sometimes made which sensationalize aromatherapy or exaggerate unwanted effects of the oils.

More to the point would be education of both the supplier and the general user in the appropriate and safe use of essential oils. That way lies a safe and sound future for the popular use of aromatherapy.

Tradition, experience and research

On the positive side, centuries of experience of essential oils worldwide has proved they are effective and safe when used knowledgeably and with care. This is true for many oils, e.g. the Egyptians proved the antiseptic powers of aromatics in the mummification process; Hippocrates fought the plague in Athens by using aromatic essences for fumigation; St. Hildegard of Bingen was using lavender oil in the 12th century; Hungary Water (a lotion scented with rosemary) began its 600 year life in the 14th century; by 1500 oils of benzoin, calamus, cedarwood, cinnamon, frankincense, myrrh, rose, rosemary, sage, spikenard and turpentine were known to the pharmacist. Essential oils were first mentioned in an official pharmacopoeia around the year 1600 in Germany (Price 1993 p. 6). Borneo camphor (an alcohol) was mentioned in Schroeder's Pharmacopoeia of 1698 as a 'prodigious alexipharmic' or antidote to poison. For others there is little historical evidence, and for almost all essential oils, while there is ample proof of their antiseptic powers, clinical trials are lacking. While this may be due in part to shortage of research funds, it is also attributable to the difficulty (even impossibility) of conducting blind trials with aromatic substances.

There is also a body of knowledge which concerns the use of essential oils on the skin by the perfumery industry, based on the impressive work carried out by the independent Research Institute of Fragrant Materials (RIFM) established in 1966. RIFM has now published over 1000 monographs on fragrance materials and almost 200 of these concern natural aromatic materials derived from plants. These include essential oils, absolutes and resins. The International Fragrance Association (IFRA) makes recommendations to the perfume industry for the safe use of such materials based on the published findings of RIFM, and these are useful guides to aromatherapists when applying essential oils to the skin.

Although some tests have been performed on humans, the majority have been carried out on animals—normally rabbits for dermal toxicity and rats for oral toxicity. However, the relevance of animal testing to humans is debatable. For instance, basil and tarragon oils may contain estragole (methyl chavicol) in high amounts and this compound has been implicated by research on animals as being a strong carcinogen. By inference, the use of these oils in aromatherapy might be considered hazardous, but research at St Mary's Hospital London indicates that the results of animal tests cannot be extended directly to humans. The carcinogenicity is due to the metabolite 1-hydroxyestragole, and the conclusion was that estragole presented little hazard to humans at normal food usage levels of 1 µg/kg/day (Howes et al 1990). The case for skin application of essential oils with a high content of estragole is still undecided. When applied to the skin, not all of the essential oil enters the body, but caution is advisable nevertheless pending investigation of the metabolization of estragole in the transdermal route.

Overdosing

When it comes to testing the toxic effects of swallowing essential oils, all studies are carried out using animals. There is currently no viable alternative because testing on humans is considered too hazardous. Occasionally some knowledge is derived from an accident involving a child or a deliberate overdose by an adult. Therefore, many of the opinions offered on this subject in the aromatherapy literature must be regarded as speculative.

Swallowing an overdose

The ingestion of a large quantity of neat essential oil produces a burning sensation in the mouth and throat, and in some serious cases nausea, vomiting and diarrhoea. If the overdose is extreme there may follow lethargy, ataxia and coma or perhaps irritability and convulsions (e.g. pennyroyal—see Ch. 8). The pupils may be dilated (e.g. camphor) or constricted (e.g. eucalyptus).

The effects of molecular shape

Carvone appears in laevo and dextro forms in different oils (for example d-carvone is present at

48-58% in caraway oil and l-carvone is the main constituent of spearmint oil). *Carum carvi* [CARAWAY] is considered to be a safe oil in all respects by Tisserand 1985 p. 19; Winter states (1984 pp. 62–63) both d- and l-carvone are nontoxic; l-carvone has an LD_{50} of 1640 mg/kg in rats (Jenner et al 1964) and d-carvone 3. 71 mg/kg in rats (Levenstein 1976).

Tyman (1990) has suggested that there are probably differences in effect between α- and β-thujone, and others have suggested the same is true for cis- and trans-anethole.

One frequently repeated statement is that all forms of ketones are neurotoxic, but this is not so (Tisserand 1985 p. 61). Thujone is not to be treated lightly whenever and wherever it occurs; however, the thujone molecule has four possible shapes, and it is not known whether they all have the same toxic potential and should all be avoided (Tyman 1990). The seed oil of *Anethum graveolens* [DILL] contains 40–60% of ketones, with a minimum of 28% d-carvone, and is considered neurotoxic by Franchomme (1990 p. 323). On the other hand, Tisserand (1985 p. 62) considers that 'carvone, which occurs in oils of caraway, dill, spearmint … is not present in sufficient quantities in the essential oils to present any risk'. There are many other anomalies such as this to be found in books on aromatherapy, which underlines the complexity of the individual chemicals and the wide variation in percentages present in essential oils and therefore in the overall effect on the human organisms.

Toxicity depends not only on the nature of the main component, but also on the relationships and synergy (see below) between this and some of the smaller (perhaps as yet unidentified) constituents, which are known to ameliorate undesirable effects in some cases.

Essential oils are very complex substances, and it is worth repeating the statement made earlier that there is no simple direct relationship between the effects of any single component of an essential oil and the effects of the complete natural essential oil—essential oils are synergistic mixes (Price 1990). This may illustrate why certain oils high in ketones are not considered toxic, or even why a

few oils which are considered toxic by some people do not appear to be so.

The study of essential oils can be a minefield, and to understand them completely would take a lifetime. For the present, it may be preferable in the current state of knowledge to continue to regard aromatherapy as much an art as a science. Nevertheless, it should be remembered that a great deal of good has been done (and no serious harm has so far been recorded) by qualified aromatherapists since the 1960s in Britain.

A nurse practising aromatherapy in a hospice some years ago was concerned to prove the safety of the oils she was administering to patients and took 5 ml of each of about 40 essential oils by mouth (one per week). In a personal communication she stated that she suffered no ill efects apart from dreaming more vividly than usual.

There is a large safety factor when using the oils in normal aromatherapy quantities, i.e. two or three drops compared with approximately 100 drops that a 5 ml teaspoon holds. The 40 oils included some that are potentially hazardous and it is advisable not to follow this extreme example. Individuals vary greatly in their reaction to different substances and such actions may produce a disastrous result.

Synergy

The word synergy is derived from two Greek words which mean 'working together'. In essential oils this is the working together of all the constituents within the whole. The effect of synergy is such that when two or more components are put together there is some extra activity greater than that of the individual components simply added together.

As discussed in Chapter 2, essential oils are complex mixtures, some containing several hundreds of different molecules, some comparatively few. Whole (or complete) essential oils have been found in practice to be more effective than their isolated principal constituent(s) and without side-effects (when used properly) on account of the synergistic effect (Hall 1904). 'It is this principle (synergy) which allows the achievement of strong effects from infinitely small doses of non-toxic products, but judiciously combined by nature herself' (Duraffourd 1982 p. 16). Constituents present in very small amounts (e.g. furocoumarins) are often found to be as, or more, active than the principal constituent.

Another complication regarding synergy is illustrated by the case of eucalyptus. Dr Pénoël writes:

Most of the eucalyptus products found on the usual aromatic market have been redistilled, rectified and refined. In reality the residue left behind in the still from the rectification of the crude oils is rich in precious molecules (like the rare phenol australol). Even if their proportion seems low, they work in synergy with the main components and should be kept in order for the essential oil to express its full healing potential.

(Pénoël 1993 personal communication)

Because of this synergistic feature, it can be difficult to assess the contribution made by any one component to the total effect of an essential oil. When tested individually they may behave differently than when in the presence of the other naturally-occuring molecules in the makeup of the oil. Tests carried out on individual components from *Eucalyptus citriodora* revealed that they were relatively inactive. However, a combination of the three major components in the same ratio found in the natural oil produced a four-fold increase in antimicrobial activity against *Staphylococcus aureus* (Low et al 1974).

Apart from the synergy produced by the components of a single oil, there is also an enhancement of effect when two or more whole oils are mixed together. For example, the bactericidal effect of several oils combined is greater than the effect of any of the individual oils.

Quenching

Quenching is another important aspect of synergy, whereby the potential unwanted side-effects of one component are nullified by the presence of other component(s). A good illustration of this is found by comparing the effects of two eucalyptus oils, *Eucalyptus globulus* [TASMANIAN BLUE GUM] and *Eucalyptus smithii* [GULLY GUM]. Both contain around 65% of 1,8-cineole (an oxide which is a skin irritant), yet the former is contraindicated for use on young children and the latter not (Pénoël 1993).

This quenching effect is well known in the perfumery industry, which turns it to advantage by adding quenching components to its perfumes to prevent skin irritation. An example is the use of d-limonene which when put together with lemongrass oil quenches the irritating effect of the aldehydes (see below).

To recapitulate, such interactions of components take place between the constituents within one oil and also between two or more essential oils, so that potentially toxic elements may be altered, enhanced or counteracted, by other constituents present. It is for this reason that aromatherapists use the whole natural oil rather than an active isolate, e.g. the eucalyptol from eucalyptus, thought to be responsible for the antiseptic, expectorant and contra-antigen action. Gattefossé, chemist and perfumer, the man who coined the term aromatherapy, wrote that eucalyptol is 'a substance with no apparent activity' and 'only an excipient' (Gattefossé 1937 pp. 41, 88). Hindsight makes wise men of us all.

Isolates are sometimes used by the medical profession in France, but they need to be used sparingly and with knowledge, and they are not used in aromatherapy as practised in this country.

Tests carried out employing the isolates phenylacetaldehyde, citral and cinnamic aldehyde—found in *Citrus aurantium* (flos) [NEROLI BIGARADE], *Cymbopogon citratus*, *C. flexuosus* [LEMONGRASS] and *Cinnamomum zeylanicum* (cort.) [CINNAMON] oils respectively—showed them to be skin sensitizers. However, the whole essential oils in which the aldehydes are present (at up to 85%) were found not to provoke sensitizing reactions. It appeared that some other component(s) of the natural oil inhibited the induction or expression of sensitization (Opdyke 1976). As a test of this hypothesis, several terpenes and alcohols, found along with the particular aldehyde in the natural composition were combined with each of the aldehydes in question. It appears now to be a consistent finding that each of these aldehydes, although producing sensitization reactions when applied alone, produces no sensitization reactions in selected simple mixtures with other compounds (Opdyke 1979) (see Table 3.1). These findings point to the difference between using a

Table 3.1 Results of quenching tests on mixtures of cinnamic aldehyde with other essential oil components. (Reprinted from Opdyke 1979 p. 255, with kind permission from Elsevier Science Ltd, The Boulevard, Langford Lane, Kidlington OX5 1GB, UK)

Second test material	Relative proportions*	Results of sensitization test
Dipropylene glycol	1 : 1	+
Phenylethyl alcohol	1 : 1	+
Eugenol	1 : 1	-
Eugenol	1 : 1[†]	-
Eugenol	2.5 : 1[†]	+
Cinnamic alcohol	1 : 1	+
Benzyl salicylate	1 : 1	+
d-limonene	1 : 1	-

* Ratio (w/w) of cinnamic aldehyde to second test material. Each mixture was tested at an overall concentration of 6% in petrolatum by the maximization procedure (Kligman 1966, Kligman & Epstein 1975).
† Duplicate tests.

single compound and the use of a natural synergistic mix with inbuilt quenching action. The above mentioned tests contrast with two earlier tests carried out by Kligman in 1971 and 1972 on 25 volunteers using cinnamon bark oil at 8% concentration and producing 18 and 20 sensitization reactions respectively (Kligman 1975). Cinnamic aldehyde is not the only component in *Cinnamomum zeylanicum* (cort.) [CINAMMON BARK] oil acting as a sensitizer, and perhaps this may be a case of synergy enhancing the unwanted effect. On the other hand, the irritation produced by the cinnamic aldehyde is completely quenched when in the whole oil. IFRA recommend that this oil is used at 1% max. on the skin.

It is believed that many natural essential oils which have not been tampered with display this quenching effect. Just because an oil contains one or more components which are thought to be hazardous in some way it does not automatically follow that the oil is unsafe, although caution must be observed. This feature can also be made use of when mixing oils. The aldehyde citral is a constituent of *Citrus limon* [LEMON] (5%) which on its own is irritating to the skin, yet the whole oil is not. Essential oil of *Cymbopogon citratus* and *flexuosus* has a high content of citral (approximately 70%) and the whole oil can therefore be irritant, but this effect can be quenched by adding an oil containing an equal amount of d-limonene (a terpene present in some citrus oils to around 80–90%).

The peel oils from *Citrus paradisi* [GRAPEFRUIT] or *Citrus sinensis* [SWEET ORANGE] when added to *Cymbopogon citratus* in a 50–50 mix successfully quench the irritant properties of the latter (Witty 1992 personal communication).

WHAT ARE WE USING?

Of the many factors involved in the safe use of essential oils, not least is the specification of the oil itself. Knowledge of such factors as where it is grown, whether it is cloned by cuttings or grown from seed, the plant variety, how produced (wild, organic or with chemicals), the part of the plant used and the chemotype leads to safe usage.

The importance of knowing what material is being used in a treatment is obvious, therefore it is imperative that the oil is precisely identified. This fact escapes the attention of many people treating others and even of some of those carrying out trials. Before embarking on a trial using essential oils it is of primary importance that a specified oil from a known source is used, and to have as a minimum a GLC analysis of the oil actually used in the test. Oil from the same harvest batch should be used throughout one test because aromatherapy oils are natural products, not standardized, and the actual composition of an oil may vary within wide limits.

The botanical name of the plant should always be used (unless talking generally about a species), because common names are imprecise and can cause confusion. The same common name can be given to different plants (such as marjoram, which might be *Origanum majorana* or *Thymus mastichina*), or more than one name is given to the same plant. An extreme example is cedarwood oil, which may be any one of the following, since all are traded as cedarwood:

- *Cedrus atlantica* [ATLAS CEDARWOOD]
- *Cedrus deodora* [DEODAR or HIMALAYAN CEDARWOOD]
- *Cedrus libani* [CEDAR OF LEBANON]
- *Chamaecyparis lawsoniana* [WESTERN WHITE CEDAR]
- *Cryptomeria japonica* [JAPANESE CEDAR]

- *Juniperus procera* [EAST AFRICAN CEDARWOOD]
- *Juniperus mexicana* [TEXAS CEDARWOOD]
- *Juniperus virginiana* [RED CEDARWOOD]
- *Thuja occidentalis* [WHITE CEDAR]
- *Thuja plicata* [WESTERN RED CEDAR].

In many cases it is not sufficient merely to specify in Latin the genus and species (and the variety if applicable), but also necessary to designate the chemotype (explained in Ch. 1) and the part of the plant used for extraction. An example is the cinnamon tree where the oil from the bark consists principally of an aldehyde, while the oil from the leaf is mainly a phenol with different effects and uses. The oil from the thuja tree, *Thuja occidentalis* (responsible for the restriction of cedarwood oils in France), is taken from the leaves—but other 'cedarwoods' from the wood. In the umbellifer family the seed oils can be significantly different from oils extracted from other parts of the same plant, e.g. in the case of *Angelica archangelica* the root oil is phototoxic while that from the seed is not. Therapists need to be aware of this and it is their responsibility to ensure that inappropriate treatment is not given.

Safe quantities

Essential oils may be applied to the body in a variety of ways, and these are discussed in Chapter 5, but usually their use involves inhalation, applying them to the skin or ingestion. Essential oils are powerful, otherwise they would be of no use therapeutically, and this means that they must be employed with care and knowledge to achieve beneficial results. Inappropriate use in whatever way can bring about undesired effects. Dosage, involving both quantity and time, is all important since too little may mean little or no result, and too much may (depending on the oils used) have a beneficial effect or create a serious problem.

The majority of essential oils may be considered less toxic than the over-the-counter medicines aspirin and paracetamol, and aromatherapy is a safe therapy provided the therapist is suitably trained. If this requirement is observed, there need be no hesitation in introducing these natural aromatic products into a hospital environment.

Many things in common use are toxic in overdose—for example, carrots, beneficial in moderation, although a surfeit will produce illness, and this is true of many other everyday foods such as tomatoes, saffron and mustard. Valnet (1980) cites the loss of eyebrows and headaches in workers handling vanilla, but vanilla ice cream is eaten and enjoyed without ill effect. An essential oil may be both safe and toxic depending on the amount administered—it all depends on the knowledge, skill and experience of the therapist. For example, we have observed that while lavender is sedative in low dose, with a high dose it can cause insomnia.

Ingestion of essential oils

N.B. This method of using essential oils in the case of pregnant women and very young children may be hazardous. See Chapter 8 for pregnancy and contraindications.

Only genuine natural essential oils should be employed for internal use, although, as we have seen, it is difficult for anyone to guarantee the purity of an essential oil, given the current state of the market. The ingestion of essential oils is therefore to be left in the hands of an aromatologist, as in the Community Health Sheffield (NHS Trust) area (see Ch. 14), or an experienced aromatherapist working under the direction of a doctor, who should exercise great care and discretion both in advising the use and procurement of essential oils. Any national legal requirements and any rules of the hospital management board will have to be observed, as also will the ethical considerations of any professional body to which the aromatherapist may belong. The therapist will take into account age, body weight, general state of health, current medication (if any) and the oils to be used.

Nevertheless, some conditions such as enteritis, irritable bowel syndrome and diverticulitis can scarcely be treated in any other way than by ingestion. If a course of treatment is embarked upon, then a rule of thumb for the *maximum* dose is 3 drops, 3 times daily for 3 weeks. Whether treating a patient or yourself, do not go beyond these limits—almost always, less is advisable. The best medium for diluting the oils for internal use is a fixed oil because the essential oils will dissolve easily and completely in it (Collin P 1994 personal communication). Runny honey is also a good diluent, with the addition of a little water.

Table 3.2 shows the lethal dose (LD50 is the dose at which 50% of the test subjects die) of some representative oils for a typical adult and a small child. These figures have been extrapolated from figures derived from animal testing and as metabolization in humans is not always the same as in animals their accuracy cannot be guaranteed (as seen above). In the absence of other information we must rely on these figures as a guide, and because the quantities used in aromatherapy are very small, there is normally an extremely high safety factor when comparing the lethal dose with the effective dose. The effective dose (ED_{50}) is the term used when some sort of response is being monitored in the experimental animal other than the death of the animal. The median effective dose is the dose at which 50% of the test subjects achieve the desired benefit.

Toxicity figures given in the aromatherapy literature do not always make it clear that these doses are per *kilogram* of body weight. This could lead to the misunderstanding that the figures given are the effective or lethal doses for a *person*. They are not; it is dependent on their weight.

For example the LD_{50} value for the oil from *Salvia officinalis* [SAGE] is 2.6 g/kg, which equates to a fatal dose of approximately 170 ml for a 60 kg person; the equivalent figure for *Chamaemelum nobile* [ROMAN CHAMOMILE] is 570 ml for a 60 kg person. The quantities involved are so great that anyone in their right mind would jib at taking them, although illness may be caused by a much lower dose.

Health professionals working in hospitals and similar establishments should secure the approval of a consultant or other suitably qualified and responsible person before giving oils by mouth, rectum or vagina. No carer without accredited training should administer oils in these ways unless under the supervision of an aromatologist. It is also important to preserve procedural safety, where prescriber, dispenser and administrator are separate persons to guard against error.

Only steam-distilled oils and the expressed citrus essences should be employed for ingestion. The following classes of oils should never be administered internally:

- oils obtained from gums (other than by distillation)
- resins (because of the solvent residue)
- absolutes (because of the solvent residue).

Dispensing and storage precautions

Labelling

As essential oils are freely available in most countries, the supplier needs to ensure that they are properly labelled, with proper cautions regarding children, eyes, pregnancy and skin. In France the sale of a few oils has been restricted since 1986 to the pharmacies: mugwort, wormwood, cedar, hyssop, sage, tansy and thuja (botanical names not given). Generally, self-regulation by an industry is to be preferred to governmental regulation and accordingly any oil which may be harmful when used injudiciously should not be offered for sale to anyone lacking adequate aromatherapy training. This would still leave a wide range of safe oils accessible for use by the general public. The Trades and Industries Board of the Aromatherapy Organisations Council (AOC), the self regulatory body for aromatherapy in Britain, requires its members to ensure that essential oil containers carry printed cautions and that hazardous oils are removed from retail shelves.

Flammability

One other aspect to be remembered when handling essential oils is that because they are so volatile, they are highly inflammable. Typical flash points for essential oils range between 43°C for citrus oils to about 70°C for peppermint. They should be stored carefully in a cool, dark area, and working areas for mixing should contain no naked flame. Smoking should not be permitted and the area should be well ventilated. It may be necessary to warn the insurer if oils are to be stocked in bulk.

Table 3.2   Lethal dose (LD50) of essential oils in animals with human lethal doses extrapolated from animal test results

	LD50 g/kg (animal)	Lethal dose 15 kg (child)	Lethal dose 70 kg (adult)
		ml	ml
Aniba rosaeodora (lig.) [ROSEWOOD]	4.30	72	334
Boswellia carteri [FRANKINCENSE]	5.00	83	389
Cananga odorata (flos) [YLANG YLANG]	> 5.00	83	389
Cedrus atlantica (lig.) [ATLAS CEDARWOOD]	> 5.00	83	389
Chamaemelum nobile (flos) [ROMAN CHAMOMILE]	8.56	143	666
Chamomilla recutita (flos) [GERMAN CHAMOMILE]	> 5.00	83	389
Cinnamomum zeylanicum (cort.) [CINNAMON BARK]	3.40	57	264
Cinnamomum zeylanicum (fol.) [CINNAMON LEAF]	2.65	44	206
Citrus aurantium var. *amara* (flos) [NEROLI BIGARADE]	> 5.00	83	389
Citrus aurantium var. *amara* (fol.) [PETITGRAIN BIGARADE]	> 5.00	83	389
Citrus bergamia (per.) [BERGAMOT]	> 10.00	167	778
Citrus reticulata (per.) [MANDARIN]	> 5.00	83	389
Commiphora myrrha [MYRRH]	1.65	28	128
Coriandrum sativum (fruct.) [CORIANDER]	4.13	69	321
Cupressus sempervirens (fol.) [CYPRESS]	> 5.00	83	389
Eucalyptus citriodora (fol.) [LEMON-SCENTED GUM]	> 5.00	83	389
Eucalyptus globulus (fol.) [TASMANIAN BLUE GUM]	4.44	74	345
Foeniculum vulgare var. *dulce* (fruct.) [SWEET FENNEL]	3.80	63	296
Hyssopus officinalis [HYSSOP]	1.40	23	109
Juniperus communis (fruct.) [JUNIPER BERRY]	8.00	133	622
Lavandula angustifolia [LAVENDER]	> 5.00	83	389
Lavandula x *intermedia* 'Super' [LAVANDIN]	> 5.00	83	389
Melaleuca alternifolia (fol.) [TEA TREE]	1.90	32	148
Melaleuca leucadendron (fol.) [CAJUPUT]	3.87	65	301
Mentha x *piperita* [PEPPERMINT]	4.50	75	350
Myristica fragrans (sem.) [NUTMEG]	2.60	43	202
Ocimum basilicum [BASIL]	1.40	23	109
Origanum majorana [MARJORAM]	2.24	37	174
Pelargonium graveolens (fol.) [GERANIUM]	> 5.00	83	389
Pimpinella anisum (fruct.) [ANISEED]	2.25	38	175
Pinus sylvestris (fol.) [PINE]	6.88	115	535
Piper nigrum (fruct.) [BLACK PEPPER]	> 5.00	83	389
Pogostemon patchouli (fol.) [PATCHOULI]	> 5.00	83	389
Rosa damascena, R. centifolia (flos) [ROSE OTTO]	> 5.00	83	389
Rosmarinus officinalis [ROSEMARY]	5.00	83	389
Salvia officinalis [SAGE]	2.52	42	196
Salvia sclarea [CLARY]	5.60	93	436
Santalum album (lig.) [SANDALWOOD]	5.58	93	434
Satureia hortensis [SUMMER SAVORY]	1.37	23	107
Syzygium aromaticum (flos) [CLOVE BUD]	2.65	44	206
Thymus mastichina [SPANISH MARJORAM]	> 5.00	83	389
Thymus vulgaris ct. thymol [THYME]	4.70	78	366

Table 3.2 *(continued)*

	LD50 g/kg (animal)	Lethal dose 15 kg (child)	Lethal dose 70 kg (adult)
		ml	ml
Vetiveria zizanioides (rad.) [VETIVER]	> 5.00	83	389
Zingiber officinale (rad.) [GINGER]	> 5.00	83	389
Compound 1,8-cineole	2.48	41	193
Compound carvacrol	0.81	14	63
Compound carvone	1.64	27	128
Compound linalool	2.79	47	217
Compound *p*-cymene	4.75	79	369
Compound pulegone	0.40	7	31
Compound safrole	1.95	33	152
Compound terpinen-4-ol	4.30	72	334
Compound thymol	0.98	16	76

Table 3.3 Flash points of some essential oils

	°C		°C
Boswellia carteri (dist.) [FRANKINCENSE]	32	*Nardostachys jatamansi* (rad.) [SPIKENARD]	>74
Cananga odorata (flos) [YLANG YLANG]	65	*Ocimum basilicum* var. *basilicum* (fol.) [EXOTIC BASIL]	75
Cedrus atlantica (lig.) [ATLAS CEDARWOOD]	110	*Ocimum basilicum* (fol.) [BASIL]	75
Chamaemelum nobile (flos) [ROMAN CHAMOMILE]	58	*Origanum majorana* (fol.) [SWEET MARJORAM]	54
Citrus aurantium var. *amara* (per.) [ORANGE BIGARADE]	43–45	*Pelargonium graveolens* (fol.) [GERANIUM]	77
Citrus aurantium var. *amara* (fol.) [PETITGRAIN BIGARADE]	68	*Petroselinum sativum* (fol.) [PARSLEY LEAF]	44
Citrus aurantium var. *amara* (flos) [NEROLI BIGARADE]	59	*Pimpinella anisum* (fruct.) [ANISEED]	90
Citrus bergamia (per.) [BERGAMOT]	58	*Pinus sylvestris* (fol.) [PINE]	38
Citrus limon (per.) [LEMON]	43–50	*Piper nigrum* (fruct.) [BLACK PEPPER]	47–58
Citrus reticulata (per.) [MANDARIN]	43–46	*Pogostemon patchouli* (fol.) [PATCHOULI]	>65
Cupressus sempervirens (fol.) [CYPRESS]	37	*Rosa damascena, R. centifolia* (flos) [ROSE OTTO]	100
Eucalyptus globulus (fol.) [TASMANIAN BLUE GUM]	38–51	*Rosmarinus officinalis* (fol.) [ROSEMARY]	49
Eucalyptus smithii (fol.) [GULLY GUM]	38–51	*Salvia officinalis* (fol.) [SAGE]	41
Eucalyptus staigeriana (fol.) [LEMON-SCENTED IRON TREE]	38–51	*Salvia sclarea* (flos, fol.) [CLARY]	77
Juniperus communis (ram.) [JUNIPER TWIG]	33	*Santalum album* (lig.) [SANDALWOOD]	>100
Juniperus communis (fruct.) [JUNIPER BERRY]	33	*Syzygium aromaticum* (flos) [CLOVE BUD]	>65
Lavandula angustifolia (flos, fol.) [LAVENDER]	75	*Thymus mastichina* (herb.) [SPANISH MARJORAM]	55
Melaleuca alternifolia (fol.) [TEA TREE]	57	*Thymus satureioides* (herb.) [MOROCCAN THYME]	55
Melaleuca leucadendron (fol.) [CAJUPUT]	45	*Thymus vulgaris* (herb.) [THYME]	55
Melissa officinalis (fol.) [MELISSA]	60	*Vetiveria zizanioides* (rad.) [VETIVER]	>65
Mentha x *piperita* (fol.) [PEPPERMINT]	67–70	*Zingiber officinale* (rad.) [GINGER]	55
Myristica fragrans (sem.) [NUTMEG]	38	*Valeriana officinalis* (rad.) [VALERIAN]	>74

UNDESIRED EFFECTS

It is undeniable that, along with the undoubted power of essential oils, there will be some unwanted effects. However, it is safe to say that these are rare, mostly only following an overdose.

The general safety of essential oils normally used in aromatherapy may be judged by the health of workers who handle and inhale significant quantities of essential oils in the course of their daily work, e.g. in the perfumery industry. Some members of our staff have been handling, bottling and breathing a wide range of oils during the whole of their working day for over a decade, with no reported bad effects. There are many therapists (including ourselves) who have been working full time with the oils over an even longer period of time who have experienced nothing but good effects, and it may therefore be inferred that aromatherapy is basically a safe therapy. However, there are one or two therapists who have developed a sensitivity to a few oils; unfortunately, if the sensitivity is due to a specific chemical in the oil, then wherever that chemical occurs, they may have a reaction. It should be noted that in some cases a reaction may be due to an adulterant rather than an essential oil component.

Therapists who do not use commercial perfumes run less risk of developing sensitivities to essential oils, as the overall quantity of synthetics employed in perfumes in day-to-day situations plays a large part in the growing number of people developing allergies and substance sensitivities (Bennett 1990)—quite an alarming fact.

In general aromatherapists do not use the expression side-effects, because of its undesirable connotations. As can be seen from the list of properties of lavender oil given on p. 37, most (but not all) of the side-effects of essential oils are desirable. For example, lavender oil may be used as part of a treatment for depression. If, as a result, there are other beneficial results such as the alleviation of insomnia and relief from rheumatic pain, this is to be welcomed. Undesired side-effects occur usually as a result of the misuse of the oils, e.g. in the attempt to produce an abortion, or by accidental overdose—typically a toddler swallowing essential oils from a bottle. If essential oils are sold only in bottles with integral droppers and sensible precautions are taken to prevent access by children to the essential oils then this can be considered an extremely low-risk therapy. In normal aromatherapy or aromatology use the dose is usually very low, but idiosyncratic reaction is a rare possibility, as with any form of treatment.

In orthodox medicine, as mentioned in Chapter 2, a single molecule 'bullet' is aimed at the symptom. In aromatherapy we point a shotgun at the problem which sprays all sorts of beneficial shot, together with the occasional unwanted effect.

Because of possible harmful effects, some oils are rarely or never used in aromatherapy (a more comprehensive list of such oils can be found in Appendix B.4). Some examples are *Juniperus sabina* [SAVIN], *Gaultheria procumbens* [WINTERGREEN], *Peumus boldus* [BOLDO LEAF], *Sassafras officinale* [SASSAFRAS], *Thuja occidentalis* [THUJA].

Dermal toxicity

This term includes irritation, phototoxicity and sensitization.

Skin irritation

This is a reaction to an irritant which produces inflammation and itchiness. Some essential oils are irritating to the skin and, usually but not exclusively, these are found to contain high proportions of either aldehydes or phenols. Oils in common use which have been found to be irritant are listed in Appendix B.6. Because there appears to be a wide tolerance variation between people, a given oil might not cause a reaction in the majority of people yet be irritant to one or two more sensitive individuals. However, dermal irritation produced by essential oils is usually localized and short-lived. Assuming one oil has a 50% presence of an offending component, this is present in the total mix at only 0.5% when the oil is used in a normal massage mix, along with two or three other oils, at the standard dilution of 3% essential oils in a carrier. When spread over a large area of skin the possibility of irritation is remote, and in any case the degree of irritation is proportional to the strength of the mixture applied.

Examples of oils containing aldehydes can be found in Appendix B.6. The phenolic oils can also be found there, but not listed separately. The essential oils which are potentially irritant to the skin include:

- *Cinnamomum zeylanicum* (fol.) [CINNAMON LEAF]
- *Origanum vulgare* [OREGANO]
- *Satureia hortensis* [SUMMER SAVORY]
- *Satureia montana* [WINTER SAVORY]
- *Syzygium aromaticum* (flos) [CLOVE BUD]
- *Syzygium aromaticum* (fol.) [CLOVE LEAF]
- *Syzygium aromaticum* (lig.) [CLOVE STEM]
- *Thymus vulgaris* ct. phenol [RED THYME]
- *Thymus capitatus* [SPANISH OREGANO]
- *Thymus serpyllum* [WILD THYME] (depending on chemotype).

Tagetes glandulifera is sometimes cited as being a skin irritant, but we have not found this to be the case in practice, although it is a photo-sensitizer. Two oils from the cruciferae family—*Brassica nigra* [MUSTARD] and *Armoracia rusticana* [HORSE RADISH] are not normally recommended for aromatherapy use, because both consist almost entirely of allylisothiocyanate. These oils applied neat to the skin will provoke severe burning and blistering. However, it has been known for these oils to be recommended at the extremely low concentration of 1 drop of essential oil in 500 ml of carrier oil for rheumatism.

A Japanese study showed that the skin of men tends to be more than twice as sensitive as that of women, and when in situations of severe stress, lack of sleep, etc., then all skins are rendered more sensitive (Hosokawa & Ogwana 1979)

Mucous membrane irritation

Generally speaking, essential oils with a substantial content of phenols (chiefly thymol, carvacrol and eugenol) can be responsible for irritating a mucous membrane. Oils containing aldehydes may also be implicated. In the past it was believed that the hydrocarbon terpenes caused mucous membrane irritation (Gattefossé 1937 p. 40) but this is now thought not to be the case. Any of the oils listed in Appendix B.6 may cause irritation of the mucous membranes of the alimentary, respiratory and genito-urinary tracts. A possible exception is lemon oil, which contains less than 5% aldehyde and consists mainly of hydrocarbon terpenes.

Phototoxicity, photosensitivity

This occurs when the essential oil reacts with the skin under the influence of ultraviolet rays, and does not occur on skin protected from natural or artificial sunlight. It may result in erythema, hyperpigmentation and perhaps vesicles, depending on the severity of the reaction. Care needs to be taken with the citrus essences, which are expressed from the peel and contain large furo-coumarin molecules which cause skin reactions. This is particularly so with bergamot. Other oils exhibiting this characteristic at aromatherapeutic doses are *Angelica archangelica* (rad.) [ANGELICA ROOT], *Juniperus virginiana* [VIRGINIAN CEDARWOOD], *Ruta graveolens* [RUE], *Lippia citriodora* [VERBENA] and *Cuminum cyminum* [CUMIN]. (See App. B.7.)

It is fortunate that the essential oils cross the skin rather quickly, and it it safe to expose the skin to sunlight 1 hour or more from application.

Contact sensitization

There are some oils which do not produce any reaction on first contact with the skin, but may do so on a subsequent application. The body's reaction involves the immune system via the cells in the basal layer of the epidermis. There are several oils which are sensitizing, and there seems to be no common denominator. Poor storage of oils containing a significant amount of mono-terpenes can lead to the formation of sensitizing hydroperoxides: an infamous example is turpentine, which is responsible for skin allergies to workers in the paint industry. Oils to be wary of in this respect are shown in Appendix B.8.

Cross-sensitization

Once a person is sensitized to one substance, then that person is more likely to be susceptible to other similar substances, although the risk is low. This need not cause concern, but any aroma-therapist who is sensitive to substances should be aware of the possibility. This is a complex topic, not well understood, but one example is when people become sensitive to benzoin after sensitization to Peru balsam or turpentine. There is a similar relationship between turpentine and peppermint (see App. B.8).

Other sensitivities and toxicities

Prolonged use

If any one oil is used for a very long period of time then there may be a risk of sensitization even though none exists for normal usage. It is relevant to note here that when eau de Cologne (which contains bergamot and other citrus essences) was much in vogue many people wore it daily over a period of years and developed raised erythematous rough skin where the Cologne was applied—usually on the neck (Berloque dermatitis). This reaction can be semi-permanent, lasting for years after cessation of use of the fragrance before disappearing (Shirley Price's personal experience). Many perfumes have ingredients in common with eau de Cologne and may produce similar reactions.

To obviate toxicity as a result of overuse of any one oil it is good aromatherapy practice to employ essential oils for short term use and to change the oils used during a treatment of long duration.

Mutagenicity and teratogenicity

There is no available evidence that any natural essential oil has ever provoked mutagenicity or teratogenicity in an embryo or developing fetus. No tests have been carried out, because the possibility of fragrant materials causing either genetic mutation or malformation is regarded as unlikely.

Carcinogenicity

A few oils have been tested for carcinogenicity on animals and the essential oil components safrole and dihydrosafrole have been implicated in the formation of hepatic tumours in rats, and calamus oil containing β-asarone produced duodenal tumours (Taylor et al 1967). For this reason

sassafras, which contains safrole as an important constituent, is not used in aromatherapy. Safrole is also significantly present in Brazilian sassafras oil, and in trace amounts in white camphor oil. β-asarone (found in calamus oil) is restricted in foods and drinks to 0.1-1 mg/kg. Despite the evidence from animal testing (where the doses used were large), it is thought that there is minimal risk in humans undergoing aromatherapy treatment.

Neurotoxicity

Special care must be taken with a few essential oils containing significant amounts of a ketone which are aggressive to nerve tissue. Not all ketones are neurotoxic (Winter 1984 pp. 62-63, Tisserand 1985 p. 61), but as a class they must be regarded as hazardous in this respect. Particular care must be exercised when using oils containing apiole (e.g. *Petroselinum sativum* (fruct.)) and ascaridole (e.g. *Peumus boldus*). (Regarding risks of using neurotoxic oils in pregnancy see Ch. 8). The molecules in essential oils are lipid-soluble and as such can pass the blood-brain barrier and access the central nervous system. The degree of lipid-solubility varies from one class of molecule to another; for example, the esters are more fat soluble than the alcohols. Once past this barrier there is a potential for toxicity: accidental overdose of *Syzygium aromaticum* produced convulsions in a child. It is thought that the ketone thujone (found in *Thuja occidentalis, Salvia officinalis, Tanacetum vulgare, Artemisia vulgaris, Artemisia absinthium*) is toxic to the CNS, as is the ketone asarone (found in *Acorus calamus*) Wenzel & Ross 1957).

Hepatotoxicity

When using essential oils having appreciable quantities of aldehydes there is a risk of toxicity due to build-up in the liver. People taking fennel essential oil over a long period of time show a colour change in the liver tissue (Franchomme & Pénoël 1990). Thujone, thymol and turpentine oil may damage the liver following oral ingestion in high doses (Schilcher 1985). Liver toxicity seems to arise when innocuous essential oil components are metabolized to toxic chemicals, as with pulegone, found in many of the mint oils. Also to be treated with caution (based largely on animal testing using very high doses) are methyl chavicol (found in *Artemisia dracunculus* [TARRAGON]), safrole (in *Sassafras albidum*), myristicin and elemicin (in *Myristica fragrans* [NUTMEG OIL]) and apiole (in *Petroselinum sativum* (fruct.)).

Nephrotoxicity

Some essential oils have an effect on the kidneys which is regarded as stimulating and beneficial in low doses, but could be classed as toxic if the quantity of oil used is excessive or it is used for too long a time. *Juniperus sabina* is mentioned by Schilcher (1985) as causing damage to the kidneys, even when applied externally. Large quantities of the ester methyl salicylate, found in

the oils of *Gaultheria procumbens* and *Betula lenta* [SWEET BIRCH], and of safrole (found in *Sassafras albidum*) are nephrotoxic. Sandalwood and turpentine taken orally in excessive doses can cause kidney damage (Tukioka 1927).

Respiratory sensitivity

See Chapter 5.

Summary

The need for a dispassionate and scientific attitude towards media charges of the dangers of essential oils has been demonstrated, as has the need for skill in their selection and prescription. Various types of potentially toxic situations have been identified. These should not occur if the guidelines for safe administration are followed.

REFERENCES

Bennett G 1990 Allergy and substance sensitivity. Shirley Price Aromatherapy College, Hinckley
Duraffourd P 1982 En forme tous les jours. La Vie Claire, Périgny
Franchomme P, Pénoël D 1990 L'aromathérapie exactement. Jollois, Limoges
Gattefossé R-M 1937 Aromatherapy (trans. 1993). Daniel, Saffron Walden p. 34
Hall C 1904 cited in Valnet J 1980 The practice of aromatherapy. Daniel, Saffron Walden
Hosokawa H, Ogwana T 1979 Study of skin irritations caused by perfumery materials. Perfumer & Flavorist 4(4): 7–8
Howes A, Chan U, Caldwell J 1990 Structure specificity of the genotoxicity of some naturally occurring alkenylbenzenes determined by the unscheduled DNA synthesis assay in rat hepatocytes. Food and Chemical Toxicology 28(8): 537–542
Jenner P M, Hagan E C, Taylor J M, Cook E L, Fitzhugh O G 1964 Food flavourings and componds of related structure. I. Acute oral toxicity. Food and Cosmetics Toxicology 2: 327
Kligman A M 1966 The identification of contact allergens by human assay. III. The maximization test, A procedure for screening and rating contact sensitizers. Journal of Investigative Dermatology 47: 393
Kligman A M, Epstein W 1975 Updating the maximization test for identifying contact allergens. Contact Dermatitis 1: 231
Levenstein I 1976 Report to RIFM 18 August. Cited in Food and Cosmetics Toxicology 16: 673

Low D, Rawal B D, Griffin W J 1974 Antibacterial action of the essential oils of some Australian Myrtacae with special references to the activity of chromatographic fractions of oil of *Eucalyptus citriodora*. Planta Medica 26: 184–189
Opdyke D L J 1976 Inhibition of sensitization reactions induced by certain aldehydes. Food and Cosmetics Toxicology 14(3): 197–198
Opdyke D L J 1979 Fragrance raw materials monographs. Food and Chemical Toxicology 17(3): 253–258
Pénoël D 1992 Winter shield. International Journal of Aromatherapy 4(4): 11
Price L 1990 Clinical practitioners aromatherapy course notes. Shirley Price International College of Aromatherapy, Hinckley
Price S 1993 The aromatherapy workbook. Thorsons, London
Schilcher H 1985 Effects and side-effects of essential oils. In: Baerheim Svendsen A, Scheffer J J C (eds) Essential oils and aromatic plants. Martinus Nijhof/Junk, Dordrecht
Tisserand R 1985 The essential oil safety data manual. Association of Tisserand Aromatherapists, Brighton
Tukioka M 1927 Proceedings. Imperial Academy Tokyo 3: 624
Tyman J H P 1990 Essential Oils Trade Association Symposium, Brunel University, June
Valnet J 1980 The practice of aromatherapy. Daniel, Saffron Walden, p. 11
Wenzel D G, Ross C R 1957 Journal of the American Pharmaceutical Association 46: 77
Winter R 1984 A consumer's dictionary of cosmetic ingredients. Crown, New York

4

Traditional use, modern research

Introduction

The use of essential oils as part of traditional plant-based medicine has led to the accumulation of a large body of empirical knowledge about their effectiveness in different conditions. This chapter looks systematically at their therapeutic properties, and shows where possible how modern science confirms traditional usage.

ORTHODOX MEDICINE AND PHYTOTHERAPY

There have always existed many different approaches to the healing of people. Today these approaches are generally viewed as being complementary and supplementary to each other rather than competitive and antagonistic. Two of the different medical approaches are contrasted here: orthodox medicine and phytotherapy.

The orthodox approach

The predominant contemporary approach is that adopted by orthodox allopathic medicine, where illness is regarded as being due to an outside agent. Throughout the ages this outside agent concept has been looked upon in various ways and illness attributed to 'evil spirits', 'ill will' or 'microbes' and, in more modern times, 'bacteria' and 'viruses'. In classical medicine the aim is to target and exterminate this outside agent, so freeing the body from further attack: the body is left to repair itself (Verdet 1989). It has, however, been estimated that 85% of all illness is self limiting (see Ch. 7).

This selective focusing on the causative agent has brought about an enormous increase in the knowledge of the separate body systems and organs. However, the sheer volume of knowledge acquired has resulted in specialization and compartmentalization becoming the norm, and it is left to the general practitioner to preserve an overview of the whole person.

For many decades now medicine, and consequently pharmacy, has lived under the reign of analysis, of simplification. This philosophy shows itself in the production of medicines which are for the most part composed of a single well defined molecule, well-known regarding its structure and properties, particularly the pharmacodynamics or therapeutic action on the organism. This style of analysis and simplification is the heritage of Descartes, who said quite rightly that to know the body better it was necessary to divide it into its constituent parts.

(Duraffourd 1982 p. 14)

This excellent principle has been pursued to such a degree that there now exists a detrimental imbalance in medical care as the large number of iatrogenic illnesses show.

The phytotherapy approach

Phytotherapy (herbal medicine, but without the old-fashioned connotation of 'herbalism') deals exclusively in whole plants or isolated plant principles, and aromatherapy may be considered to be one of its branches (unlike homoeopathy which uses plant, animal and mineral materials). It is essentially an empirical medicine, which recognizes the importance of the individual, and that each person lives their own ill health. This means that each person must receive individual treatment and care in their own environment, which may take longer than orthodox medicine but has a long-lasting effect. As well as treating illness, phytotherapy and aromatherapy are valuable for everyday prophylactic use, reinforcing weak points in the person to maintain good health. The following theoretical comparison illustrates the different approaches taken by orthodox and complementary practitioners in treating a person.

- Allopathy: Should an apparently healthy person suddenly develop a gastroenteric problem, a gastroenterologist will investigate only the digestive system and not pay too much attention to neighbouring organs and systems. The offending bacteria will be identified in the laboratory and an antidote will be prescribed, most probably an antibiotic. After treatment the symptoms will disappear and the client is said to have regained health.
- Aromatherapy: The therapist will look at the patient and will say that the defence system has broken down and this is the cause of the illness, allowing the bacteria to enter and thrive. The weakness will be considered in relation to other systems—kidneys, liver, lungs, skin—and all this is then studied in the context of the living environment. It may be a problem relating to food, a stressful experience or climate. A balance must be sought; and the therapist using the properties of essential oils has the necessary weapons to effect this.

Recent history of plant-based medicine

At the beginning of this century many medicines were based on plants and plant extracts. One reason for the former popular use of plants in healing was their easy availability in a still largely rural environment—people could gather plants and process their own medicines. Another reason for their use was the prevailing poverty at the time. In many areas of Europe money was scarce, there was little state assistance and private health insurance was practically unknown. Bonnelle (1993) quotes some older people's memories:

Before the social security, when people had to pay, they didn't call the doctor out. ...That's why people used to treat themselves with plants then. My mother had 50 plants which she used to dry. ...The doctor never came to our house. 20 franc pieces came in but never went out, except to buy a field.

However, after the Second World War, orthodox medicine took advantage of recent developments in science and technology. This resulted in an accelerating shift in emphasis from natural to rapidly-acting drugs.

Decline and fall of popular plant medicine

As part of the fresh start after the Second World War, state medicine was introduced in some Western European countries, including France and Britain. This was one of the greatest advances in civilization the world has seen, and we should all be very much the worse off, both as individuals and as a society, if it did not exist. Unwittingly, this wonderful step forward struck a near-mortal blow at folk plant medication because, with the availability of free treatment and advice from doctors, the knowledge of centuries was discarded or at best put to one side and little used. People were no longer content with the gentle use of plants which took rather a long time both to prepare and to bring about healing. They had great expectations of the new synthetic drugs, which genuinely appeared then to produce immediate and startling results without any real effort on the part of the sufferer.

Nowadays, speaking for myself, plants are not strong enough. I used nothing else before ... but now you have to get the doctors' medicines. When they discovered the new drugs, everyone forgot about the plants.

(Bonnelle 1993)

Both doctors and vets have used antibiotics extensively and liberally since 1945, and people's expectations of medical practice have changed in that instant cures are asked for, without any effort or responsibility on the part of the sufferer. In a broad sense the relationship of people to their own health has changed and, as plant remedies have fallen into disuse and lost ground to high-tech instant medicine, popular knowledge has disappeared inexorably. The older generation who used to practise self-healing with plants, talk about plants but no longer use them and do not pass on their knowledge to their successors.

In the flower-power and Beatles age of the 1960s and 1970s there was a resurgence of many ideas, including caring for the ecological balance of nature, the use of natural as opposed to synthetic products, and the idea of eating organically-grown foods. This new vision also encompassed the field of medicine and as a result many alternative (as they were viewed then) approaches to healing took root and flourished.

These are now known as energetic, parallel or complementary approaches and, in contra-distinction to the idea of conquering the illness by destroying the disease, there is much attention paid to a holistic style of treatment, of strengthening the body's own natural defences to cope with attacks by pathogens, of helping a person to live in harmony with their own body, with other people and with the environment. When a person is successful in this, then good health is enjoyed, and illness strikes when the balance of the person within the environment is disturbed.

Today plant remedies are beginning to become more popular again, chiefly for small problems (such as headaches and twinges) which are too insignificant to warrant troubling the busy doctor and for chronic complaints (which by definition are not easily susceptible to orthodox treatment). Here, people are prepared to try at their own expense alternative procedures for the 'you must learn to live with it' conditions. It is significant that the most popular aromatherapy treatment and therefore one which might be regarded as successful is, in our experience, for chronic arthritis and rheumatism.

Modern research and traditional usage

Huge sums are spent on research, clinical trials and licensing for each orthodox medicine, pill or tablet which appears on the market. This is done with the best will in the world—to help alleviate suffering and disease—but medical science is now faced with the situation, despite all the care and time spent on research, that there are still many serious side-effects. Essential oils have not been clinically tested in this way because it would cost billions, not millions, of pounds to test each oil and synergistic mix for each therapeutic effect of which it is capable. In the absence of scientific proof, orthodoxy finds it difficult to accept a discipline such as aromatherapy, which is still more art than science. Nevertheless essential oils have been used traditionally for hundreds of years to good effect. Had they manifested serious side-effects their use would certainly not have survived to the present day; yet in the recent past clinical tests on animals (which have a different physiology from humans) have allowed the creation of drugs which have had disastrous effects on humans: Thalidomide and Opren passed such recognized tests. The enormous beneficial advances made in the field of orthodox medicine should not be underestimated, but appreciation and inclusion of the available natural ways are needed too—there is room for more than one approach in the healing arena.

Acceptance of aromatherapy

Litigation in all fields of medicine has increased dramatically over the last decade and it has now reached a significant level of cost. Where midwifery is concerned, the Congenital Disabilities (Civil Liabilities) Act 1976 provides for a child to be entitled to recover damages where he has suffered as a result of a breach in duty of care, and litigation can be instigated up to 21 years after the event. With this in mind it is understandable to a degree that 'unproven' complementary treatments and medicaments are viewed with a certain amount of caution. Nevertheless, the intrinsically safe practice of aromatherapy is finding acceptance in many hospital departments today. The following comparison may help to explain why.

- **Orthodox drugs:** These are predominantly synthetic but may include isolated natural components, and are mostly used in a symptomatic way. Side-effects (iatrogenic disease) are always present to some degree and may necessitate further medication. The drugs themselves are usually available only on prescription, but less powerful drugs and tablets are sometimes available over-the-counter. The clinical testing of drugs is rigorous but carried out over a comparatively short timescale compared with traditional plant usage.
- **Essential oils:** These are completely natural, only whole unadulterated oils being used. As a general rule the dose used is extremely small and side-effects are rare in practice. It is usual for ample time to be devoted by the aromatherapy practitioner for discussion with the client and for the treatment. Individual treatment is necessary because clients are regarded as individuals. Germs do not necessarily produce the same reaction in different hosts, and it may be necessary to specify different oils

to tackle the same infection in different people (Valnet 1980 p. 42). With one mix of essential oils it is possible to care for more than one problem.

THE THERAPEUTIC PROPERTIES OF ESSENTIAL OILS

There are many reasons why essential oils need to be included in the armoury of weapons in the fight against disease. They have many positive properties and effects which are desirable and few drawbacks. They are capable of being anti-inflammatory, antiseptic, appetite-stimulating, carminative, choleretic, circulation-stimulating, deodorizing, expectorant, granulation-stimulating, hyperaemic, insecticidal, insect-repelling and sedative (Schilcher 1985 p. 217). They are natural antimicrobial agents able to act on bacteria, viruses and fungi, and many trials have been performed in this field (see below). Tropical countries have traditionally used lots of spices in their cuisines, not only for the flavour, but also to kill the microbes which flourish in hot climates. It is thought that the antiseptic powers of essential oils are due to their lipid solubility (Malowan 1931) and their surface activity (Rideal et al 1928).

Essential oils are applied to the skin by various methods, ingested or inhaled (see Ch. 5), and all of these are harmless unless used incorrectly. A significant point in their favour is their pleasant aroma. They are much used in products for the home (examples are lemon and lavender) and are well accepted—they are much pleasanter and safer in use than bleach or carbolic acid. The aroma itself has effects on the person using them (see Ch. 7).

The healer should have precise control over and full knowledge of the substances being employed in the treatment. If this is the case, and the healer determines the therapeutic materials to be used, not some faraway laboratory, the medicine may be tailored precisely to the individual patient. Generally speaking there is an absence of unwanted side-effects arising from the use of essential oils in a healing situation (see Synergy in Ch. 3), and plant extracts are ecologically sound, causing no pollution, unlike the antibiotics which are flushed down the drain to pollute the land (Verdet 1989).

Case 4.1 Aromatologist: Dr D Pénoël, France

A's case is a 'princeps' one because it was the first time that a full medical aromatherapeutic treatment was undertaken in Australia, and it completely succeeded where all the other therapies, official or alternative, had failed.

1 month after her premature birth, A began to suffer from recurrent ENT infections that were repeatedly treated by antibiotics. Her parents, very worried by this situation, which seemed to become worse every time, consulted a renowned homoeopath in Auckland. However, this treatment did not prevent the recurrence of the infections, together with very high fever, so the homoeopath reluctantly turned to antibiotics.

At 18 months, the condition was so bad that the parents decided to leave the wet climate of New Zealand and to settle in 'the driest state of the driest continent of the world'—South Australia. This change did not help A's internal condition, and again she received lots of antibiotics, each time worsening her state of health. Tetracyclines had rotted her teeth and her knees hurt whenever the weather was wet. After repeated infections artificially suppressed, her immune system was beginning to turn against her own organism.

When A was 7 years old, the ENT children's specialist asked for an X-ray of the sinuses. The radiography showed a complete blockage of the left maxillary sinus, a thickening of the wall of the right maxillary sinus and an infectious condition of the enlarged adenoids. The specialist decided to perform a surgical operation, under general anaesthesia, in order to flush the pus out of the sinuses. Beforehand, A was to receive another course of antibiotics over 15 days and a fresh X-ray examination. A's parents refused this procedure and announced to the specialist that they had decided to try aromatherapy. The specialist said: 'Do it at your own risk and I will see you in a fortnight'.

A's condition was miserable. She had tubes in her ears and impaired hearing, frequent pains in her knees and her breathing was affected by her permanent chronic infection. She was skinny, pale, permanently tired and sad, and she was backward at school due to absence from illness.

I had 2 weeks to prove the worth of medical aromatherapy, compared with 7 years of continuous disease and allopathic treatments. A complete programme of treatment was established, involving 2-hour sessions in the surgery each day and treatments at home. A's diet was corrected and nutritional advice was scrupulously followed by the family.

When dealing with a chronic and complex medical situation, it is of crucial importance to consider essential oils from an analytical perspective, i.e. knowing the molecules they contain and their percentages and linking this data with the different pathological aspects of the case and the capacity of the aromatic molecules to fight and correct these.

In A's case, the pathology included infection, mucus production and stagnation. The chronic inflammatory state of the mucous membrane was the result of the first two factors. The essential oils were carefully selected in relationship to how they could enter her body. Here, two errors have to be avoided: thinking only of the local treatment and forgetting the general one, and believing that correcting the overall state of health will be sufficient to clear the local situation.

Local treatment. High-tech aerosol equipment, using sonic vibrations, penetrated deeply into the sinuses (a drop of *Mentha* × *piperita* in some liquid honey, kept 30 seconds in the mouth as a pre-treatment, helped to open the nostrils). The essential oil used in the aerosol was *Inula graveolens*, which contains a small percentage of sesquiterpenic lactones, endowed with a strong mucolytic power. Besides, it contains an antiinfectious and immunoregulator monoterpenic alcohol (borneol) plus an antiinflammatory and antispasmodic ester (bornyl acetate) which work in conjunction, making an excellent synergy within a single oil.

Cutaneous treatment. Here, essential oils were applied neat on different parts of the body—mainly on the back and thoracic area. The blend, 10 ml of which was used neat daily, included: *Rosmarinus officinalis* ct. cineole (respiratory), *Rosmarinus officinalis* ct. verbenone (mucolytic and antiinflammatory), *Melaleuca alternifolia* (antiseptic) and *Thymus satureioides* (antiinfectious, antiinflammatory, immunobalancing).

Internal treatment. Orally, 5–6 drops of the following essential oils were blended in honey and taken 4 times a day with warm water, like a herbal tea: *Melaleuca alternifolia, Mentha* × *piperita, Thymus satureioides, Satureia montana*. Other complementary techniques used were: Swiss reflex massage on the feet, dynamic drainage of the face area by suction cups and magnetic field therapy on the face, liver, spleen and kidney areas.

After 2 weeks, A had received 11 sessions in my practice and it was clear that an overall and local improvement had taken place. When the new X-ray was taken it showed that the sinus and adenoid infections had totally cleared.

The ENT specialist, on seeing the X-ray, simply said 'cases of spontaneous healing are known among children'. Nevertheless, medical aromatherapy had won the first battle, in a case where everything else had failed.

4 months later, during winter, A had acute tonsillitis. Looking at the case holistically, we did not conclude that a 'bug' had jumped into A's throat, but that her whole organism had won enough strength, through the continued aromatherapeutic treatment, to expel toxins and waste matters coming from all the medications and accumulated infections, that had been locked inside until then. Every morning for 4 days an enormous quantity of thick brown mucus had been found on A's pillow. To keep this acute elimination process under control (but not to counteract it!), essential oils were used in the same intensive way as before, and after a battle of 4 days, her throat was completely cleansed, the fever stopped, and A was feeling like a new child! Whenever the acute stages of disease are dealt with successfully by implementing natural medicine treatments, it really marks a turning point in the evolution of the underlying illness.

A is now 15 years old and has taken no antibiotics since she was 7. She is strong, healthy, excels at school (especially in French!), in art and in sport and believes that the intervention of medical aromatherapy thoroughly changed her life.

Antiseptic and antibacterial

Essential oils have multiple actions and effects, e.g. when used for a respiratory infection an oil may be not only antiseptic, but also mucolytic, antiinflammatory and so on (Duraffourd 1987 p. 17). Another example is the use of oils on the digestive system, where the oils are antiseptic but do not act unfavourably on the flora and on the digestive secretions, in contrast to the unwelcome effects of antibiotics.

The molecules of essential oils occur naturally and are not inimical to the human body. They support the immune system and can be considered as pro- and eubiotic as opposed to the synthetic antibiotics. There is a natural variation in the chemical composition and physical characteristics of essential oils from year to year but this variation does not seem materially to affect their antiseptic properties, although it is always necessary to be aware of the analysis of the actual sample being tested. It is possible to have two factors for the one essential oil, depending on the method of use, e.g. the antiseptic use of liquid or vaporized oil.

Essential oils are especially valuable as antiseptics because their aggression towards microbial germs is matched by their total harmlessness to tissue—one of the chief defects of chemical antiseptics is that they are likely to be as harmful to the cells of the organism as to the cause of the disease. ... It is very important to remember that [chemical] antiseptics will destroy not only the micro-organisms but also the surrounding cells.

(Valnet 1980 p. 44)

The use of essential oils is a sure way of avoiding the phenomenon of developed resistance in microbes as experienced with antibiotics, because the aromatic essences are able to destroy even the resistant strains selectively (Pellecuer et al 1974). Germs resistant to synthetic antibiotics are susceptible in certain cases to some essences in dilutions as low as 1 in 16 000, e.g. *Satureia montana* (Belaiche 1979 p. 31). (See Table 4.1.)

It is wise to avoid any possible resistance on the part of a germ by always prescribing the use of 3 or 4 essential oils in combination. This multimix approach will tend to minimize any risk of acquired resistance to any oil, and it is unlikely that bacteria will be resistant at the same time to the other oils in the mix. This is one of the reasons

Table 4.1 Antibacterial spectrum of *Satureia montana* on some species and strains resistant to antibiotics (after Pellecuer et al 1976)

Bacteria tested	Origin of bacteria	Type of resistance	Active dose in mg/ml
Staphylococcus aureus	IP 6454	penicillin	0.250
Staphylococcus aureus	IP 6455	penicillin streptomycin tetracycline	0.250
Staphylococcus aureus	IP 52149	penicillin streptomycin tetracycline	0.250
Staphylococcus aureus	IP 52150	streptomycin	0.250
Sarcina lutea	natural	100γ of tetracycline	0.062
Bacillus subtilis	natural	streptomycin	0.250
Escherichia coli	natural	ampicillin colomycin	0.250
Staphylococcus pathogen	natural no. 1	⎱	0.062
Staphylococcus pathogen	natural no. 2	⎰	0.062
Staphylococcus pathogen	natural no. 3	Resistant	( )
( )		to 500γ of	0.062
Staphylococcus pathogen	natural no. 5	virginiamycin	0.125
Staphylococcus pathogen	natural no. 8		0.250
Staphylococcus pathogen	natural no. 10		0.125

Case 4.2 Aromatherapist: Ulrike Rädlein SRN, Germany

A 45-year-old woman had a motor vehicle accident, resulting in a comminuted fracture of the ankle. It was operated on but the operation site became infected, and was open for 4 months. At this stage I was asked if I could try and treat the wound with essential oils. The orthopaedic surgeon gave his permission and before I started I took a wound swab for microscopy, culture and sensitivity. On the wound swab *Staphylococcus aureus*, *Streptococcus pseudomonas* and *Escherichia coli* were isolated and from this I formulated my programme. The treatment consisted of a daily footbath with 3 drops each of *Thymus vulgaris* ct. alcohol, *Citrus limon* and *Melaleuca alternifolia* (the essential oils were put on a small spoon of salt as an emulgator and then put into the water). The wound was then cleaned with dry compresses, and a gauze (on which was put 3 drops of tea tree) put on. This acted as a compress and was covered with a mull bandage; this change was carried out once daily.

During this treatment the patient was given no antibiotics and only 20 drops Tramal when it was needed for her pains. After 3 days she no longer needed any analgesics. 2 weeks later, when a wound swab was tested none of the original bacteria were present. The wound closed after 3 weeks of using aromatherapy.

---

why the authors strongly advise using a powerful synergistic mix of oils in any treatment. Moreover this risk is further reduced, even though the metabolism of the microbe changes continually, because essential oils are natural products and their composition varies with each fresh batch.

Testing for antiseptic and antibacterial activity

Tests have been carried out on the antiseptic and antibacterial properties of essential oils for more than a century. Two of the first were Chamberland's in 1887, concerning the activity of cinnamon oils, angelica and geranium (Valnet 1980 p. 33), and Koch's 1881 investigation of turpentine with respect to the anthrax bacillus. Since then the antiseptic and bactericidal powers of well-grown natural essential oils have been tested many times in laboratories across the world using the aromatogram technique (see below). This is a recognized standard test and the results obtained are repeatable (provided the essential oils themselves are repeatable) and are universally acceptable: it is virtually the same as the antibiogram test.

Tests proving the antiseptic effects of essential oils are numerous, and the following are cited as examples: Belaiche (1985a, 1985b), Beylier (1979), Bonnaure (1919), Carson & Riley (1993), Cavel (1918), Chamberland (1887), Courment et al (1938), Deans & Svoboda (1988), Deans & Svoboda (1990a, 1990b), Gattefossé (1919, 1932), Gildemeister & Hoffmann (1956), Hinou et al (1989), Holland (1941), Jalsenjak et al (1987), Jasper et al (1958a, 1958b), Kienholz (1959), Low et al (1974), Martindale (1910), Onawunmi (1988, 1989), Onawunmi & Ogunlana (1986), Onawunmi et al (1984), Pellecuer et al (1974, 1975, 1976), Raharivelomanana et al (1989), Ramanoelina et al (1987), Ritzerfeld (1959), Shemesh & Mayo (1991), Tukioka (1927), Yousef & Tawil (1980).

There is a wide variation in the antiseptic and bactericidal effects between different individual essential oils as shown by their phenol coefficients (Rideal et al 1930, Martindale 1910, Poucher 1936). This is illustrated in Table 4.2.

It is well known that essential oils provide a very pleasant and effective means of disinfecting the air in an enclosed area (Kelner & Kober 1954, 1955, 1956) and are therefore ideal for use in sick rooms, burns units, reception areas, waiting rooms, etc. A test describing the use of a blend of

Table 4.2 The phenol coefficients of some essential oils and their isolated compounds (from Schilcher 1985 p. 221 reprinted by permission of Kluwer Academic Publishers). The phenol coefficient gives an indication of the antiseptic strength or weakness of a substance compared with that of phenol (which has a coefficient of 1.0)

Whole essential oil	Compound	Phenol coefficient
aniseed		0.4
peppermint		0.7
	menthol	0.9
lavender		1.6
lemon (Java)		2.2
	cinnamaldehyde	3.0
	citral	5.2
	camphor	6.2
clove		8.0
	eugenol	8.6
fennel		13.0
thyme		13.2
	thymol	20.0
	synthetic chlorothymol	75.0

pine, thyme, peppermint, lavender, rosemary, clove, and cinnamon essential oils for the bacteriological purification of the air concluded that 'the atmospheric dispersion of the prepared liquid brought about a very marked disinfection of the air, as demonstrated by the considerable reduction in the number of pre-existing microorganisms, some types being destroyed completely' (Valnet 1980 pp. 36–38).

Poucher (1936) quotes the results of an early investigation of the effect of 33 essential oils and phenol on beef tea which had been infected with water taken from a sewage tank. The trial referred to was originally carried out by Cavel (1918) and a selection from the results are shown in Table 4.3. The figures denote the dilution (per) 1000 at which the oils no longer showed effective antiseptic action, hence the lower the figure the greater the antiseptic power. It is interesting to note that phenol (the standard for comparison) appears fairly low in the following table.

Table 4.3 Antiseptic effect of essential oils in sewage water (from Poucher 1936 vol. 2 p. 361 with permission)

Essential oil	Dilution
Thyme	0.70
Origanum	1.00
Orange (sweet)	1.20
Verbena	1.60
Cassia	1.70
Rose	1.80
Clove	2.00
Peppermint	2.50
Vetiver	2.70
Eucalyptus	2.25
Gaultheria	3.00
Palmarosa	3.10
Spikenard	3.50
Star anise	3.70
Cinnamon (Ceylon)	4.00
Anise	4.20
Rosemary	4.30
Cumin	4.50
Neroli	4.75
Lavender	5.00
Melissa	5.20
Ylang ylang	5.60
PHENOL	5.60
Fennel (sweet)	6.40
Lemon	7.00
Angelica	10.00
Patchouli	15.00

Antibiogram and aromatogram

An antibiogram can test the validity of an antibiotic agent for the treatment of, say, a chest infection. A sample of sputum is taken and a culture grown in a dish. The antibiotic is introduced into the centre of the culture and its activity against the offending microorganism may be measured by the appearance of a clear killing zone. The diameter of this clear area indicates the power of the antibiotic: the greater the diameter, the greater the effectiveness of the antibiotic agent. The aromatogram is carried out in exactly the same way as the antibiogram, except essential oil is used instead of an antibiotic. Both methods are subject to the proviso that in vitro activity is not always echoed in vivo, which is modified by absorption, metabolism, bioavailability, etc. Finding the most effective and appropriate essential oil to counteract any particular germ can be a lengthy undertaking: if there is no previous experience to go on, it will be necessary to test all the oils in the therapist's repertory, perhaps 60 or more. It goes without saying that the essential oils used in the treatment should be from the same batch as the sample tested, because essential oils from different sources can vary in chemical composition. This testing procedure has confirmed the antiseptic powers of many oils but at the same time has revealed in some other oils antiseptic powers which were hitherto unsuspected, or at least underrated. At one time in aromatherapy fennel (*Foeniculum vulgare* var. *dulce*) was known only for being an appetite stimulant, nutmeg (*Myristica fragrans*) as a stomachic and tarragon (*Artemisia dracunculus*) as an antispasmodic, but now the antiseptic qualities of these oils are also recognized. These tests allow essential oils to be used precisely and effectively, without the consequences which sometimes follow the use of antibiotics (such as tiredness, lowered immune system and destruction of intestinal flora). Because of the huge number of aromatogram results which have now been published, it is possible to list the major essential oils by their antimicrobial properties (Roulier 1990 p. 55)—see Table 4.4.

Table 4.4 Antibacterial properties of essential oils according to Belaiche P 1979, Franchomme & Pénoël 1990, Valnet J 1980, Deans & Ritchie 1987, Deans & Svoboda 1988, 1989. Not all the oils in this table have been tested for all the bacteria shown. The x's indicate effectiveness—xxx is the most effective

	Bacillus subtilis	Candida albicans, Monilia albicans	Clostridium sporogenes	Corynebacterium diphtheriae	Diplococcus pneumoniae	Enterobacter aerogenes	Enterococci	Escherichia coli	Klebsiella	Myobacterium tuberculosis	Neisseria meningitidis	Neisseria gonorrhoeae
Artemisia dracunculus [TARRAGON]		x			x		x	x	x			
Carum carvi [CARAWAY]						xx		x	x			
Cedrus atlantica ? (not specified) [CEDARWOOD]								x				
Cinnamomum zeylanicum (cort.) [CINNAMON BARK]		xx			xxx		xxx	xxx	xxx			
Citrus aurantium var. amara (flos) [NEROLI BIGARADE]							x	x	x			
Citrus aurantium var. amara (fol.) [PETITGRAIN BIGARADE]		xxx			x		x	x	x			
Citrus aurantium var. bergamia (per.) [BERGAMOT]						x			x			
Citrus limon (per.) [LEMON]					x		x	x		x	x	
Coriandrum sativum (fruct.) [CORIANDER]					x	x		x	xx			
Cupressus sempervirens [CYPRESS]								x		x		
Eucalyptus globulus [TASMANIAN BLUE GUM]					xxx		x	xx	xx			
Foeniculum vulgare var. dulce (fruct.) [FENNEL]					x							
Hyssopus officinalis [HYSSOP]					xx					xxx		
Lavandula angustifolia [LAVENDER]		xx	x		xx	xx	xx	xx	xx			
Melaleuca alternifolia [TEA TREE]		xxx	xx		xx	x		xxx	x			x
Melaleuca leucadendron [CAJUPUT]		xx			xxx		xx	xx	xxx			
Melaleuca viridiflora [NIAOULI]							x	x	x			
Mentha × piperita [PEPPERMINT]	xx	x			x			xx	xx	xx		
Myristica fragrans (sem) [NUTMEG]						x		xx	xx			
Ocimum basilicum var. album [BASIL]					x	x		x				
Origanum majorana [MARJORAM]			xx		x	xx		xx	xx			
Ormenis mixta [MOROCCAN CHAMOMILE]								xx				
Pelargonium graveolens, P. × asperum [GERANIUM]		x			xx	xx	x		x			
Pimpinella anisum [ANISEED]												
Pinus sylvestris [PINE]		xx			xx		xx	xx	xx			
Piper nigrum [BLACK PEPPER]								x				
Rosa damascena [ROSE OTTO]												
Rosmarinus officinalis [ROSEMARY]		x	xx		x	xx		x	xx			
Salvia officinalis [SAGE]					x			xx	x			
Satureia hortensis & S. montana [SAVORY]		xx			xxx		xx	xx	xx	x		
Syzygium aromaticum (flos) [CLOVE BUD]		xx			xxx	xx	xxx	xx	xx			
Thymus capitatus [SPANISH OREGANO]		xxx			xxx		xxx	xxx	xxx			
Thymus serpyllum [WILD THYME]		x			x		x	x	x			
Thymus mastichina [SPANISH MARJORAM]										xx		
Thymus vulgaris ct. thymol [RED THYME]		xxx			xxx	xxx	xxx	xxx	xxx			

Table 4.4 (*continued*)

	Proteus	Pseudomonas aeruginosa	Salmonella pullorum	Salmonella typhi, Eberthella typhosa	Sarcina	Staphylococcus albus	Staphylococcus aureus	Staphylococcus faecalis	Streptococcus beta-hemolyticus, S. pyogenes	Streptococcus faecalis	Vibrio cholerae	Yersinia enterocolitica
Artemisia dracunculus [TARRAGON]		x	x			x	x		x			x
Carum carvi [CARAWAY]	xx		x				xx					x
Cedrus atlantica ? (not specified) [CEDARWOOD]												
Cinnamomum zeylanicum (cort.) [CINNAMON BARK]	xxx	x	xxx			xxx	xxx		xxx	x		xx
Citrus aurantium var. amara (flos) [NEROLI BIGARADE]	x								x			
Citrus aurantium var. amara (fol.) [PETITGRAIN BIGARADE]						x	xx		x			
Citrus aurantium var. bergamia (per.) [BERGAMOT]			x				x			x		
Citrus limon (per.) [LEMON]					x		x					
Coriandrum sativum (fruct.) [CORIANDER]	x		x				x					xx
Cupressus sempervirens [CYPRESS]									x			
Eucalyptus globulus [TASMANIAN BLUE GUM]	xx		x			xx	xx		?			x
Foeniculum vulgare var. dulce (fruct.) [FENNEL]	x		x				x					
Hyssopus officinalis [HYSSOP]						x	x	x	x			
Lavandula angustifolia [LAVENDER]	x		x	x		x	xx		xxx	xx		x
Melaleuca alternifolia [TEA TREE]	x	xx		xxx		x	xxx		x			
Melaleuca leucadendron [CAJUPUT]	xx					xx	xx		x			
Melaleuca viridiflora [NIAOULI]	x						x		x		x	
Mentha × piperita [PEPPERMINT]	xx	xx	xx				xx	x	x	x		xx
Myristica fragrans (sem) [NUTMEG]	x		x									x
Ocimum basilicum var. album [BASIL]		x	x				x			x		x
Origanum majorana [MARJORAM]	xx	x	xx				x			xx		xx
Ormenis mixta [MOROCCAN CHAMOMILE]												
Pelargonium graveolens, P. × asperum [GERANIUM]	x	x	xx			xx	x		xx			xx
Pimpinella anisum [ANISEED]					x	x	x	x			x	
Pinus sylvestris [PINE]	xx					xx	xx		xx			
Piper nigrum [BLACK PEPPER]			x									x
Rosa damascena [ROSE OTTO]												x
Rosmarinus officinalis [ROSEMARY]	x		x			x	x		x	xx		
Salvia officinalis [SAGE]		x	x				xx		x	x		
Satureia hortensis & S. montana [SAVORY]	x	xx	xx			xxx	xxx		xxx			xx
Syzygium aromaticum (flos) [CLOVE BUD]	xx	xx	xx			xxx	xx		xx	x		xx
Thymus capitatus [SPANISH OREGANO]	xxx					xxx	xxx		xxx			
Thymus serpyllum [WILD THYME]	x						x		xx			
Thymus mastichina [SPANISH MARJORAM]												
Thymus vulgaris ct. thymol [RED THYME]	xxx	x	xxx		xxx	xxx	xxx		xxx	xxx		xxx

Other properties

Analgesic

Many essential oils have this property to some degree and there seems to be no single reason why they do, just as pain itself is complicated. It is thought that it is partly due to the antiinflammatory, circulatory and detoxifying effects of some oils and to the anaesthetic effect of others. The phenol eugenol found in the oil of clove is well known for its use to calm dental pain, wintergreen oil (containing methyl salycilate, an ester) has traditionally been used in rubs for muscle pain, and menthol has been used specifically for headaches. On the skin oils rich in terpenes have an analgesic effect, especially those containing paracymene (Franchomme & Pénoël 1990 p. 86). Many aromatherapists report that the oil of *Alternifolia melaleuca* has this effect. Azulene and chamazulene (found in the chamomiles) can be used on the skin also.

Some essential oils have a universal sedative or soporific action leading to an easing of pain, e.g. *Chamaemelum nobile, Cananga odorata, Citrus reticulata* (fol.) (Rossi et al 1988), *Citrus bergamia* (per.) and (fol.) (Franchomme & Pénoël 1990 p. 86).

Case 4.3   Aromatherapist; Jill Baxter SEN, UK

Jim's main problem area is on the sciatic nerve, left hand side. He has had several operations and the deep creases, puckering and scar tissue on the site means that surgeons would be against further incisions—in fact they say there is little they can do, apart from giving morphia for the pain.

Jim has told me the history from 4 years ago, when a wart first needed surgery and was found to be benign. Following that, a severe injury against the angle of a piece of furniture was thought to trigger malignant growths. When I first saw him he moved very stiffly indeed and lay on the couch most awkwardly. I massaged his back, shoulders, legs and feet with lavender and rosemary in a blend of wheatgerm and grapeseed oil and afterwards I applied lavender (neat) freely to the site of the wound.

Jim tells me he would never have believed the measure of relief he has found since having aromatherapy treatments. He says he gains immediate relief from constant aching, has a greater range of movement and a good night's sleep. He has noticed his skin is more supple and is looking forward to being able to sit more squarely in an easy chair, instead of sideways, one leg extended, as at present.

Case 4.4   Aromatherapist: R.A.H. RGN, RM, UK

Mr H. had acute back pain in July after lifting heavy weights at work. He was treated with conventional drugs by his GP and returned to work fairly quickly. However, the pain recurred and he was off sick from work in September, again not benefiting from conventional treatment, which consisted of analgesics, antiinflammatory drugs and physiotherapy. He developed an allergy to Ibuprofen, an antiinflammatory drug, but this was detected before any harm was done to him. Several of the doctors in the practice had been called out to administer analgesia, by tablet, injection or suppository. Obviously, this could not go on and he was admitted to hospital over Christmas with chronic back pain.

I was asked to see whether aromatherapy could bring him some relief. The essential oils selected were: 3 drops *Chamaemelum nobile*, 2 drops *Lavandula angustifolia* and 1 drop *Origanum majorana* in 10 ml grapeseed oil. Having given him a full back massage, I gave special attention to his lower legs and feet, as I had observed how rigid his feet were, with virtually no flexibility in his ankles. I taught him foot exercises, massaging his lower extremities and counselling him. That night he slept very well without sedation.

26–29 December.   Massaged as before. Now walking better during day and pain less. Being apprehensive as I was to be off duty for several nights, I prepared white lotion containing the same essential oils so that the other night nurses could stroke this on his back every night. He promised to continue his foot exercises.

7–11 January.   Massaged back and feet as before. Excellent effect. Mr. G. was confident and talking about the possibility of going on holiday. Had been to physiotherapy and had used the exercise bike, but disliked it (legs aching). He had continued with his leg- and foot-exercises, and on 29 January said he was pain-free.

According to Roulier (1990), the analgesic and antalgic essential oils are white birch, chamomile, frankincense, wintergreen, clove, lavender, mint (common names only given). (See Appendix B.9 for a list of effective oils.)

Antifungal

Many essential oils have been reported as having an antifungal effect and many investigations have taken place, some more than half a century ago (Schmidt 1936) showing the fungicidal and fungistatic effects of cinnamon, clove, fennel, and thyme; these were active against *Candida albicans*, *Sporotrichon* and *Trichophyton* species (Gildemeister & Hoffmann 1956 p. 140). The fungicidal activity of the oil of *Chamomilla recutita* and its components including chamazulene and (-)-α-bisabolol has been well investigated and shown to be effective against *Trichophyton rubrum*, *T. mentagraphytes*, *T. tonsurans*, *T. quinckeanum* and *Microsporum canis* in concentrations of 200 mg/ml (Szalontai et al 1975a, 1975b, 1976, 1977, Janssen et al 1984, 1986). *Satureia montana* has also been found to be active against candida (Pellecuer et al 1975). A general review of some essential oils with antifungal properties has been carried out (Pellecuer et al 1976) and in other trials a number

of compounds found in essential oils, especially the aldehydes and esters, are effective against various fungi, including candida infection (Maruzella 1961, Thompson & Cannon 1986, Larrondo & Calvo 1991). The oil of *Melaleuca alternifolia* has been investigated with regard to vaginal infection with candida and found to be effective (Belaiche 1985c, Pena 1962, Shemesh & Mayo 1991). Rosemary, savory and thyme have antifungal properties (Pellecuer et al 1973) and *Ocimum basilicum* has antifungal and insect-repelling properties (Dube et al 1989).

Table 4.5 Antifungal effects of essential oils

	General antifungal properties*	Candida albicans	Microsporon canis	Sporotrichon species	Tinea pedis	Trichophyton species	T. mentagraphytes T. quinckeanum T. rubrum, T. tonsurans
Cinnamomum zeylanicum (cort) [CINNAMON BARK]		x		x		x	
Chamomilla recutita [GERMAN CHAMOMILE]			x				x
Eucalyptus globulus [TASMANIAN BLUE GUM]		x					
Foeniculum vulgare var. *dulce* [FENNEL]		x		x		x	
Lavandula angustifolia [LAVENDER]		x			x		
Lavandula × *intermedia 'Super'* [LAVANDIN]					x		
Melaleuca alternifolia [TEA TREE]		x					
Melaleuca leucadendron [CAJUPUT]		x					
Ocimum basilicum [BASIL]	x						
Pelargonium graveolens [GERANIUM]		?					
Pinus sylvestris [PINE]		x					
Rosmarinus officinalis [ROSEMARY]	x						
Satureia montana [WINTER SAVORY]	x	x					
Syzygium aromaticum (flos) [CLOVE BUD]		x		x		x	
Tagetes glandulifera, T. patula [MARIGOLD]					x		
Thymus mastichina [SPANISH MARJORAM]		x					
Thymus vulgaris ct. carvacrol [RED THYME]	x	x		x		x	
Thymus vulgaris ct. thymol [RED THYME]	x	x		x		x	
Aldehydes constituent		x					
α-bisabolol constituent		x					
Chamazulene constituent		x					
Esters constituent		x					

* Oils having antifungal properties but without mention of a specific fungus

Case 4.5 Aromatologist: Alan Barker, UK

In July 1990 Mrs F (aged 40) was referred to a consultant, suffering from a continuous urinary tract infection (with inflammation, incontinence and pain) which antibiotics failed to control. She was given intermittent self-catheterization (ISC) and by April 1992 major surgery (removal of the bladder) was considered. She also developed a vaginal inflammation—thrush. By September 1992, Mrs F was unable to perform the ISC due to thrush and inflammation and a cystectomy was again discussed.

In November, the sister suggested to the consultant that aromatherapy should be tried, and as Mrs F was interested, the consultant gave his permission. I was asked if I was happy to start treatment and a meeting was finally arranged between myself, the continence adviser, Mrs F and her husband in March 1993.

Mrs F complained of constant pain and swelling of the abdomen (caused by having to have residual catheterization using microcatheters). She felt (and it was apparent on inspection) that her vagina was the consistency of 'raw liver' and she suffered frequent discharges. Intercourse was impossible. I had asked her husband to attend with her so that I could check him over, as this side of the partnership, although important, is often overlooked. Mrs F had had this recurrent form of candida for about 15 years with very few periods of respite—the relationship was beginning to suffer and credit was due to the couple for the level of understanding shared.

The couple's normal diet plan for an average week was looked at and changes arranged to help the body balance itself. These changes were to be gradual, over a period of time, so as not to add to the stress of the situation. Because of the latter, massage was to be part of Mrs F's treatment. A colonic massage was decided upon, with essential oils to benefit the swelling, pain and infection: *Citrus bergamia* (per.), *Eucalyptus globulus*, *Melaleuca alternifolia* and *Melaleuca viridiflora*. These were mixed together in equal quantities and a 15-minute massage given. At the first treatment a high concentration of 2.5 ml of the essential oils was put into 5 ml grapeseed oil—a 50% dilution.

I taught Mr F how to perform a simple abdominal massage in a clockwise direction consisting of very few strokes, to be carried out once daily to aid Mrs F's constipation. This was a good morale booster for him, as he had previously felt helpless—and he now became part of her recovery process. For this, he was given a 3% mix of: *Zingiber officinale* (antispasmodic and laxative), *Foeniculum vulgare* var. *dulce* (appetite stimulant, laxative and circulation stimulant) and *Mentha* × *piperita* (analgesic, antiinflammatory and stomachic).

Treatment with live yogurt and essential oils was discussed; this could not be carried out by using a tampon as the client was too swollen. It was decided to pour the yogurt mixture into the vagina, the client being propped up, legs raised, to allow the mix to penetrate. Mrs F found this was messy and difficult. However, after several days the swelling had reduced enough to insert a tampon soaked in the mixture, changing it morning and night.

Colonic massage treatment at the hospital involved using different strengths of essential oil: for 3 days a dilution of 5 drops in 5 ml was used. Several weekly treatments followed, using only 1 drop of the synergistic blend in 5 ml grapeseed oil.

Treatment at home involved the following: marigold flowers used for making tea (plus 1 drop *Citrus bergamia* 3 times a day for 3 weeks); acidopholus tablets (6 daily); a combination of essential oils to be used in the bath; abdomen massage oil—3% mix for F to use at home as above; yogurt treatment—5 drops *Melaleuca alternifolia* was put with 10 ml yogurt—used as above

By the end of the month Mrs F was already beginning to feel the benefits from the treatment. In June 1993, the abdominal swelling was going down; the yogurt treatment was changed to oral yogurt tablets as insertion was sometimes difficult. By the end of July the urinary tract was almost clear. Mrs F was on 3 acidopholus tablets (daily), marigold tea, occasional yogurt and *Melaleuca alternifolia* taken internally. Abdomen massage was still carried out by husband once or twice a week with a reduced concentration of 1.5%.

The couple's relationship is now close once more, partially due to Mr F's eagerness to help by giving his wife a daily massage.

Antiinflammatory

The oils of *Lavandula angustifolia* and *Chamomilla recutita* are widely used to soothe minor inflammations such as sunburn, small burns and insect bites, and plenty of people can testify to their effectiveness in this respect. Jakovlev et al (1983) showed the antiinflammatory effect of yarrow, chamomile containing chamazulene, arnica flower and turpentine.

Azulenes are sesquiterpene derivatives and have the empirical formula $C_{15}H_{18}$. While chamazulene and (-)-α-bisabolol found in chamomile oils are antiinflammatory agents (Weiss 1988 p. 24), other azulenes which may be added to antiinflammatory preparations are not so effective, e.g. guaiazulene (manufactured from guaiol) and elemazulene (from elemol). Also (+)-α-bisabolol and synthetic (-)-α-bisabolol are not as effective as the natural form.

There do appear to be differences in some cases between the natural and synthesized molecule: synthetic myristicin does not produce hallucinations (D'Arcy 1993) unlike natural myristicin extracted from nutmeg oil (in which it is present at 4%). (See Appendix B.9 for a list of effective oils.)

Antitoxic

Chamomile oil has been found to be capable of inactivating toxins produced by bacteria. The amount of oil obtained by distilling 0.1 g of chamomile is sufficient to destroy, within 2 hours, 3 times that amount of staphylococcal toxins—the highest concentration of toxin so far found in the human organism. Streptococcal toxins proved even more sensitive (Weiss 1988 p. 26).

Antiviral

Most people practising aromatherapy have reported success in the control of herpes simplex virus I but there is no consistency in choice of oils used (as can be seen from Table 4.6 below). Speaking from personal experience, we have always found the oils of *Melissa officinalis* and *Eucalyptus smithii* to be helpful for HSV I. The use of melissa agrees with tests showing this plant to be antiviral

Table 4.6 Essential oils mentioned as having antiviral effects (from various authors)

	Adenovirus	Glandular fever	Herpes simplex	Influenza	Viral enteritis	Viiral enterocolitis	Viral hepatitis	Viral neuritis	Zoster
Cinnamomum zeylanicum (cort.) [CINNAMON BARK]									
Citrus aurantium var. *amara* (per.) [ORANGE BIGARADE]									
Citrus aurantium var. *bergamia* (per.) [BERGAMOT]			x						
Citrus limon (per.) [LEMON]			x	x					
Commiphora molmol [MYRRH]							x		
Cupressus sempervirens [CYPRESS]				x					
Eucalyptus globulus [TASMANIAN BLUE GUM]				x					
Eucalyptus smithii [GULLY GUM]				x					
Hyssopus officinalis [HYSSOP]									
Lavandula latifolia, L. spica [SPIKE LAVENDER]						x			
Melaleuca alternifolia [TEA TREE]			x		x	x			
Melaleuca leucadendron [CAJUPUT]								x	
Melaleuca viridiflora [NIAOULI]			x	x			x		
Melissa officinalis [MELISSA]			x						x
Mentha × *piperita* [PEPPERMINT]							x	x	
Ocimum basilicum [BASIL]								x	
Pelargonium graveolens, P. × *asperum* [GERANIUM]			x						x
Pimpinella anisum [ANISEED]									
Piper nigrum [BLACK PEPPER]	x			x	x		x		
Ravensara aromatica [RAVENSARA]				x	x		x		
Rosa damascena [ROSE OTTO]			x						x
Rosmarinus officinalis [ROSEMARY]			x				x		
Satureia montana [WINTER SAVORY]						x			
Salvia officinalis [SAGE]		x		x	x			x	x
Syzygium aromaticum (flos) [CLOVE BUD]							x		
Thymus serpyllum [WILD THYME]				x					
Thymus vulgaris ct. phenol [RED THYME]		x		x					
Thymus vulgaris ct. alcohol [SWEET THYME]									x

(Cohen et al 1964, Herrman & Kucera 1967, Kucera & Herrman 1967). For herpes zoster (shingles) the oil of *Pelargonium graveolens* is specifically recommended, but it is best applied at the first sign of an attack to prevent the viruses from replicating. Used early it prevents blisters from forming and damps down the pain. Although attempts have been made to treat HSV II—the many oils suggested include *Melaleuca alternifolia*, and *Melaleuca viridiflora* (Franchomme & Pénoël 1990)—little success has been reported. Despite the lack of scientific support, many aromatherapists still feel that HSV II and other viral infections such as glandular fever and influenza do respond to essential oil treatment. There is also some research to support the use in this area of black pepper oil (*Piper nigrum*) (Lembke & Deininger 1988). The oils of *Cymbopogon flexuosus*, *Mentha arvensis* and *Vetiveria zizanioides* (Pandey et al 1988) and *Eucalyptus viminalis*, *E. macarthurii*, *E. dalrympleana* appear to be effective in vitro and in ovo on two strains of influenza virus (Vichkanova et al 1973). There have been other papers published on this topic in India, Russia and China and a Swiss patent was filed in 1979 for an antiviral preparation using essential oils.

Table 4.6 on page 66 shows the essential oils which have been recommended for antiviral use. The information has been culled from many sources, which often used only the common name for the plant volatile oil. The sources include Wabner, Tyman, Franchomme & Pénoël, Roulier and Price.

The following oils are also mentioned as having antiviral properties, but without specific indications (Franchomme & Pénoël 1990):

Aniba rosaeodora, Cinnamomum camphora var. *glavescens Hayata, Cinnamomum cassia, Cinnamomum zeylanicum, Cinnamomum zeylanicum* ct. eugenol, *Cistus ladaniferus* ct. pinene, *Cistus ladaniferus, Citrus limon* (per.), *Corydothymus capitatus, Cymbopogon martinii* var. *motia, Cymbopogon martinii* var. *sofia, Eucalyptus polybractea* ct. cryptone, *Eucalyptus radiata, Hyssopus officinalis* var. *decumbens, Hyssopus officinalis, Lantana camara* ct. davanone, *Lavandula × intermedia* 'Reydovan', *Ocimum gratissimum* ct. eugenol, *Ocimum gratissimum* ct. thymol, *Origanum compactum, Origanum heracleoticum, Ravensara*

aromatica, Satureia hortensis, Thymus vulgaris ct. geraniol, *Thymus vulgaris* ct. linalool, *Thymus vulgaris* ct. thujanol-4, *Trachyspermum ammi.*

Several constituents which are found naturally in a wide range of essential oils (anethole, β-caryophyllene, carvone, cinnamic aldehyde, citral, citronellol, eugenol, limonene, linalool, linalyl acetate, α-sabinene, γ-terpinene) were found to be active against HSV (Lembke & Deininger 1985, 1988). The above lists show that there is no one molecule or even one class of molecule involved. If the oils are effective it could well be because of some property common to all of them—perhaps lipid-solubility.

Balancing

Aromatherapists are well aware of the remarkable balancing powers of the essential oils. At times this can cause puzzlement because of the apparently contradictory effects of the oils, but essential oils are complex mixtures of many natural constituents, some of which are stimulating and others sedative, so a single oil may demonstrate an arousing effect on one occasion and a sedative effect on another. This is known as the adaptogenic effect.

Hyssop essential oil contains the ketone pinocamphone and is said to be toxic in high doses, causing epileptic attacks in those so predisposed (Valnet 1980). Yet this oil is used in the following case study (and has been used by the authors in

---

Case 4.6 Aromatologist: Alan Barker, UK

M is 7 years old. He is hyperactive and epileptic: in a few seconds he went from daydreaming to petit mal convulsions. He is on a high dose of Epanutin, which his mother is not very happy about.

I used essential oils in high concentration as recommended in Valnet (1980). The essential oils used were: *Hyssopus officinalis, Salvia officinalis* and *Ocimum basilicum*, altogether 60 drops in 30 ml of carrier oil (10% dilution). The mix was used only on the kidney area on the back, therefore the quantity of essential oils being applied was in reality quite small.

The convulsions ceased within a week. M. is now on a minimum dose of Epanutin, the massage oil concentration reduced to 1.5% and treatments to one a month. M's mother is now looking at withdrawing conventional drug therapy.

an epilepsy case) with beneficial effects. *Lavandula angustifolia* is well-known for its sedative effect but rather less known for its ability to prevent sleep at high doses (observed and experienced by many aromatherapists). Similarly hawthorn berries (used in herbal medicine) can lower blood pressure in some but raise it in others (Mabey 1988 p. 179). In aromatherapy this balancing of blood pressure is often ascribed to *Cananga odorata* but is not proven. The skill of the aromatherapist lies in using such effects in skilful blends to the best advantage of the client.

Deodorant

Bad smells sometimes arise from the disease process, and the sweet-smelling oils act to prevent degradation, replace the odours and tackle the bacteria causing these effects. The use of sweet-smelling and familiar essential oils is more acceptable to the client (who may be in a weakened state) than the imposition of harsh synthetics. This attribute is also helpful in a healing situation where bad smells are generated, for example in some severe burns injuries. Essential oils do not merely disguise these unpleasant odours which clients and nurses have to suffer, but actually cancel them out. 'The odour of essential oils does not cover up the bad smells of infected gangrenous or cancerous wounds; it suppresses them by physicochemical action' (Valnet 1980 p. 44).

We have supplied a mixture of essential oils designed for this purpose for a number of years to a burns unit at the request of the consultant surgeon. The nurses find it particularly useful when bathing patients with burns. Essential oils find a similar use in incontinence cases, making life a great deal more pleasant for all concerned. Bad-smelling wounds can be deodorized by the use of hypericum oil (see below), thyme, and citrus oils (Schilcher 1985 p. 222). Chamomile preparations are also known for their deodorizing effect.

Because of the deoderizing effect of some fragrant materials they are useful in underarm and foot deodorants. Compounds and oils recommended as effective against b.o. are eugenol, linalool and the essential oil *Pogostemon patchouli*

(Decazes 1993). Elsewhere *Salvia sclarea*, *Cymbopogon flexuosus*, *Zingiber officinale* and *Myristica fragrans* are also mentioned in this respect.

Digestive

Essential oils have strong effects on the digestive system and are used in appetite-stimulating and digestive drinks as carminatives and stimulants for the stomach, liver and gall bladder. The carminative effect of many essential oils is strong, and there are other benefits, such as increased secretory activity of the stomach and gall bladder, antiseptic and spasmolytic effects. The essential oils concerned are mainly from the umbellifer botanical family—*Carum carvi, Coriandrum sativum, Foeniculum vulgare* var. *dulce, Pimpinella anisum,* and also *Mentha × piperita, Ocimum basilicum* and the chamomiles (Schilcher 1985 p. 224). Wild thyme (*Thymus serpyllum*) has been shown to stimulate bile production (Chabrol 1932), and essential oils containing the alcohols menthol and thujanol-4 seem to be beneficial to liver function (Gershbein 1977, Zara 1966).

The citrus oils generally have a favourable effect on the digestive system, being mildly appetite stimulating and digestive. *Citrus aurantium* var. *amara* (per.) is given as a treatment for constipation as it encourages intestinal peristalsis and also acts as a cholagogue (Duraffourd 1982 p. 95) and for dyspepsia, flatulence and gastric spasm (Franchomme & Pénoël 1990 p. 337). *Rosmarinus officinalis* has always been associated with improving the liver function. In animals an intravenous infusion of rosemary doubled the volume of bile secreted (Valnet 1980 p. 177), and it is given as a carminative and cholagogue (Lautié & Passebecq 1984 p. 74) and to stimulate hepato-biliary secretions (Duraffourd 1982 p. 107).

Diuretic

Just as rosemary oil is traditionally associated with the liver, so juniper berry oil—*Juniperus communis* (fruct.)—is associated with the kidneys. At normal dosage it is a beneficial stimulant, although it has a toxic effect on inflamed kidneys. There is a diuretic effect (Franchomme & Pénoël

Table 4.7 Essentials oils and the digestive system. Sources same as for Appendix A

	Properties								Indications										
	Antispasmodic	Aperitive	Astringent	Carminative	Choleretic	Hepatic stimulant	Litholytic (g=gall, k=kidney, u=urinary)	Pancreatic stimulant	Colic	Colitis, gastroenteritis	Constipation	Diarrhoea	Digestion painful	Digestive stimulant	Diverticulitis	Enteritis, gastritis	Indigestion	Nausea	Ulcers (duodenal, gastric)
Achillea millefolium [YARROW]				x			k							x					
Carum carvi [CARAWAY]	x			x	x				x								x		
Chamaemelum nobile (flos) [ROMAN CHAMOMILE]		x		x					x		x						x		
Chamomilla recutita (flos) [GERMAN CHAMOMILE]	?													x	x			x	d,g
Citrus aurantium var. *amara* (flos) [NEROLI BIGARADE]						x		x											
Citrus aurantium var. *amara* (fol.) [PETITGRAIN BIGARADE]																	x		
Citrus aurantium var. *amara* (per.) [ORANGE BIGARADE]						x			x		x					x	x		
Citrus bergamia (per.) [BERGAMOT]	x	x	x						x					x			x		
Citrus limon (per.) [LEMON]	x	x	x	x			g,u	x	x				x	x	x		x	x	
Citrus reticulata (per.) [MANDARIN]				x		x						x					x		
Commiphora myrrha [MYRRH]																x			
Coriandrum sativum [CORIANDER]	x			x							x			x					
Cupressus sempervirens [CYPRESS]	x		x									x							
Eucalyptus smithii [GULLY GUM]														x					
Foeniculum vulgare var. *dulce* [FENNEL]				x	x		u				x			x			x		
Hyssopus officinalis [HYSSOP]							u		x					x			x		
Juniperus communis (fruct.) [JUNIPER BERRY]		x	x	x		x	u,k	x	x	x					x				
Melaleuca alternifolia [TEA TREE]										x									
Melaleuca leucadendron [CAJUPUT]	x																		
Melaleuca viridiflora [NIAOULI]				x		x	g			x		x				x	x		d,g
Melissa officinalis [MELISSA]	x				x	x			x					x			x	x	
Mentha x *piperita* [PEPPERMINT]	x			x	x	x			x	x			x	x	x	x	x	x	
Myristica fragrans (sem.) [NUTMEG]	x			x										x					
Nepeta cataria [CATNEP]							g												
Ocimum basilicum var. *album* [BASIL]	x			x		x			x	x				x			x		
Origanum majorana [MARJORAM]	x			x					x	x	?	x		x			x	x	d,g
Pelargonium graveolens [GERANIUM]			x		x			x	x		x				x				
Pimpinella anisum [ANISEED]	x	x		x					x					x			x	x	
Pinus sylvestris [PINE]							g												
Piper nigrum [PEPPER]						x						x		x					
Rosmarinus officinalis [ROSEMARY]				x	x	x	g		x				x	x	x	x	x	x	
Salvia officinalis [SAGE]		x	?	x					x					x			x		
Santalum album [SANDALWOOD]			x									x							
Satureia montana, S. hortensis [WINTER AND SUMMER SAVORY]	x			x	x				x		x	x	x	x					
Syzygium aromaticum (flos) [CLOVE BUD]	x																		
Thymus serpyllum [WILD THYME]									x										
Thymus vulgaris [THYME]				x										x					
Zingiber officinale [GINGER]				x					?		x	x	x	x				x	

1990 p. 361, Duraffourd 1982 p. 67, Viaud 1983, Lautié & Passebecq 1984 p. 51) although this is denied by Schilcher (1985 p. 226) and omitted by Roulier (1990). However, one authority (Gattefossé 1937 p. 71) states that nearly all essences are diuretic and endorses juniper oil. It is also claimed that terpene-free oil containing mainly terpinen-4-ol has marked diuretic effects (Schneider 1975), although juniper oils consist of more than 90% hydrocarbon monoterpenes and the level of this alcohol may be only 2–5%.

Energizing

Plants capture electromagnetic energy from the sun and some of this is stored in the essential oil. The biosynthesis of the terpenes has as a starting point acetyl coenzyme A (Hay & Waterman 1993 p. 52) and in certain plants this process of synthesis goes beyond terpenes to finish at the production of steroids with hormonal properties. Plant metabolic mechanisms have much in common with those of man, and this starting-point of acetyl coenzyme A is analogous to the process in the human body by which steroids are synthesized—cortisone, vitamin D, cholesterol. The phenyl propanoids are another building block of essential oils and provide another example. They are in effect the precursors of some of the amino acids, the basic elements for the synthesis of proteins. Proteins are the building blocks of the human body, the agents for transformation and energy transfer which maintain the fabric of the body and all the physiological activity (Duraffourd 1987 p. 26). This may help us in understanding the special nature of essential oils: they can, because of their molecular energy and because they have elements in common with human physiology, help to put in order deficits or energy blockages (Duraffourd 1987 p. 27).

Granulation-promoting

This helps in healing where there has been damage or removal of tissue. Probably the best known use is lavender oil for minor burns, which yields positive and rapid results (Gattefossé 1937). Hypericum oil and chamomile oils have been used traditionally for wound healing, and

---

Case 4.7 Aromatherapist: Lynne Reed, UK

A community colleague of mine was called out one evening to see a client (a medical practitioner) with extremely sore nipples. On arrival, the nipples were cracked, bleeding and extremely painful—made worse by the application of a nipple cream which the client said had caused stinging. The baby was unable to be latched on. My colleague hand-expressed the mother and the baby was fed. She then left her with a small bottle of the nipple oil which is used in the hospital and arranged to call back the following morning.

When she revisited, the baby was back feeding on the breast and both client and colleague were surprised by the amount of healing that had taken place. The mother said that she had felt instant relief as soon as she applied the nipple oil.

Nipple Oil

Chamaemelum nobile, *Lavandula angustifolia* and *Rosa damascena* 1 drop each in 30 ml carrier oil made up of: 20% calendula, 80% sweet almond. The blend is divided into 10 ml bottles for use in hospital. Apply to sore nipples after feeding the baby, remembering to wash the breasts with warm water just before the next feed.

The oils used are analgesic, antiseptic, bactericidal, antiinflammatory, granulation stimulating, haemostatic and anti-depressant (rose). The analgesic effect has had a response of 7+ on a scale of 0–10 from patients using this oil in a small study.

---

the validity of this has been borne out by studies in the case of chamomile (Glowania et al 1987, Thiemer et al 1973). Red oil of hypericum is available: it is a fixed oil—usually with a base of olive oil or sunflower oil—in which the flowers of St. John's Wort (*Hypericum perforatum*) have been macerated. This oil contains as active constituents not only the essential oil but also hypericin and was much used in the past for the external treatment of wounds and burns (Weiss 1988 p. 296).

Hormonal

Some essential oils have a tendency to normalize hormonal secretions, and it is thought that this action may be direct or is effected via the hypophysis (Franchomme & Pénoël 1990). No work has so far been done to establish precisely how the oil molecules could do this, and there is little likelihood of this being carried out in the forseeable future. For the present, treatment is easy and pleasant for the client and, so far as is known, without any side-effects. The hormone-like action of some plant extracts has been widely noted. Extracts of fennel seed have a slight oestrogenic effect in animal experimental models (Foster 1993). Bernadet (1983) and others advise the use of essential oils for such disorders as dysmenorrhoea and amenorrhoea. The essences of pine (needles), borneol, geranium, basil, sage, savory and rosemary stimulate the cortex of the suprarenal gland; anise excites the anterior pituitary body, as does mint (Valnet 1980).

Valnet also writes that the essence of cypress seems to be the homologue of the ovarian hormone. There are compounds in some volatile oils which have structures similar to natural human hormones, and these promote efficient endocrine gland activity by natural means. Sclareol, viridiflorol and trans-anethole are examples of compounds which have structures similar to folliculin or analogous to oestrogen. Other compounds found in *Pinus sylvestris* are similar to cortisone (Franchomme & Pénoël 1990) (see Table 4.8).

Table 4.8 The influence of essential oils on the hormonal system (from various authors)

	Adrenal (cortex)	Adrenal (medulla)	Anaphrodisia	Emmenagogic	Hypophysis	Hypophysis (gonads)	Hypophysis (ovarian)	Hypophysis (pancreas)	Hypophysis (suprarenal cortex)	Hypothalamus	Lactogenic	Oestrogenic	Pancreas (diabetes)	Pituitary (anterior)	Pituitary (posterior)	Reproduction (ovaries)	Sex hormones (testes)	Thymus	Thyroid	Thyroxine production	Uterotonic
Chamomilla recutita [GERMAN CHAMOMILE]				?																	
Citrus aurantium var. *amara* (per.) [ORANGE BIGARADE]					x					x				x							
Citrus limon (pericarp.) [LEMON]					x					x					x						
Commiphora myrrha [MYRRH]			x	?															x		
Cymbopogon citratus, C. flexuosus [LEMONGRASS]																	x				
Foeniculum vulgare var. *dulce* [FENNEL]					x						x	x									x
Melaleuca leucadendron [CAJUPUT]					?																
Melaleuca viridiflora [NIAOULI]					x	x	x			x											
Mentha × piperita [PEPPERMINT]					?											x					x
Pelargonium graveolens [GERANIUM]														x							
Pimpinella anisum [ANISEED]					x						x	x									x
Pinus sylvestris [PINE]						x		x	x								x				
Rosa centifolia, R. damascena [ROSE OTTO]				?																	
Rosmarinus officinalis [ROSEMARY]	x			?																	
Salvia officinalis [SAGE]			x	x						x											
Salvia sclarea [CLARY]				?						x											
Santalum album [SANDALWOOD]																x					
Syzygium aromaticum (flos) [CLOVE BUD]																				x	
Thymus vulgaris ct. geraniol [THYME]																				x	
Thymus vulgaris ct. thymol [RED THYME]	x																				
Vetiveria zizanioides [VETIVER]				?												x					

Hyperaemic

Essential oils promote local peripheral circulation due to a primary irritation of the skin, and the effects of this are twofold:

* the freeing of mediators (e.g. bradykinin) which cause vasodilatation
* humoral reactions resulting in the antiinflammatory effect.

On the skin there is a sensation of warmth, comfort and pain relief following the use of rubefacients such as *Eucalyptus globulus*, *Rosmarinus officinalis* and *Juniperus communis* which cause increased local blood circulation. Local skin irritation may also have some effect on internal organs (e.g. cardiac ointment used in angina). Some essential oils are vesicants e.g. *Brassica nigra* and *Armoracia lapathifolia* due to the principal constituent allyl isothiocyanate. Croton oil is also a vesicant, and its use is proscribed by the Medicines Act 1968.

Immunostimulant

Melaleuca viridiflora has been reported to have an immunostimulant effect by increasing the level of immunoglobulins (Pénoël 1981), and many other oils have been mentioned by various writers as strengthening the immune system. There is a wide variety and no common agreement, and this may be so because many oils possess a range of properties (antifungal, antiseptic, antiviral, etc.) that are beneficial to the immune system (see Ch. 13). (See Appendix B.9 for a list of effective oils.)

Insecticidal and repellent

Plant volatile oils may be used over a long period of time without promoting resistance. Some plants use essential oils to repel attacking insects, and they are still effective after millions of years. In the south of France citronella is universally used as an insect repellent, and tests show other oils to have

this property too, e.g. *Ocimum basilicum* (Dube et al 1989). Of a number of essential oils and some of their components investigated for insecticidal activity, only a few demonstrated this attribute— *Cinnamomum camphora* , *Cinnamomum zeylanicum*, *Cymbopogon nardus*, *Syzygium aromaticum* and *Eucalyptus* oils, and two aldehydes and a ketone (cinnamic aldehyde, citral and carvone) (Gildemeister & Hoffmann 1956). Our past experience indicates that *Thymus vulgaris* ct. thymol and *Melaleuca alternifolia* are effective parasiticides (head and pubic lice), and tests that we are involved in at the time of writing tend to confirm this.

Mucolytic and expectorant

The accumulated secretions in the mucous linings can hold germs and it is necessary to break down the mucus in order to kill them. Many oils are mucolytic thanks to their content of powerful ketones (carvone, menthone, thujone, pino-camphone, etc.) and in some cases lactones. The expectorant effect is due to the breaking down of secretions and cilial activity, and several oils have in the past been tested to determine expectorant properties (Gordonoff 1938, Boyd & Pearson 1946, Schilcher 1985 p. 223). Besides *Eucalyptus globulus* and other essential oils containing the oxide 1,8-cineole, *Pimpinella anisum*, *Foeniculum vulgare* var. *dulce*, *Pinus sylvestris*, *Pinus mugo* var. *pumilio*, *Thymus vulgaris* ct. phenol and *Thymus serpyllum* are also expectorants. These oils, whether used by external application or by inhalation, reach the bronchi and are eliminated from the lungs in the exhaled air.

Sedative

In the past there has been little apart from anecdotal evidence for the sedative properties of essential oils, but now several oils have been investigated and found to be effective. They include *Melissa officinalis* which is calming to the CNS because of its citronellal and other mono-terpene content (Becker & Förster 1984, Mills

Table 4.9 Effects of fragrance compounds and essential oils on the motility of mice after a 1 hour inhalation period (from Buchbauer et al 1993 p. 661)

Compound	Effect on Motility %[a]	Effect on Motility after Caffeine %[b]
Anethole	-10.81	-1.26
Anthranilic acid methyl ester	+17.70	+38.22
Balm leaves oil (Austria)	-5.21	+16.29
Benzaldehyde	-43.69	-34.28
Benzyl alcohol	-11.21	-23.68
Borneol	-3.05	-1.88
Bornyl acetate	-7.79	+2.27
Bornyl salicylate	-17.29	-2.99
Carvone	-2.46	-47.51
Citral	-1.43	+17.24
Citronellal	-49.82	-37.40
Citronellol	-3.56	-13.71
Coumarin	-15.00	-13.75
Dimethyl vinyl carbinol	+5.36	-2.11
Ethylmaltol	+9.73	+2.09
Eugenol	+2.10	-38.73
Farnesol	+5.76	+36.34
Farnesyl acetate	+4.62	-30.71
Furfural	+3.04	-4.51
Geraniol	+20.56	+1.20
Geranyl acetate	-29.18	-7.46
Isoborneol	+46.90	-11.23
Isobornyl acetate	+3.16	-22.35
Isoeugenol	+30.05	-74.34
ß-Ionone	+14.20	-27.97
Lavender oil (Mont Blanc)	-78.40	-91.67
Lime blossom oil (France)	-34.34	+30.41
Linalool	-73.00	-56.67
Linalyl acetate	-69.10	-46.67
Maltol	+13.74	-50.04
Methyl salicylate	+16.64	-49.88
Nerol	+12.93	+29.31
Neroli oil	-65.27	+1.87
Orange flower oil (Spain)	-4.64	-14.62
Orange terpenes	+35.25	-33.19
Passion flower oil (USA)	+8.15	-27.93
2-phenyl ethanol	+2.67	-30.61
2-phenylethyl acetate	-45.04	+12.42
α-pinene	+13.77	+4.73
Rose oil (Bulgaria)	-9.50	+4.31
Sandalwood oil (East India)	-40.00	-20.70
α-terpineol	-45.00	-12.50
Thymol	+33.02	+19.05
Valerian root oil (China)	-2.70	-12.01

a motility of untreated control animals = 100%

b motility of control animals after pretreatment with 0.1% caffeine solution (0.5 mL, ip) = 100%

1991), and the valerian oils which contain small amounts of valepotriates (Becker & Reichling 1981, Becker 1983, Boeters 1969, Schmiedeberg 1913). *Valeriana officinalis* contains about 1.5% of these but this figure can rise to 12% in other species, and the valerian plant was used as the blueprint for the drug valium. Recently other tests have been carried out which prove for the first time the sedative, calming effects of other oils, such as *Citrus aurantium* var. *amara* (flos) and *Passiflora incarnata* (Buchbauer et al 1992, Buchbauer 1993, Buchbauer et al 1993). The aromatic water collected during the distillation of the orange flowers (orange flower water) also has sedative properties, and more effective still is the essential oil of petitgrain *Citrus aurantium* var. *amara* (fol.) (Duraffourd 1982 p. 97). Lavender is recognized as a calming oil (Guillemain et al 1989) and is now used in many hospital wards to aid sleep (see Ch. 12). It is thought that the sedative effect of *Lavandula angustifolia* is due in part to the presence of coumarins in the oil, even though the content is low at 0. 25% (Franchomme & Pénoël 1990 p. 364) (see Table 4.9).

Spasmolytic

Essential oils have been found to relieve smooth muscle spasm (Debelmas & Rochat 1964, 1967a, 1967b, Taddei et al 1988), hence their usefulness for some problems of the digestive tract. The oils with this property are chamomile oils containing (-)-α-bisabolol (Achterrath-Tuckerman et al 1980, Melegari et al 1988) *Carum carvi, Cinnamomum zeylanicum* (cort.), *Citrus aurantium* var. *amara* (per.), *Foeniculum vulgare* var. *dulce, Melissa officinalis, Mentha × piperita* (Schilcher 1985 p. 225).

There is value in successful practical experience, and essential oils have been used to ease spasm in skeletal muscle also, despite the lack of clinical trials. We have used *Ocimum basilicum* and *Origanum majorana* successfully over the years, and a fuller list has been published (Price 1993 p. 278). *Cupressus sempervirens* is also credited with this property (Franchomme & Pénoël 1990 p. 346).

Other considerations

Essential oil effects on other treatments

Essential oils are composed of chemicals which are known to be active, gain access to cells by virtue of being fat soluble, and are metabolized by the body. It has been found by experience that some oils are relaxing, some sedative, some sharpen the memory, some promote the circulation and so on. Therefore it may be assumed that as active agents they may react with other drugs present in the body, although there has been no evidence so far which would imply any adverse significant reaction between essential oils and allopathic drugs, and they have been used together successfully in hospitals (Barker 1994 personal communication).

Nevertheless this is a cloudy area and, until laboratory investigations into possible reactions between essential oils and other drugs have been carried out and results made known, it is only possible to surmise what may happen. If sedative pills to help sleep are being prescribed then it may be unwise with our present level of knowledge to use an essential oil such as rosemary which keeps the mind alert. It would be better to choose oils like lavender, vetiver and valerian, which are known to aid relaxation and sleep. It has been suggested that when a person is on medication the drugs involved could possibly affect metabolization of essential oil molecules. In some cases metabolism may be increased, e.g. with clofibrate (blood lipid level reducer), steroids and phenobarbitones (anti-epileptics). In other cases the drugs involved may reduce the metabolism of essential oil molecules, e.g. imidazole (antifungal), plant drugs, caffeic acid, myristicin or tannic acid.

Some essences have been found to complement the action of antibiotics. Laboratory tests have shown that the essence of niaouli will increase the activity of streptomycin, cocaine and, more especially, of penicillin (Quevauviller & Panousse-Perrin 1952a, 1952b). Reporting the results obtained when using turpentine derivatives in conjunction with antibiotics, Mignon has shown, from tests *in vitro* and on mice, the action of the antibiotics to be considerably augmented by being administered in a solution of oxygenated turpentine derivatives. There are, however, some constituents of some essential oils (aldehydes, ketones and some alcohols) which inactivate antibiotics and so limit their use in ointment form.

(Valnet 1980 p. 39)

Homoeopathy. For many years now we have been questioning practitioners of homoeopathy as to whether homoeopathic treatment is affected in any way by the concurrent use of essential oils, and the answers have varied from the total prohibition of all essential oils to the unrestricted use of any. However, the chief common ground is that peppermint should be avoided and probably eucalyptus and camphor as well, and this is what is advised in the absence of a definitive answer.

Molecular structure

A possible relationship between the molecular structure of the essential oil components and their therapeutic effect has been studied and published

(Franchomme & Pénoël 1990). This is an interesting piece of work and although not proven rigorously is nevertheless very useful to therapists when studying and choosing oils; the principles involved are to be found in Price (1993 pp. 49–55). 'It is based on the presence of key chemical groups in the oil molecules. If this approach is valid, then it may well be that essential oil molecules are interacting with the same receptors on nerve cells and in other tissues which respond to drugs' (Balacs 1991).

British Pharmacopoeia

Mabey (1988 p. 190) points out that no less than 80% of the medicines in the BP were plant-based at one time (e.g. aspirin)—and even today 30% are still plant-based (e.g. digitalis). Current pharmaceutical formulae demonstrate that essential oils and oleoresins derived from spices and herbs are valued not only as flavouring agents but also for other properties they possess: for instance, they stimulate the appetite by increasing salivation, they relieve gastric discomfort and flatulence by acting as carminatives, and they counteract the griping action of purgatives. In cough mixtures and pastilles they contribute as mild expectorants and in inhalants they check profuse secretion and relieve congestion of the bronchioles. Formulated as ointments, creams and liniments they act as counter-irritants and rubefacients, for the chest in bronchitis and pleurisy, and for the relief of rheumatic pain. As flavouring agents, essential oils are acceptable for repeated dosage, e.g. in tablets to be chewed and for repeated usage in such products as toothpaste. As perfumes they are essential in a variety of cosmetics which are used daily over long periods of time.

The essential oils as specified in the BP are not suitable for use in aromatology or aromatherapy because the specification is too broad or does not reflect the materials currently available. In fact 'the analytical figures for the present English lavender oil do not correspond with the existing BP standards' (Trease & Evans 1983). There are many different varieties of eucalyptus used in aromatherapy, each with its own characteristics, but many are lumped together in the BP where eucalyptus essential oil is given as *E. globulus* Labill., *E. fruticetorum* F von Muell., *E. polybractea* R T Baker, or *E. smithii* R T Baker. Each of these indeed has 1,8-cineole as its major component but the other constituents modify the effects of the whole oil. The BP gives the results of thin layer chromatography on some of the oils listed, but for some there is not even this specification: a critical commentary on the BP monograph for peppermint oil can be found in Hay & Waterman (1993).

Lemon is listed as *Citrus limon* (L) Burm, f. with not less than 2.2% w/w and not more than 4.5% w/w of carbonyl components (calculated as citral) $C_{10}H_{16}O$. Also listed as *Citrus limon* is terpeneless lemon oil containing not less than 40% w/w of aldehydes (calculated as citral) $C_{10}H_{16}O$. However, the deterpenated essence is not used in aromatology as defined today because only unadulterated and unrectified oils may be used. Some of the oils mentioned in the BP lack any complete specification: anise, caraway, cardamom, cedarwood, cinnamon, clove, coriander, dill, eucalyptus, lemon, nutmeg, orange, peppermint, spearmint and turpentine.

A survey of the European pharmacopoeia (Bischof et al 1992) shows that only a few oils are common to the major pharmacopoeia—caraway, eucalyptus, lemon, peppermint. Surprisingly, lavender is not one of them, but the *Pharmacopoeia Helvetica* does allow synthetic lavender. The *Formulaire National de France* has three monographs on lavender.

Summary

The numerous therapeutic properties of essential oils have been examined in some detail, and scientific confirmation of traditional wisdom given where possible. It is to be hoped that more controlled trials take place, and the importance of the totality of effects of any essential oil will be given precedence over the activity of its components. There is also an urgent need for official sources such as the British Pharmacopoeia to be revised to take into account modern botanical and therapeutic knowledge of essential oils.

REFERENCES

Achterrath-Tuckerman V et al 1980 Pharmacological investigations with compounds of chamomile. V. Investigations on the spasmolytic effect of compounds of chamomile. Planta Medica, Stuttgart 39: 38–50

Balacs T 1991 Essential issues. International Journal of Aromatherapy 3(4): 24

Becker H 1983 Deutsche Apotheker Zeitung 123: 2470

Becker H, Förster W 1984 Biologie, Chemie und Pharmakologie pflanzlicher Sedativa. Zeitschrift Phytotherapie Stuttgart 5: 817–823

Becker H, Reichling J 1981 Deutsche Apotheker Zeitung 121: 1185

Belaiche P 1979 Traité de phytothérapie et d'aromathérapie, 3 vols. Maloine, Paris.

Belaiche P 1985a L'huile essentielle de Melaleuca alternifolia (Cheel) dans les infections cutanées. Phytothérapie 15 September: 15–18

Belaiche P 1985b L'huile essentielle de Melaleuca alternifolia (Cheel) dans les infections urinaires colibacillaires chroniques idiopathiques. Phytothérapie 15 September: 9–12

Belaiche P 1985c L'huile essentielle de Melaleuca alternifolia (Cheel) dans les infections vaginales à candida albicans. Phytothérapie 15 September: 13–14

Bernadet M 1983 La phyto-aromathérapie pratique. Dangles, St-Jean-de-Braye

Beylier M F 1979 Bacteriostatic activity of some Australian essential oils. Perfumer & Flavorist 4(23) April/May: 23–25

Bischof C, Holthuijzen J, Löwenstein C, Stengele M, Stahl-Biskup E, Wilhelm E 1992 Essential oil analysis in the European Pharmacopoeia. 23rd International Symposium on Essential Oils, West of Scotland College, Ayr, Scotland. Copies available from Lehrstuhl für Pharmakognosie der Universität Hamburg, Bundesstrasse 43, D-2000 Hamburg 13

Boeters M 1969 Behandlung vegetativer Regulationsstörungen mit Valepotriaten (Valmane). Münchner Medizin Wochenschrift 11: 1873–1876

Bonnaure F 1919 Essais sur les propriétés bactericides de quelques huiles essentielles. Parfumerie Moderne 12: 151

Bonnelle C 1993 Des hommes et des plantes. Editions du Parc Naturel Régional du Vercors, Lans-en-Vercors, p. 32

Boyd E M, Pearson G L 1946 The expectorant action of volatile oils. American Journal of Medical Science 211: 602–610

Buchbauer G 1993 Biological effects of fragrances and essential oils. Perfumer & Flavorist 18 January/February: 19–24

Buchbauer G, Jirovetz L, Jäger W 1992 Passiflora and lime blossoms: motility effects after inhalation of the essential oil and of some of the main constituents in animal experiment. Archiva Pharmaceutica (Weinheim) 325: 247–248

Buchbauer G, Jirovetz L, Jäger W, Plank C, Dietrich H 1993 Fragrance compounds and essential oils with sedative effects upon inhalation. Journal of Pharmaceutical Sciences 82(6) June: 660–664

Carson C F, Riley T V 1993 Antimicrobial activity of the essential oil of Melaleuca alternifolia. Applied Microbiology 16(2): 49–55

Cavel L 1918 Sur la valeur antiseptique de quelques huiles essentielles. Comptes Rendus Académie des Sciences, p. 827

Chabrol E, Charonnat R, Maximum M, Busson A 1932 Le serpolet: cholagogue. Comptes Rendus Société Biologie 109: 275–276

Chamberland M 1887 Les essences au point de vue de leurs propriétés antiseptiques. Annales Institut Pasteur 1: 153–154

Cohen R A, Kucera L S, Herrman E C 1964 Antiviral activity of Melissa officinalis extract Proceedings of the Society of Experimental Biology and Medicine, p. 431–434

Courmont P, Morel P, Bay I 1938 The antiseptic action of essential oils. Parfumerie Moderne 21: 161

D'Arcy P F 1993 Drug reactions and interactions. International Pharmacy Journal 7(4) July/August: 140–142

Deans S G, Ritchie G A 1987 Antibacterial properties of plant essential oils. International Journal of Food Microbiology 5: 165–180

Deans S G, Svoboda K P 1988 Antibacterial activity of French tarragon (Artemisia dracunculus L) essential oil and its constituents during ontogeny. Journal of Horticultural Science 63: 135–140

Deans S G, Svoboda K P 1989 Antibacterial activity of summer savory [Satureia hortensis L] essential oil and its constituents. Journal of Horticultural Science 64: 205–211

Deans S G, Svoboda K P 1990a Essential oil profiles of several temperate and tropical aromatic plants: their antimicrobial and antioxidative properties. Proceedings 75th International Symposium of Research Institute for Medicinal Plants, Budakalasz, Hungary pp. 25–27. Copies obtainable from authors at Scottish Agricultural College, Ayr

Deans S G, Svoboda K P 1990b The antimicrobial properties of Marjoram (Origanum marjorana L.) volatile oil. Flavor & Fragrance Journal 5(3): 187–190

Debelmas A M Rochat J 1964 Etude comparée sur la fibre lisse des solutions aqueuses saturées d'essence de thym, de thymol et de carvacrol. Bulletin des Travaux. Société de Pharmacie de Lyon 4: 163–172

Debelmas A M, Rochat J 1967a Action des eaux saturées d'huiles essentielles sur la musculature lisse. 25th International Congress of Pharmaceutical Science. Butterworth, London pp. 601–607

Debelmas A M, Rochat J 1967b Activité antispasmodique étudiée sur une cinquantaine d'échantillons différents. Plantes Médicinales et Phytothérapie 1: 23–27

Decazes J-M 1993 The masking effect of perfume ingredients. Symposium at Stoke-on-Trent: Fragrance— more than just a pleasant smell? Society of Cosmetic Chemists

Dube S, Upadhyay P D, Tripath S C 1989 Antifungal, physiochemical, and insect-repelling activity of the essential oil of Ocimum basilicum. Canadian Journal of Botany 67(7): 2085–2087

Duraffourd P 1982 En forme tous les jours. La Vie Claire, Périgny, p. 107

Duraffourd P 1987 Les huiles essentielles et la santé. La Maison du Bien-Etre, Montreuil-sous-Bois

Franchomme P, Pénoël D 1990 L'aromathérapie exactement. Jollois, Limoges

Gattefossé R M 1919 Propriétés bactéricides de quelques huiles essentielles. Parfumerie Moderne 13: 152

Gattefossé R M 1932 Rôle antiseptique de la lavande. Parfumerie Moderne 26: 543–553

Gattefossé R M 1937 Aromatherapy (trans 1993). Daniel, Saffron Walden, p. 87

Gershbein L E 1977 Regeneration of rat liver in the presence of essential oils and their components. Food and Cosmetics Toxicology 15: 173–181

Gildemeister E, Hoffmann F 1956 Die ätherischen Öle. Akademie Verlag, Berlin, vol. 1: 119

Glowania H J, Raulin C, Swoboda M 1987 Effect of chamomile on wound healing—a clinical double-blind study. Zeitschrift für Hautkrankheiten, Berlin 62(17): 1262, 1267–1271

Gordonoff T 1938 Ergebnisse der Physiologie, biologischen Chemie und experimentallen Pharmakologie 40: 53

Guillemain J, Rousseau A, Delaveau P 1989 Neurodepressive effects of the essential oil of Lavandula angustifolia Mill. Annales Pharmaceutiques Françaises 47(6): 337–343

Hay R K M, Waterman P G 1993 Volatile oil crops. Longman, Harlow, p. 52

Herrman E C junior, Kucera L S 1967 Antiviral substances in plants of the mint family (Labiatae). II. Nontannin polyphenol of Melissa officinalis. Proceedings of the Society for Experimental and Biological Medicine: 369–374

Hinou J B, Harvala C E, Hinou E B 1989 Antimicrobial activity screening of 32 common constituents of essential oils. Pharmazie 44(4) April: 302–303

Holland E H 1941 Results of a series of investigations carried out on the germicidal, disinfectant and bacteriostatic action of Melasol (Melaleuca alternifolia). Unpublished paper, Sydney University

Jakovlev V, Isaac O, Flaskamp E 1983 Pharmacological investigations with compounds of chamomile. VI. Investigations on the antiphlogistic effects of chamazulene and matricin. Planta Medica 49: 67–73

Jalsenjak V, Peljnjak S, Kustrak D 1987 Microcapsules of sage oil: essential oils content and antimicrobial activity. Pharmazie 42(6) June: 419–420

Janssen A M, Scheffer J J C, Baerheim Svendson A, Aynehchi Y 1984 Pharmazeutisch Weekblad (Scientific Edition) 6: 157

Janssen A M, Chin N L J, Scheffer J J C, Baerheim Svendsen A 1986 Screening for antimicrobial activity of some essential oils by the agar overlay techniques. Pharmazeutisch Weekblad (Scientific Edition) 8: 289–292

Jasper C, Maruzella J C, Laurence Liguori L 1958a The in vitro antifungal activity of essential oils. Journal of the American Pharmaceutical Association 47(4): 294–296

Jasper C, Maruzella J C, Percival A, Henry P A 1958b The antimicrobial activity of perfume oils. Journal of the American Pharmaceutical Association 47(7): 471

Kellner W, Kober W 1954 Möglichkeiten der Werwendung ätherischer öle zur Raumdesinfektion. I. Mitteilung: Die Wirkung gebräuchlicher ätherischer Öle auf Testkeime. Arzneimittel-Forschung [Drug Research] 4(5): 319

Kellner W, Kober W 1955 Möglichkeiten der Werwendung ätherischer Öle zur Raumdesinfektion. II. Arzneimittel-Forschung [Drug Research] 5(4): 224

Kellner W, Kober W 1956 Möglichkeiten der Werwendung ätherischer Öle zur Raumdesinfektion. III. Arzneimittel-Forschung [Drug Research] 6(12): 768

Kienholz M 1959 Action antibactérienne des huiles essentielles. Arzneimittel-Forschung [Drug Research] 9(8): 518–519

Kucera L S, Herrman J C Jr 1967 Antiviral substances in plants in the mint family (Labiatae). 1. Tannin of Melissa officinalis. Proceedings of the Society for Experimental and Biological Medicine 124: 865

Larrondo J V, Calvo M A 1991 Effect of essential oils on Candida albicans: a scanning electron microscope study. Biomed Letters 46(184): 269–272

Lautié R, Passebecq A 1984 Aromatherapy. Thorsons, Wellingborough, p. 74

Lembke A, Deininger R 1985 Preparation and method for stimulating the immune system. German Patent 3508875 A 1 21 November 1985

Lembke A, Deininger R 1988 Virus inactivating pharmaceutical containing formates and black pepper oil. European Patent (EP) 259617 A 2 16 March 1988

Low D, Rowal B D, Griffin W J 1974 Antibacterial action of the essential oils of some Australian Myrtaceae. Planta Medica 26: 184

Mabey R 1988 The complete new herbal. Elm Tree, London

Malowan S L 1931 Zeitschrift für Hygiene 1(1): 93

Martindale W H 1910 Antiseptic powers of essential oils. Perfumery & Essential Oil Record 1: 266, 274

Maruzella J C 1961 Antifungal properties of perfume oils. Journal of the American Pharmaceutical Association 50: 655

Medicines Act 1968 HMSO, London

Melegari M et al 1988 Chemical characteristics and pharmacological properties of the essential oil of Anthemis nobilis. Fitoterapia 6: 449–455

Mills S Y 1991 Essential book of herbal medicine. Penguin, London, p. 452

Onawunmi G O 1988 In vitro studies on the antibacterial activity of phenoxyethanol in combination with lemongrass oil. Pharmazie 43(1) January: 42–43

Onawunmi G O 1989 Antifungal activity of lemongrass oil. International Journal of Crude Drug Research 27(2): 121–126

Onawunmi G O, Ogunlana E O 1986 A study of the antibacterial activity of the essential oil of lemongrass Cymbopogon citratus (DC) Stapf. International Journal of Crude Drug Research 24(2): 64–68

Onawunmi G O, Yisak W A, Ogunlana E O 1984 Antibacterial constituents in the essential oil of Cymbopogon citratus (DC) Stapf. Journal of Ethnopharmacology 12(3): 279–286

Pandey M P, Prasad J, Awasthi L P, Kaushik P 1988 Antiviral effect of the essential oils from lemongrass (Cymbopogon flexuosus), mint (Mentha arvensis) and vetiver (Vetiveria zizanioides). Indigenous Medicinal Plants 47–49

Pellecuer J, Roussel J L, Andary C 1973 Propriétés antifongiques comparatives des essences des trois Labiées méditerranéennes: romarin, sarriette et thym. Travaux de la Société de Pharmacie de Montpelier 33(4): 587

Pellecuer J, Allegrini J, De Buochberg S 1974 Etude in vitro de l'activité anti-bactérienne et antifongique de l'essence de Satureia montana L. Labiées. Journal de Pharmacie de Belgique 29(2): 137–144

Pellecuer J, Allegrini J, De Buochberg S, Passat J 1975 Place de l'essence de Satureia montana L. Labiées dans l'arsenal thérapeutique. Plantes Médicinales et Phytothérapie. 9(2): 99–106

Pellecuer, J Allegrini J, Seimeon M, De Buochberg S 1976 Huiles essentielles bactéricides et fongicides. Revue de l'Institut de Lyon 01 (2): 135–159

Pena E F 1962 Melaleuca alternifolia oil—its use for trichomonal vaginitis and other vaginal infections. Obstetrics and Gynecology, June: 793–795

Pénoël D 1981 Phytomédecine. CIMP, La Courtête 1/2: 63

Poucher W A 1936 Perfumes, cosmetics and soaps. Chapman & Hall, London, 3 vols

Price S 1993 The aromatherapy workbook. Thorsons, London, pp. 49–55

Quevauviller A, Panousse-Perrin J 1952a Exaltation du pouvoir anesthétique local de la cocaïne par l'essence de Niaouli purifiée. Anesthésie 9: 421

Quevauviller A, Panousse-Perrin J 1952b Influence du Gomenol sur l'activité in vitro de certains antibiotiques. Revue de Pathologie Comparée et Hygiene Générale 637: 296

Raharivelomanana P J, Terrom G P, Bianchini J P, Coulanges P 1989 Study of the antimicrobial action of various essential oils extracted from Malagasy plants. II: Lauraceae. Archives Institut Pasteur de l'Afrique (Madagascar) 56(1): 261–271

Ramanoelina A R, Terrom G P, Bianchini J P, Coulanges P 1987 Antibacterial action of essential oils extracted from Madagascar plants. Archives Institut Pasteur de l'Afrique (Madagascar) 53(1): 217–226

Rideal S, Rideal E K, Sciver A 1928 An investigation into the germicidal powers and capillary activities of certain essential oils. Perfumery and Essential Oil Record 19: 285

Rideal E K, Sciver A, Richardson N E G 1930 Perfumery and Essential Oil Record 21: 341

Ritzerfeld W 1959 Arzneimittel-Forschung 9: 521

Rossi T, Melegari M, Bianchi A, Albasini A, Vampa G 1988 Sedative, antiinflammatory and antidiuretic effects induced in rats by essential oils of varieties of Anthemis nobilis: a comparative study. Pharmacol Res Commun 5, December 20: 71–74

Roulier G 1990 Les huiles essentielles pour votre santé. Dangles, St-Jean-de-Braye

Schilcher H 1985 Effects and side effects of essential oils. In: Baerheim Svendson A, Scheffer JJC (eds) Essential Oils and Aromatic Plants. Martinus Nijhof/Junk, Dordrecht

Schmidt P W 1936 Zentralblad für Bakteriologie, Parasitenkunde und Infektionskrankenheiten 138: 104

Schmiedeberg O 1913 Grundriss der Pharmakologie, 7th edn. Pharmokologie, Leipzig

Schnaubelt K 1994 Aromatherapy and chronic viral infections. In: Aroma 93 Conference Proceedings. Aromatherapy Publications, Brighton, pp. 34–41

Schneider G 1975 Pharmazeutische Biologie. Wissenschaftsverlag, Mannheim, p. 128

Shemesh A U, Mayo W L 1991 Tea tree oil—natural antiseptic and fungicide. Journal of Alternative and Complementary Medicine 12 December 9: 11–12

Szalontai M, Verzar-Petri G, Florian E, Gimpel F 1975a Pharmazeutische Zeitung 120: 982

Szalontai M, Verzar-Petri G, Florian E, Gimpel F 1975b Deutsche Apotheker Zeitung 115: 912

Szalontai M, Verzar-Petri G, Florian E 1976 Acta Pharmaceutica [Hungary] 46: 232

Szalontai M, Verzar-Petri G, Florian E 1977 Contribution to the study of antimycotic effect of biologically active components of Matricaria chamomilla L. Parfümerie und Kosmetik [Hungary] 58: 121

Taddei I, Giachetti D, Taddei E, Mantovani P, Bianchi E 1988 Spasmolytic activity of peppermint, sage and rosemary essences and their major constituents. Fitoterapia 59: 463–468

Thiemer K, Stadler R, Isaac O 1973 Arzneimittel-Forschung 23: 756

Thompson D P, Cannon C 1986 Toxicity of essential oils on toxigenic and nontoxigenic fungi. Bulletin of Environmental Contamination and Toxicology 36(4) April: 527–532

Trease G E, Evans W C 1983 Pharmacognosy, 12th edn. Baillière Tindall, London, p. 424

Tukioka M 1927 Proceedings. Imperial Academy Tokyo 3: 624

Valnet J 1980 The practice of aromatherapy. Daniel, Saffron Walden

Verdet 1989 Why phytotherapy? Aromatherapy Study Trip Lecture notes. Price Publishing, Hinckley, p. 10

Viaud H 1983 Huiles essentielles. Présence, Sisteron

Vichkanova S A, Dzhanashiya N M, Goryunova L V 1973 Antiviral activity displayed by the essential oil of Eucalyptus viminalis and of some frost-hardy eucalypti. Farmakol Toksikol 339–341

Weiss R F 1988 Herbal medicine. Arcanum, Göteborg, p. 296

Yousef R T, Tawil G G 1980 Antimicrobial activity of volatile oils. Pharmazie 35(11) 698–701

Zara M 1966 Association atoxique de dérivées terpéniques d'huiles essentielles possédant une triple action en hépatologie (cholérétique, antispasmodique, lipotrope). Vie Méd 47(10): 1549–1553

The foundations of practice

5

How essential oils enter the body

Introduction

Essential oils follow three main pathways to gain entry to the body: ingestion, olfaction and absorption through the skin (Fig. 5.1). Ingestion is little-used in the UK. Of the two remaining pathways, inhalation is a very effective method and indeed is regarded by some (e.g. Buchbauer 1988) as the only method truly deserving the name aromatherapy. However, topical application via the skin has also been found to be effective—the route selected depends on the problem being helped.

INGESTION

Ingestion is the main route employed by aromatologists and doctors in France, but is not usually used by aromatherapists in other countries. This is because in the UK and elsewhere there are wide variations in training standards, ranging from those designed for simple beauty therapy to that enabling a therapist to practise clinical aromatherapy/aromatology. Therapists who have successfully completed an advanced aromatology training course are in a position to advise the use of essential oils per os. Most of the research carried out by medical aromatologists in France has involved internal use of essential oils. In this case every drop of oil used reaches the body systems, unlike inhalation, when only a tiny amount of essential oil vapour enters the body, and external application, where some of the essential oils are lost by evaporation.

Methods of ingestion

Per os

When essential oils are taken by mouth, knowledge of the constituents of the oils is of paramount importance. This is not to say that an oil containing a potentially hazardous component cannot be ingested—these components are sometimes the most effective for certain disorders. It simply means that knowledge of the strength of concentration, the nature of the diluent and the length of time for which it is to be taken is essential. Alcohol and honey water are the most usual diluents (Valnet 1980) though vegetable oils (such as hazelnut and olive oils) are excellent for this purpose and are preferred by many doctors and naturopaths practising in France (Collin 1994 personal communication), who have studied phytotherapy and are experienced in prescribing essential oils for internal use.

Although higher doses can be found in aromatherapy books (particularly those written by French authors) a guide to the maximum safe dose is 3 drops, 3 times a day, for 3 weeks (see Ch. 3), although the individual and the particular oils used must be taken into consideration. As mentioned above, all the oil is taken into the body via ingestion. Although this is not harmful when used correctly, continual ingestion for too long a period of time can eventually lead to toxic build up in the liver. This is particularly true of the powerful oils. It is for this reason that after 3 weeks, several days rest from the oils is indicated, to allow the liver the opportunity to eliminate any toxic matter.

Because they are usually tasteless and do not cause irritation, many conventional drugs are given by mouth. However, essential oils often taste quite bitter and may irritate the mucous lining, so most aromatherapists are cautious about using this method, particularly as there is much greater danger of an excessive dose reaching the liver than in external application. Further, there is the possibility of change in the essential oil molecules by digestive enzymes, strong acids and metabolization. Nevertheless, the authors have used essential oils in this way

for nearly two decades for sore throats, stomach upsets etc., with no reported adverse effects. After specialized training in this field, therapists should be confident in using this method.

Per rectum or vagina

Another method of internal use is by means of suppositories and pessaries, which can be useful in cases of irritable bowel syndrome, haemorrhoids, vaginal infections and candida. Suppositories, though not much favoured in Britain, allow the essential oils direct access to the bloodstream with little chance of metabolization. The maximum dose for for suppositories and pessaries is 6 drops (Collin 1994 personal communication). Toxic or irritant essential oils should not be used.

OLFACTION

Access via the nasal passages is indisputably the quickest effective route in the treatment of emotional problems such as stress and depression (and also some types of headache). This is because the nose has direct contact with the brain, which is responsible for triggering the effects of essential oils regardless of the route they use to gain access to it. The nose itself is not the organ of smell, but simply modifies the temperature and humidity of the air inhaled and collects any foreign matter which may be breathed in. The first cranial (olfactory) nerve is responsible for the sense of smell and serves the receptor cells, of which there are two groups of about 25 million each occupying a small area (of about 4 cm^2) at the top of the nostrils (van Toller 1993).

When essential oils are inhaled, the volatile molecules in the oils are carried by eddy currents to the roof of the nose, where delicate cilia protrude from the receptor cells into the nose itself. When the molecules lock onto these 'hairs' an electrochemical message is transmitted via the olfactory bulb and olfactory tract to the limbic system (amygdala and hippocampus). This may trigger memory and emotional responses which can, via the hypothalamus acting as relay and regulator, cause messages to be sent to other parts of the brain and the rest of the body. The received messages are converted into action, resulting in the release of euphoric, relaxing, sedative or stimulating neurochemicals as appropriate. It is worth remembering that the limbic system developed 70 million years ago and that it used to be called the rhinencephalon (Greek, *rhis* = nose, *enkephalon* = brain). The limbic system is heavily implicated in the expression of emotion, although whether it generates emotion or merely integrates it is not clear (Stoddart 1990). The body can replace olfactory nerve cells, underlining their importance.

Michael Shipley, a neurophysiologist at Cincinnati University, has demonstrated that fibres from the olfactory nerve carry impulses to two small but significant parts of the brain, the locus ceruleus and the raphe nucleus. Noradrenaline is concentrated in the locus ceruleus and serotonin in the raphe nucleus.

(Godfrey-Hardinge 1993 personal communication)

Godfrey-Hardinge goes on to say that sedative aromas such as *Origanum majorana*, *Lavandula angustifolia*, *Chamaemelum nobile*, *Chamomilla recutita* and *Citrus aurantium* (flos) cause stimulation of the raphe nucleus, which then releases the neurochemical serotonin; stimulating aromas such as *Rosmarinus officinalis*, *Citrus limon* (per.), *Ocimum basilicum* and *Mentha × piperita* will affect the locus ceruleus which then releases noradrenalin. (See Ch. 7.)

Anosmia

Not everyone can smell every aroma. Unlike vision (where differences between people can be as obvious as the need for spectacles or a white stick), there is no easy means of recognizing differences in ability to smell. Aromas are made up of individual chemicals and each cilia is equipped with uniquely contoured depressions into which a single aroma molecule can fit, somewhat like a jigsaw puzzle. However, if the appropriate 'docking' depression for the molecule being inhaled is absent, that smell will not be registered. Only when the molecule is keyed in is a specific signal generated.

Total, specific and temporary anosmia

Anosmia, the absence of sense of smell, can be total (nothing is smelt at all), or specific (inability to register certain smells). Almost everyone suffers from some form of this, and probably each of us has about five of these specific anosmias. It is interesting that about 5% of people are blind to the sweaty smell notes, and while about 50% of people are anosmic to androstenone, musk is almost universally noticed. Some aromas have exceptionally low detection thresholds (e.g. those of grapefruit and green pepper).

Temporary anosmia may be caused by colds, rhinitis and sinusitis. I (S. Price) remember a case of chronic sinusitis (suffered for 17 years), when even after an operation the client was unable to smell his wife's cooking—his main cause for concern! After three treatments he was able to detect *Mentha × piperita*, one of the essential oils in the mix (which also included *Eucalyptus globulus* and *Ocimum basilicum*). After 6 months he had recovered his sense of smell sufficiently to recognize some of the gastronomic aromas greeting him on his return from work.

Does anosmia negate aromatherapy?

If a person is incapable of smelling an aroma, does this mean that aromatherapy will not be effective? There is no definitive answer to this question, but many aromatherapists believe that prolonged use of essential oils will restore the sense of smell in some cases. This is in line with some surprising recent findings which indicate that in man and animals presenting specific anosmia, the sensitivity to some odours can be restored by repeated exposure to these odours (van Toller & Dodd 1992, Holley 1993). This may suggest that aromas are having some effect on the human system even if the aroma is not being consciously registered (see above case).

Smell adaptation

It is a common assumption that the sense of smell, more than other modalities, is readily affected by adaptation as a result of continued exposure to a stimulus. For example, a room one has just entered may have a noticeable odour, but presumably the odour quickly disappears because receptors fatigue and decrease their rate of firing in the presence of odorous molecules in the mucus.

(Engen 1982)

If the receptors do indeed stop firing, then the question arises whether aromas can bring about changes in the client. Engen goes on to say that although olfactory adaptation is apparently commonly experienced, its effect has been exaggerated. He points out that animals using olfactory cues to find a mate would be rather frustrated if the cue should disappear half-way there. Broad experience in the field of aromatherapy massage says that the aromas are indeed effective throughout the treatment, even though the quality of perception at the end of the treatment may well be different from that at the beginning.

Inhalation and the mucous membranes

When inhaling any vapour, some molecules from it inevitably travel down the pathway to the lungs where, if they are appropriate essential oils, they can have an immediate and beneficial impact on many breathing difficulties. In the nose the endothelium is thin and the site is close to the brain, therefore it must be assumed that essential oil molecules reach the local circulation and the brain fairly easily and quickly. On their journey to the lungs some molecules are undoubtedly absorbed by the mucous linings of the respiratory pathways and the bronchi and multitudinous bronchioles, where access is very easy. Arriving at the point of gaseous exchange in the alveoli, the tiny molecules are transferred to the blood circulating the lungs. It can be seen that deep breathing will increase the quantity of essences taken into the body by this route. Fortunately, ill effects from inhalation of essential oils normally used in aromatherapy are rare.

Methods of inhalation

Inhalation is an unobtrusive way of using essential oils in a healthcare setting. They may be given via a tissue, the hands (in an emergency), a vaporizer, etc., and all are effective in the appropriate situation. To choose oils for particular conditions, see the tables in Chapter 4 and Appendix B.9.

Tissues

Inhalation from a tissue with 5-6 drops of essential oil (3 drops for children, the elderly and pregnant women) is most effective for immediate results, requiring two or three deep breaths to ensure good contact with the cilia. To give further benefit, and easier with children and the elderly, the tissue can be placed inside the shirt, blouse or nightwear so the effects may continue as the heat of the body causes the oil molecules to evaporate and float upwards to the nose. Firm tissues such as kitchen towels hold the aroma longer than paper handkerchiefs.

Q-tips

This method uses less essential oil than a tissue, because it is concentrated in a small area. The Q-tip is held against the dropper and one drop allowed to wet it. Unlike a crumpled tissue, it cannot be placed next to the skin, but has the advantage of slower evaporation, so the patient/client can use it for longer.

Hands

This is an excellent method, but should be confined to emergencies only and is not suitable for children. A solitary drop of essential oil (single, or from a mix) should be put into the palm of one hand, which is then rubbed briefly against the other to disperse and warm the oil. With the patient's eyes closed, the cupped hands should be placed over the nose, avoiding the eye area, and the patient asked to take a deep nasal breath. It is usually respiratory or stress conditions which require this sort of help.

Steamers

Allowing a client/patient to hold a basin of hot water is not acceptable in many hospital situations, on account of the Health and Safety Act. Even if the nurse holds it there is always the possibility that people, especially those with learning difficulties, may strike out (involuntarily or otherwise) and knock the scalding water over themselves or the nurse. Home-visiting health professionals may find in certain circumstances and with people whose movements are stable that the method can be used safely, but it is our opinion that dry inhalation is preferable for those not enjoying full health, for whatever reason.

Nebulizers are safer but unfortunately the essential oils can attack some kinds of plastic, so care must be taken not to damage the equipment. A precautionary test is advisable for any plastic which may come into contact with essential oils. This applies also to facial steamers.

These methods are normally used for respiratory problems and the common cold, though any problem which can benefit from inhalation may obtain speedier relief when steam is used. The heat of the water evaporates the oil molecules more quickly, increasing the strength of the vapour and for this reason only half the number of drops are needed compared with inhalation from a tissue (2 drops for a child, elderly person or pregnant woman).

The following cautions may be helpful:

- Ensure the patient's eyes are kept closed and watch carefully for any adverse reaction such as choking or coughing, which can happen if too many drops have been used or too deep a breath is taken.
- 1 drop only is adequate for asthmatics because the overpowering effect of the vapour (stronger because of the speedy evaporation referred to above) may have an adverse effect.

Baths

For details, see Methods of percutaneous absorption below.

Spray bottle

A quick way of freshening the air when dressings are being changed for patients with bed sores, gangrene, etc. is by using 10-12 drops of essential oil in 250 ml of water, shaking the bottle well before spraying the room. The essential oils to use in this case are *Pinus sylvestris*, *Thymus vulgaris* (all chemotypes, though phenolic thymes are the most powerful antiseptics), *Syzygium aromaticum*, *Eucalyptus smithii* and *Mentha × piperita*.

Vaporizers and diffusers

Possibly the most favoured way of using inhalation in a healthcare setting at the moment is from a vaporizer. This liberates the lightest molecules from the oil first, releasing the heavier ones progressively. Although there are many different types of vaporizers available, only electric ones are considered completely safe where patients are concerned (the British Safety Standard mark should be looked for on the model to be used). Electric vaporizers should be thermostatically controlled at a low temperature, preventing the essential oils from becoming too hot. If this occurs, not only are they used up too quickly to be economical but the residual heaviest molecules may burn off, producing an unpleasant acrid smell.

Diffusers (units with a small blown glass container for the essential oils) are more efficient in that they push out all the differently-sized molecules at the same time. Unlike vaporizers using heat, there is no burning of residue when the essential oil is used up. Their only disadvantage is their price, which can be up to three times greater than that of an electric vaporizer. One diffuser on the market has a time switch, ideal for hospital use (see Useful Addresses).

Ethical considerations. It is the policy of Community Health Sheffield to use vaporizers and diffusers in single-occupancy rooms only— not in general ward areas. It is felt unethical to impose aromas (which may be disliked by some) on other occupants, and we agree with this. Nevertheless, when the effects required for a whole ward are the same as for each occupant, e.g. when conducting a trial or keeping a ward free from infection, the method is viable and effective. It can also be useful in the reduction of stress and insomnia as well the destruction of germs.

However, available now for commercial use in offices, hotels and hospitals are large units which will condition large rooms. The most efficient release essential oils in timed doses so that the air does not become overloaded. Unfortunately, the operators of these large units use commercial-grade essential oils and aromas to keep costs down, without taking into account what effect long-term exposure may have on people's health. It is already known that artificial perfumes and adulterated essential oils cause sensitivities in asthmatics and skin reactions in those susceptible to such effects. 'Environmental fragrancing', as this practice is termed, is most advanced in the United States of America, where there is growing concern at the use of synthetic aromas (see Ch. 15). The liberty of the individual is an important consideration and, unlike shoppers irritated by muzak or 'fragrancing' designed to alter their mood, hospital patients are not free to walk away from an environmental influence which they may not like.

ABSORPTION VIA THE SKIN

Until the second half of the 20th century the skin was thought to be almost impermeable (Stoughton 1959, Maibach & Marzulli 1977). This old idea still persists, even though the skin is now known to be a poor barrier to lipophilic substances (Brun 1952). It is slightly permeable both to water soluble substances and water itself, even though the skin has developed as a barrier specifically to resist water. This protection is vital because water comprises 90% of any cell.

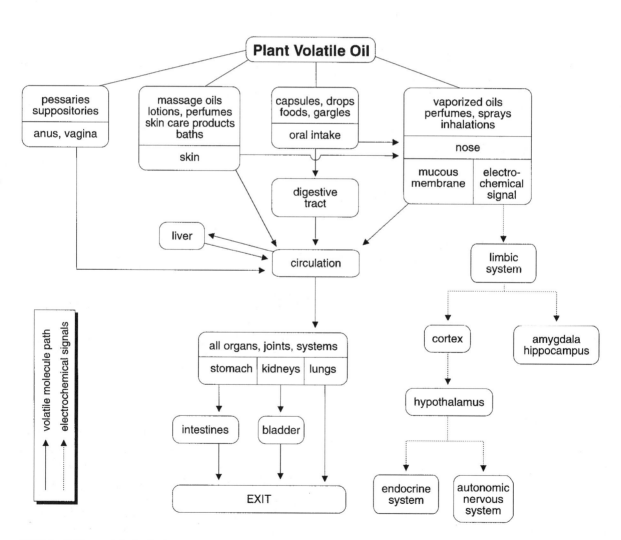

Fig 5.1 Pathways into the body

There has been a considerable amount of research regarding pesticides and the skin. Pesticides, which dissolve in essential oils, are lipid-like and can therefore get through the skin—every farmer is aware of this health hazard, and thousands of people are killed each year by pesticides, mostly in third-world countries. The skin's success as a barrier is due in the main to the stratum corneum, the tough and durable, self-repairing keratinized layer, which is only about 10 μm thick. Once a chemical gets past the epidermis—the only great obstacle—the rest of the journey into the body is easy, because the presence of lipids in all cell membranes negates the dermis's effectiveness as a barrier. For example, the antibacterial hexachlorophene is absorbed through the skin, and was shown in 1969 to cause microscopically-visible brain damage in rats (Winter 1984), and causes chloasma in humans. There are many factors which dictate the rate and quantity at which any given substance penetrates the skin, but it is now generally recognised that the skin is a semi-permeable membrane susceptible of penetration by substances to a greater or lesser degree (Lexicon Vevy 1993a). Obviously the physico-chemical properties of the molecules such as the molecular weight and spatial arrangement, liposolubility, coefficients of diffusion and dissociation are fundamental to skin penetration.

The skin as a barrier

On account of their solubility in the lipids found in the stratum corneum, lipophilic substances (such as essential oils) are considered to be easily absorbed. The absorption of organic compounds with anionic or cationic groups (weak acids and alkalis) takes place when they are found in undissociated form—more lipophilic than those dissociated: it depends however on their dissociation constant and on the pH of the substance and of the skin. Most essential oils used in aromatherapy pass through the skin and the organism and can be detected in exhaled air within 20–60 minutes (Katz 1947).

Once the essential oil constituents have passed the epidermis and entered the complex of lymph and blood vessels, nerves, sweat and oil glands, follicles, collagen, fibroblasts, mast cells, elastin and so on (known as the dermis), they are then carried away in the circulation to pervade every cell in the body.

The main factors affecting the penetration of the skin by essential oils are grouped together below.

Intrinsic factors

Area of skin. The very large area of the skin—in the region of 2 m² —makes it possible for a significant quantity of essential oils to be applied to the skin and so taken into the body. If a set quantity of essential oil in a carrier is applied to a smaller area of skin, then less will enter than if the same quantity were to be applied to a greater area.

Thickness and permeability of the epidermis. On palmar and plantar skin, because the epidermis is quite thick and there are no oil glands, the time taken to cross the skin is longer, especially for any lipid-soluble components. There is less resistance to water-soluble components however, and garlic placed on the feet is soon detected on the exhaled breath for instance. Easy penetration may occur on parts of the body where the skin is thinner e.g. behind the ears, eyelids and inside wrist. The skin regions of the legs, buttocks, trunk and the abdomen area are less permeable than those of the soles, palms, forehead, scalp, and armpits (Balacs 1993).

Gland openings and follicles. Hydrophilic molecules can find a path through the skin using the sweat glands; lipophilic molecules may use the sebaceous glands as a pathway, also travelling between the cells through the fatty cement and through the cells themselves, all of which contain lipids (Lexicon Vevy 1993b). The skin of the forehead and scalp contains numerous oil glands, and here the epidermis is thinner. This again makes for easy penetration of lipophilic substances although the water layer on the skin must present a partial barrier for the lipophilic molecules. The number of follicles and sweat glands is another factor: generally speaking, the more openings the speedier the access.

Reservoirs. It is possible essential oils may be sequestered (stored apart) in the body, as happens in the plants that produce them. If so, there would be reservoirs of essential oils (or at least of some of their molecules) in the outer layers of the epidermis and subcutaneous fat, and these may persist for some time. It might be considered that lipophilic components can, at least temporarily, be retained in this layer and consequently will not be available for rapid diffusion to other adjacent levels (Lexicon Vevy 1993b). Subcutaneous fat has a poor blood supply and although essential oils are slow to enter they probably tend to stay there for a long time.

A Dutch Government Commission report in 1983 showed that many MAC (maximum acceptable concentrations) for toxic chemicals failed to take into account the significant physiological differences between the sexes. Women's skin is more permeable to toxic chemicals than that of men and because they carry more fat their body levels of fat soluble chemicals are generally higher and take longer to disperse (Eisberg 1983).

Enzymes. Enzymes in the skin can activate and inactivate many drugs and foreign compounds. They can also activate and inactivate the body's own natural chemicals such as hormones, steroids and inflammatory mediators. The activities of these skin enzymes may vary greatly between individuals and with age (Hotchkiss 1994).

The skin contains many enzymes and therefore provides a 'laboratory' where metabolism can take place. Certainly some enzymes will effect a change in some essential oil molecules and even a slight change of shape in an essential oil molecule will mean a change in the effect on the body. Bacterial action breaks down the triglycerides in sebum to organic free fatty acids and incompletely esterified glycerol derivatives, and it is reasonable to suppose that similar sorts of processes may happen with the essential oils.

Damaged skin. Broken, inflamed and diseased skin is no barrier and ingress is rapid through cuts, abrasions, ulcers, psoriasis, burns, etc.

Other physiological factors

Rate of circulation. Where there is an increase in the rate of blood flow, perhaps due to rubbing (massage) or inflammation, there is an increased rate of absorption. Massage not only increases the speed of blood flow (causing hyperaemia) but also raises the local skin temperature, hence we can expect an increased rate and degree of absorption of essential oils due to the lowering of the viscosity. Proof that essential oils in a base oil applied to the skin are absorbed into the bloodstream has been provided by Jäger et al (1992) by the detection of linalyl acetate and linalool in a blood sample taken 5 minutes after the oil was applied.

Rate of distribution. As far as distribution is concerned the speed of the lymph and blood circulation is a limiting factor because the circulation is slower in the capillary loops than in the veins. The speed may be increased for example by massage, or by warmth (e.g. infrared). Both these methods may be used to increase the rate of distribution of essential oils. It has been proved that the blood vessels constantly resorb and expel terpenes so that a flowing balance results (Schilcher 1985, Römmelt et al 1974).

External factors

Hydration. Hydrated skin is very permeable, hence the effectiveness of what the authors term aromabalneotherapy (the use of essential oils in a bath). It has been shown that in a bath the essential oils penetrate the skin 100 times faster than water and 10 000 times more quickly than the ions of sodium and chloride (Römmelt et al 1974). Conversely, if the stratum corneum is dehydrated its permeability is decreased.

Degreased skin. Although detergents, degreasants, soaps, etc., increase the permeability of the skin to essential oils they are not necessarily recommended.

Warmth. Warm room, warm oils, warm hands and body all help speed up absorption. Care must be taken that the body is not made too warm (e.g. after a sauna) as the body is then exuding and eliminating, making ingress of oils difficult.

Occlusion. Occlusion due to a covering, e.g. a compress, has a sealing-in effect—it decreases the ability of the essential oils to volatilize, and it also aids warming. Oils applied under occlusion, as with all other substances, have an enhanced effect because of the increase in the quantity absorbed, due probably to local warming, and no loss of molecules through evaporation. Clothing may be regarded as being partially occlusive.

Oil-related factors

Viscosity. All essential oils have a low viscosity, but some oils with a relatively high viscosity, e.g. sandalwood, which is composed of 90% alcohols, will still cross the skin at a rate similar to other oils. Viscosity plays a more important part with regard to the carrier oils because some such as hazelnut are quite viscous and others such as grapeseed and sunflower are less so. If the molecular weight exceeds 500 then it is unlikely to pass the skin. Essential oils, being products of distillation, are limited to a maximum molecular weight of 225 (rarely reaching 250). In some cases it may be worth considering the use of a carrier which is partially hydrophilic even if only to a small extent (e.g. wheatgerm oil, walnut oil).

Molecular size. The size and shape of the individual essential oil molecules also have a bearing on their speed of penetration of the skin. Small molecules pass easily down the follicular and sebaceous ducts, and the smaller the molecule the faster they penetrate. Dissociation may also be relevant. When dissolved in a carrier the essential oil molecules may split into ions, thus becoming even more tiny. The bigger molecules, being less volatile, are less likely to be lost to the atmosphere, stay on the skin longer and therefore have a longer opportunity for penetration.

Frequency of use. There is some evidence that repeated use of the same oil makes the skin more permeable (see Ch. 3).

Saturated carriers. Lard, woolfat and mineral oil (e.g. baby oil) all prevent or seriously delay absorption: the higher the degree of unsaturation the easier the absorption process becomes.

Methods of percutaneous absorption

Many of the techniques used on the skin entail the use of water, vegetable oil or a bland lotion to dilute and spread the essential oils over an area of skin.

Compresses

Compresses are sometimes required on open wounds such as leg ulcers, bedsores, boils etc., and on bruising or areas of severe localized pain such as arthritis, stomach pain, fractures, etc. Nonadherent dressings such as Release should be used on open wounds. The size of compress, number of drops of essential oils and amount of water used is dependent upon the size of the area to be treated. A septic finger requires only a minuscule square of the dressing material chosen, and an eggcupful of water to which 2 drops of essential oil have been added, whereas a swollen rheumatic knee would require a piece of cloth large enough to cover the swelling, and a small basinful of water (about 200 ml) containing 5–6 drops of essential oils. As always, the quantities of essential oil should be halved for children and the elderly.

The chosen material should be immersed in the mixture of water and essential oil, squeezed gently and placed over the required area. It should be covered in the normal manner, and a piece of cling film can be ideal as a first layer to prevent evaporation of the essential oils. The compress should be left on for about 2 hours, or overnight if practicable.

During the 1914–18 war, other media used for wet dressings for large wounds with considerable tissue loss were ether and ointment bases, into which the essential oils were mixed (Valnet 1980 p. 67). If a cream or lotion base is used for open wounds (see Useful Addresses), this can be applied directly onto the dressing.

Gargles and mouthwashes

After the removal of tonsils or complicated dental surgery, gargling with essential oils helps to relieve any pain or inflammation, stem blood flow and aid healing. At the same time the oils are antiseptic to the mucous surfaces. 2–3 drops in quarter of a tumbler of water is all that is needed—the most important rule to follow being that the water should be stirred before each mouthful to disperse the essential oils each time. For children, blend only 1 drop of essential oil in a teaspoonful of honey before adding the water. *Syzygium aromaticum* (flos) is the most used for pain in this context, but see appendices also.

Sprays

The spray method mentioned above (see Methods of inhalation) can also be used as a method of application when the client is unable to be touched, for example in the case of severe burns, zoster or wounds. A higher concentration is needed when treating burns this way, e.g. 15–20 drops in 50 ml of distilled or sterilized water. Appropriate essential oils in this case are *Citrus limon, Lavandula angustifolia, Lavandula × intermedia* 'Super', *Chamomilla recutita, Melaleuca viridiflora* and *Pelargonium graveolens*.

Baths

A valuable method of use involving water and inhalation is the addition of 6–8 drops of essential oils to the bath water after running it to the correct temperature. There are those who advise adding the essential oils to another medium first, such as vegetable oil, dried milk, high proof vodka, bath bubble mix, etc. While useful for certain skin conditions, vegetable oil is not necessary in most circumstances (and it can leave an oily ring on the bath). Although the essential oils are not completely soluble in water, it is a simple matter to disperse them by vigorously agitating the water (efficiently, so no globules can get into the eyes). For water births the essential oils are best dissolved first in a small amount of powdered milk (adding enough water to make a thin paste).

Inhalation plays a valuable part in an aromatherapy bath, and there is a great deal of skin penetration as well. For maximum benefit, the patient should remain in the bath for 10 minutes if possible. Blend 3–4 drops in honey or dried milk for children and the elderly.

Foot-, hand- and sitz-baths

It is sometimes easier to use a washing-up bowl for bathing individual areas—the sitz-bath, for example, is ideal for haemorrhoids and stitches after childbirth. 3–4 drops of essential oils are needed, and a kettle should be available, to keep the bath warm during the 10 minutes. This method may not be found necessary for children but, should the occasion arise, remember to follow the recommendation above for baths.

Topical application

Application means the 'putting on' of oils—for self use or via a third party. Treatment by massage employs an organized routine using specific movements to achieve specific aims, e.g. lymph drainage, relaxation, etc. Professional aromatherapists mostly employ essential oils with massage, and this subject is covered in detail in Chapter 6 together with massage techniques suitable for nurses to administer without having qualified in whole-body-massage.

Unless aromatherapists are paid by the health authority or the patient concerned, or they are offering their services voluntarily, there is not usually time in a busy nursing schedule for a nurse to spend an hour or more with a patient requiring an aromatherapy treatment. However, nurses do have time to apply a ready-diluted oil or lotion on the relevant area daily as an embrocation. It takes no longer than giving more usual forms of medication and adds the magic of touch and care to the prescription.

The normal dilution is 15–20 drops in 50 ml of suitable carrier oil or lotion, but for the very young, elderly, heavily medicated, or those with learning difficulties, half this amount is advised. When essential oils are to be applied daily, it is less messy to dilute them in a nongreasy lotion base of emulsified oil and water (garments and bed linen can become permanently soiled by vegetable oil). A number of rheumatology wards, including the Royal Devonshire Hospital, Buxton, now apply an aromatherapy lotion as part of the daily treatment, resulting in a reduction in the use of painkillers (see Ch. 12). For effectiveness in certain conditions, e.g. lowered immune system or toxic build-up, an essential oil lotion should be applied liberally to the lymph areas such as the armpits and groin.

The significance of macerated carrier oils

It is well worth taking care to select a carrier which is of holistic and/or symptomatic use, i.e. one of the macerated oils such as calendula. Lime blossom carrier oil can help to induce sleep or soothe rheumatic pain, carrot or hypericum carrier oils will help to reduce skin inflammation or accelerate the healing of burns, calendula or hypericum carrier oils will help to soothe and heal bruising and calendula, hypericum or rose-hip carrier oils to relieve skin rashes, etc. (Price 1993). The quantity of essential oil added should be the same as if using a plain carrier oil.

Summary

This chapter has identified the principal routes by which essential oils can enter the body—and the principal hindrances. Detailed information has been given so that the aromatherapist can select the optimum pathway to achieve the desired therapeutic effect.

REFERENCES

Balacs T 1993 Essential oils in the body. In: Aroma '93 Conference Proceedings. Aromatherapy Publications, Brighton

Brun K 1952 Les essences végétales en tant qu'agent de pénétration tissulaire. Thèse Pharmacie, Strasbourg

Buchbauer G 1988 Aromatherapy: do essential oils have therapeutic properties? In: International Conference on Essential Oils, Flavours, Fragrances and Cosmetics, Beijing. International Federation of Essential Oils and Aroma Trades, London

Eisberg N 1983 Male chauvinism in toxicity testing? Manufacturing Chemist July 3: 3

Engen T 1982 The perception of odours. Academic Press, New York

Holley A 1993 Actualité du mécanisme de l'olfaction. In: 12ièmes Journées Internationales Huiles Essentielles. Istituto Tetrahedron, Milano

Hotchkiss S 1994 How thin is your skin? New Scientist January 25

Jäger W, Buchbauer G, Jirovetz L, Fritzer M 1992 Percutaneous absorption of lavender oil from a massage oil. Journal of the Society of Cosmetic Chemists 43(1) January-February: 49–54

Katz A E 1947 Parfüm mod 39: 64

Lexicon Vevy 1993a La peau: siège d'absorption et organ cible. In: Skin care instant reports. Vevy Europe, Genova, 10(4): 35–41

Lexicon Vevy 1993b La peau: siège d'absorption et organ cible. In: Skin care instant reports. Vevy Europe, Genova 10(6): 68

Macht D 1938 The absorption of drugs and poisons through the skin and mucous membranes. Journal of the American Medical Association 110: 409–414

Maibach H I, Marzulli F N 1977 Toxicologic perspectives of chemicals commonly applied to skin. In: Drill V A, Lazar P (eds) Cutaneous toxicity. Academic Press, London

Price S 1993 The aromatherapy workbook. Thorsons, London

Römmelt H, Zuber A, Dirnagl K, Drexel H 1974 Münchner Medezin Wochenschrift 116: 537

Römmelt H, Drexel H, Dirnagl K 1978 Heilkunst 91(5): 21

Schilcher H 1985 Effects and side effects of essential oils. In: Baerheim Svendsen A, Scheffer J J C (eds) Essential oils and aromatic plants. Kluwer Academic Publishers, Dordrecht

Stoddart D M 1990 The scented ape. Cambridge University Press, Cambridge, p. 132

Stoughton R B 1959 Relation of the anatomy of normal and abnormal skin to its protective function. In: Rothman S (ed.) The human integument, normal and abnormal. American Association for the Advancement of Science

Valnet J 1980 The practice of aromatherapy. Daniel, Saffron Walden

van Toller S 1993 The sensory evaluation of odours. Paper on Clinical Practitioners Course. Shirley Price International College of Aromatherapy, Hinckley

van Toller S, Dodd G 1992 Fragrance: the psychology and biology of perfume. Elsevier, Barking, pp. 99–101

Winter R 1984 A consumer's dictionary of cosmetic ingredients. Crown, New York, pp 138–139

6

Touch and massage

Introduction

Many studies exist to show the importance of touch in the development of healthy human beings. This chapter considers the reintroduction of touch to healthcare settings, and gives a practical grounding in simple massage.

TOUCH

Touch is a basic human behavioural need (Sanderson et al 1991), and its importance for both mental and physical health has been well researched (Montagu 1986). Animals and humans alike thrive and remain in better health when stroked or touched caringly. 'Take it away from the baby and the baby will not thrive' (Anckett 1979). Even the carer derives benefit—stroking a pet regularly can effectively reduce a person's blood pressure. 'We all have great technical skills, but forget how much good we can do with just ten minutes of holding someone's hand' said one nurse in an interview (Waller 1991). Executed with love, the effect of this simple action on the recipient is a feeling of pleasure and eventual relaxation of body and mind. This is especially so during the experience of sudden stressful situations. 'We need to touch each other in ways besides aggression or sex' (Rouse 1993).

Nurse/patient contact

As research and scientific developments in the efficacy of drugs forged ahead, so close patient contact diminished until, in the 1960s, massage more or less lost its therapeutic status in medical care. A senior nurse at Battle Hospital in Reading summed up the feeling among many nurses when she said: 'I felt more of a super-technician than anything else; my caring role was just not being fulfilled' (Waller 1991).

This unfortunate situation is now changing. In recent years nurses have shown a renewed interest in the value of touch where patients are concerned and massage has been introduced to several hospitals for general relaxation, relief of side-effects and to encourage recovery.

At a nursing conference at St. Catherine's College, Oxford on November 16 1991, the subject was Essential Oils and Massage. Sister Helen Passant spoke of their use on the elderly, and how massage provided nursing staff with a new way of communicating with their patients. Senior Nurse Chrissie Dunn outlined the study carried out at Battle Hospital, Reading in the Intensive Therapy Unit, where blood pressure and heart rate had both been reduced by the use of essential oils and massage. Sheena Hildebrand described how they were used on oncology patients at the Royal Marsden Hospital, London (Sutton branch), where essential oils and massage brought about relief of tension, promoting peace and tranquillity. (Chs 11, 12 and 13 discuss these fields in detail.)

The Churchill Hospital, Oxford, was possibly the first hospital (well before 1987) to introduce massage for the care of the elderly, and Sister Helen Passant has been using aromatherapy there for many years (Wise 1993). Others followed closely, including the Royal Marsden Hospital, Sutton and Battle Hospital, Reading. All the nurses involved have been extremely encouraged by the results, and, on the strength of patient satisfaction, up to 60% of the costs at the Marylebone Health Centre are now met by the local health authority (Waller 1991).

Massage has been further enhanced in many hospitals by the addition of essential oils, converting the treatment into one of aromatherapy. The benefits can not only be augmented by the choice of oil used—increased energy levels, side-effects of drugs lessened, symptoms not being treated by the hospital relieved and emotional problems eased—but the effects themselves last longer due to the therapeutic action of the essential oil components (see Chs 11, 12 and 13).

Benefits

The physiological benefits of massage may easily be assessed—it increases the circulation of both blood and lymph (helping in the elimination of toxins from the body), slows the pulse rate, lowers blood pressure, releases muscle tension, tones underworked or weak muscles and relieves cramp. The psychological benefits, though perhaps not so easy to evaluate, are also notable and play their part in the holistic healing effect: relaxing an apprehensive mind, uplifting depression and despair, relieving panic or anger and, importantly, giving a person the feeling that someone cares enough to spend time giving the specialized contact brought by touch and massage.

Many aromatherapy schools, including the authors' own, teach a specialized massage, now termed an aromatherapy massage. However, patients can also benefit greatly from:

• professional massage given by a physical therapist without essential oils

• professional massage given by a physical therapist using essentials oils ready-mixed by an aromatherapist or aromatologist

• a caring nurse with no professional training in massage, but with sound theoretical knowledge of essential oils (or under the direction of an aromatherapist or aromatologist), using them with touch and gentle, non-manipulative massage movements.

Sharon MacNish, who practised aromatherapy once a week at a London hospice, said:

The techniques I was in the habit of using were totally inappropriate in a hospice setting, so I had to revise completely the way I work with an individual. It became a case of re-learning what I knew, so that instead of using textbook massage, I was free to work with the gentlest touch and the most loving attitude.'

(MacNish 1991)

MASSAGE—A THERAPY IN ITS OWN RIGHT

The relationship of massage to aromatherapy

It would be preferable, and prevent misunderstanding of the word aromatherapy, if qualifications in professional massage were totally separate from qualifications in essential oil knowledge. Those people who have studied aromatherapy are at the moment called aromatherapists, though their massage training is not usually as thorough as that of a physical therapist. Aroma*tology* training involves full theoretical knowledge of essential oils, their chemistry and all their holistic possibilities and methods of use (to at least the standard required by the Aromatherapy Organisations Council) plus internal use, plus *simple* techniques for hand, foot, scalp, back, abdomen and shoulder massage (but not full-body-massage). Aromatology is practised by health practitioners who do not have the time either to learn—or to give—a 90 minute massage. We agree with Caroline Stevensen who believes that it is not in any case necessary to spend an hour massaging patients in order to be effective: 'Patients can benefit from a very short period of high-quality time' (quoted in Tattam 1992). Perhaps in the near future aromatology will be the accepted path in the UK for health professionals wishing to use essential oils at a professional level, but who do not wish to use full-body-massage in their work.

The aromatology approach not only modifies the idea that treatment with essential oils necessarily implies a specialized aromatherapy massage, but also eradicates the unfortunate popular association of aromatherapy with bath bubbles, soap and even tobacco.

Massage training

Massage therapists have a slightly different problem with the status of their therapy, which in the past has had other, unsavoury, connotations. Numerous books have been written for the general public on the subject, and several colleges teach short courses which are not sufficiently comprehensive to confer a recognized full massage qualification. Only bona fide massage schools can do this.

Beard and Wood (1964) considered that to be recognized as a physical therapist, one must be trained in an accredited educational programme, which was adequate to meet both the medical and the physical therapy professions' definition of professional standards:

A physical therapist who gives massage must know human anatomy and physiology. He must understand the relationship between the structure and function of the tissues being treated and the total function of the patient. He must know pathology, so that he can understand how to use massage to obtain the effects that are desired to alleviate the pathological condition being treated. He must be skilled in the proper manipulation of tissues, so that he can accomplish this aim and at the same time not cause further damage to the tissues or harm to the patient.

(Beard & Wood 1964 p.1)

However, the main object of an aromatologist using simple massage with essential oils is to enable the oils to penetrate the skin. For the layperson, or the busy nurse, knowledge of a few of the simpler techniques is an extremely valuable asset which can only bring benefit to those needing care. Aromatologists (and many aromatherapists) are not qualified to give remedial massage and further training would be required in order to incorporate this into their work.

Beneficial effects of massage

Massage is widely recognized as providing the following benefits:

- induces deep relaxation, relieving both mental and physical fatigue
- releases chronic neck and shoulder tension and backache
- improves circulation to the muscles, reducing inflammation and pain
- relieves neuralgic, arthritic and rheumatic conditions
- helps sprains, fractures, breaks and dislocations heal more readily
- promotes correct posture and helps improve mobility

- improves, directly or indirectly, the function of every internal organ
- improves digestion, assimilation and elimination
- increases the ability of the kidneys to function efficiently
- flushes the lymphatic system by the mechanical elimination of harmful substances, especially toxins from bacteria and waste matter
- helps to disperse many types of headache (or migraine) originating from the gall bladder, liver, stomach and large intestine, and also those of emotional origin (including PMS)
- stimulates both body and mind without negative side-effects
- helps to release suppressed feelings, which can be shared in a safe setting
- as a form of passive exercise, partially compensates for lack of active exercise.

These combined benefits not only result in increased body awareness, but also produce better overall health. Furthermore, studies carried out in hospitals and private practice have shown that massage with essential oils greatly enhances and prolongs the health-giving effects.

Touch and the emotions

Before forging ahead with enthusiasm, it should be remembered that close contact with patients can become 'a psychologically daunting commitment. Staff may need training to deal with the emotions massage may bring up for the patient' (Tattam 1992). In order not to take on board the patient's anxieties, the therapist (in this case, the nurse) should endeavour to be empathetic, rather than sympathetic, and a course in counselling could be of great benefit here.

It must be said that not everyone enjoys the thought of being touched (or even of touching others)—perhaps lack of love in childhood or a bad experience is responsible for this. As Burnside said (1973), 'Adults find it difficult to be asked to be touched'. However, with the right approach, once a small non-intrusive movement is made, both the giver and the receiver can come to love the care they are sharing and open up, becoming not only more relaxed in body, but also happier in mind.

SIMPLE MASSAGE SKILLS

The most easily acquired skills of massage are:

- Stroking, coming under the heading effleurage movements (perhaps the most important for hospital use), for which the whole of both hands from fingertips to wrist are usually used. Stroking is simply an extension of touch and, as well as one of the simplest, is one of the most important movements in massage.
- Frictions, under the heading of petrissage (a deeper and more energetic series of movements than effleurage), in which either the thumb or one or more fingers are employed. 'Rubbing it better' is nothing other than a simple friction movement. The Hippocratic writings (ca. 400 BCE) contain the remark that 'the physician must be experienced in many things, but assuredly also in rubbing … for rubbing can bind a joint that is too loose and loosen a joint that is too hard'.

All of us have an innate ability to perform these two movements correctly and safely without the necessity of long training and both are taught thoroughly on an aromatology course. Two further techniques, requiring greater skill and best learned under practical tuition on an accredited massage course, may be mentioned:

- Kneading (a form of petrissage), involving use of the palm, palmar surface of the fingers, the thumb, or thumb and fingers working together, is a squeezing movement.
- Percussion, including all movements in which the hands and fingers continually make and break contact with the body in a definite rhythm—like the percussion group in an orchestra or band. Vibratory and shaking movements are sometimes included in percussion movements.

These two movements are usually used on healthy individuals and have little place in the treatment of pathological conditions (Beard &

Wood 1964 p. 45). They are not normally employed by aromatherapists, though they are occasionally used by massage therapists, together with essential oils, to good effect—another reason for keeping the two therapies separate as far as qualifications are concerned. Lymph drainage is also a specialized form of massage, only briefly covered in an aromatherapy training programme.

Effleurage

Effleurage is the basis of all good massage, used not only in its own right, and to begin and end massage on a given area, but also in between other types of movements. It consists of two types of stroking movement and normally uses the whole hand or hands, which should mould themselves to the shape of the part of the body being massaged. The strokes are either deep (i.e. with pressure) or superficial (without pressure). Sometimes only part of the hand is used— perhaps only two fingers on a small area.

Deep stroking with both hands is accomplished by moving up the body with pressure, usually towards the heart (see below) and its purpose is to assist the venous and lymphatic circulation by its mechanical effects on the tissues.

Superficial stroking is effected without pressure of any kind, and in any direction (the pressure is so light that the circulation is not directly affected). The perfection of this technique can require skill and long practice. However, in simple massage, superficial effleurage is mostly used as the return movement of deep effleurage, moving away from the heart back to the starting position.

Effleurage is used mainly to relax the recipient both mentally and physically and to improve the vascular and lymphatic circulation. Many different strokes come under this heading, but all should follow the basic principles above.

Frictions

Frictions are another form of compression massage, or kneading. They may be performed with the whole or proximal part of the palm of the hand, or with the palmar surface of the distal phalanx of the thumb or of the fingers which carry out circular movements over a restricted area. There are two types of frictions:

- Fixed frictions move the superficial tissues over the underlying structures—i.e., the part of the hand used is 'stuck' firmly to the client's skin, which is moved over the tissues beneath by the act of making circles.
- Gliding frictions move part of the hand over a small area of the skin surface and may also progress along a specific path.

Frictions are primarily used to break down fibrous knots, loosen adherent skin, loosen scar tissue, relieve tension nodules in the muscles and increase the circulation in a specific area.

Other considerations

Learning the different types of movement is only part of massage. Equally important is the way in which these movements are performed. Essential factors to consider are the direction of movement, the amount of pressure, the rate and rhythm of the movements, the medium used, the position of both patient and therapist and the duration and frequency of the treatment (Beard & Wood 1964 pp. 37-40). Further factors include the need for full contact with the patient and complete relaxation of the masseur/euse's own hands and arms because hard, tense hands transfer tension (and possibly pain) to the recipient. The mind should also be cleared of any intruding, disruptive thoughts.

The following principles need to be absorbed at the same time as the actual movements are learned.

Contact

No part of the human body is flat; nevertheless, when using effleurage (stroking movements) there should be full hand contact with every part of any large area to be massaged. Hands and fingers when fully relaxed can maintain this contact by following the body's contours closely, draping themselves over the body like silk. The hands should remain in contact with the body for both outward and return journeys of all movements made in sequence. Neither should the hands be lifted off between changes in movements, because this disrupts the flow of the massage as a whole (Price 1993 pp. 202–203).

Pressure

In effleurage, when using the whole hand on a large area, pressure should always be concentrated on the palm of the hand (Price 1993). The fingers should be kept completely relaxed because pressure from them at this time does not provide the relaxation required from effleurage, and finger pressure should be kept for friction movements only. Palm pressure should only be applied when moving towards the heart, with none on the return journey. One of the aims of massage is to stimulate the circulation, and the return of the venous blood is not as easily accomplished by the pumping action of the heart as is the movement of the arterial blood— therefore pressure towards the heart increases the rate of circulation. The lymphatic flow is also increased, ridding the body more quickly of any harmful substances.

Pressure in frictions, using the thumb or finger pads as described above, needs to be firm, but care must be taken to use the whole pad and not to dig with the tip.

In Japanese shiatsu massage, pressure usually follows the acupuncture meridian lines and can therefore sometimes be applied moving away from the heart. This kind of massage works on body energy—not necessarily the circulation of blood and lymph—and its technique should be learned independently from western techniques.

Speed

This depends to a certain extent on the effects to be achieved. Generally speaking, massage is given to relax the recipient, and a rate of approximately 15 strokes a minute for a long stroke (e.g. hand to shoulder) is considered correct (Mennell 1945). Anything faster than this can induce a state of agitation, and is used only if the massage is intended to be stimulating.

Rhythm

Uneven or jerky movements are not conducive to relaxation and care should be taken to maintain an unbroken rhythm (Price 1993). While practising, relaxing music with a regular gentle beat can be of great help in sustaining continuous, fluent and flowing effleurage movements. Frictions should also be performed rhythmically (Beard & Wood 1964 pp. 10–11).

Continuity

Nothing breaks the relaxing effect of massage more than the constant lifting off of the hand or hands. Because most massage is carried out to relax both mind and body, the movements themselves (and the changeover from one movement to another) should be smooth and unnoticeable to the recipient. The whole area receiving massage should be covered without a break in continuity, contact or rhythm. Nevertheless, should a stimulating effect be required then staccato-type massage can be effective.

Duration

The duration of a massage session depends on how much of the body is to be massaged, the age of the individual, the size of the body and by no means least, the enjoyment level of the recipient. The massage sequences suggested in this book last between 5 and 15 minutes, taking into consideration only the size of the area to be massaged. 10 minutes of massage should provide sufficient relaxation to induce a good night's sleep (Breakey 1982).

Frequency

The frequency of massage treatment depends to a great extent on the pathological condition of the patient, as does the type of massage given. 'It is generally believed that massage is most effective daily, although some investigators have suggested that it is more beneficial when administered more frequently and for a shorter duration than … a once daily treatment' (Beard & Wood 1964 p. 39).

CONTRAINDICATIONS FOR MASSAGE

Contraindications for massage depend very much on the type of condition suffered. The lists below should be consulted to determine whether massage of any kind is appropriate or not.

Illness

Whole-body-massage is not taught in this book (see Recommended Reading) and is contra-indicated in the situations described below. Although whole-body-massage should not be given, specific-area-massage (e.g. shoulders, hands and arms, feet and lower legs, face and scalp) is acceptable in most instances.

Infection. The advice of the microbiologist or the infection control nurse should be sought if considering any type of massage for the infectious or contagious patient.

Pyrexia. If the client feels well enough an appropriate specific area could be massaged gently, using oils to give a cooling effect.

Severe heart conditions. Permission from the doctor or specialist must be obtained for whole-body-massage.

Medication. If on strong (and/or many types of) medication, specific-area-massage only.

Cancer. There is some controversy regarding massage where this condition is present, and reports from aromatherapists show that consultants can give conflicting advice. Some of the latter say that it is not advisable to encourage movement of the lymph, because this may promote the cancer in another area of the body. Others say that to move the lymph and therefore encourage the elimination of toxins, and possibly some of the cancer cells also, could be beneficial (see Ch. 13). Horrigan (1991) offers the opinion that: 'Surface massage will not make the cancer grow due to an increased blood supply; not make the cancer spread; not interfere with chemotherapy and radiotherapy; not cure cancer by natural means'.

Localized damage

In the following situations, the site of any trauma should be avoided, although other areas can be massaged.

Inoculations. The site of an inoculation given within the previous 24 hours should not be massaged.

Recent fractures and recent scar tissue. However, the healing of scar tissue can be hastened by the gentle application of essential oils in a carrier oil or lotion, or spraying them in a water carrier onto the site if it cannot be touched.

Bruises, broken skin, boils and cuts. However, if small, they can be covered with thin transparent tape and treated as normal.

Normal physiology

In the following situations, whole-body-massage is contraindicated, although specific-area-massage is allowed.

Hunger. If 6 hours or more since any food intake, or if the patient feels hungry, fainting may occur with whole-body-massage.

Digestion. Immediately following a heavy meal, the digestive system is working full-time and whole-body-massage could cause either nausea or fainting.

Alcohol. After recent alcohol intake, massage and certain essential oils can intensify the effects of alcohol, possibly causing dizziness, or a floating feeling. Specific-area-massage does not have this effect, and the amount of any essential oil used (in the recommended dilution) would be too small to make their use contraindicated.

Perspiration. Immediately after exertion, sport, a long hot bath or sauna, the body absorbs essential oils with difficulty. It is advisable to wait 30-60 minutes before whole-body-massage, although a wait of 10-15 minutes is adequate for specific-area-massage.

Menstruation. During the first two days of menstruation, bleeding could be accelerated by whole-body-massage. However, specific-area-massage can help to relieve congestion and soothe any pain or discomfort.

Varicose veins and oedema

These two conditions are often believed to be unsuitable for massage. In fact, they can both be alleviated by massage with essential oils. However, special care is needed in the execution of the massage, and only gentle, almost super-ficial, *upward* effleurage strokes should be used.

Varices. The area above the damaged valve should be cleared first with deep, firm, upward effleurage strokes.

Oedema. This condition must be treated by a precise technique. When it is present in an extremity, then the massage should begin with the proximal portion, because it is important to improve the circulation in this area first before attempting to relieve the oedema. Treatment of the distal part should then be carried out, returning to the proximal part at intervals during the massage and to finish with. The affected part must be elevated while giving the massage. (Beard & Wood 1964 pp. 38, 60, 104).

MASSAGE SEQUENCES

The following are simple techniques, easily carried out after attending an introductory course.

Introducing massage

The hand is a good place to begin a massage, because few people have a hang-up about shaking hands—we all do it as a matter of course when the occasion arises. At the same time, the 'handshake' technique described below can be used to introduce the aromas of essential oils. To prepare to give such a handshake, add to a carrier oil a blend of two or three relaxing essential oils which have an aroma you feel would be acceptable to your client or patient. Place a little of this oil in your hands, rubbing them briefly together to distribute the oils evenly, then follow steps 1-3 below.

1. Take your patient's right hand in yours as if about to give a firm handshake (palm to palm—see Fig. 6.1a) and place your left hand over the dorsum of the hand, relaxing your fingers to 'cradle' your patient's hand (Fig. 6.1b). While you are holding his/her hand, ask your usual questions such as 'Did you have a good night? How is your back this morning?'. Your patient is bound to notice the aroma and comment on it. As you explain, you can say essential oils are used for massage too, and if the interest is there, you can demonstrate by continuing as follows.
2. Gently raise the patient's forearm slightly, leaving the upper arm resting on the bed. Keeping your fingers in complete contact with the arm, begin to move your left hand up the outer side of the lower arm firmly (Fig. 6.1c); turn at the elbow towards the lateral epicondyle, moving your palm underneath the arm and return gently to the wrist down the inner side of the arm (Fig. 6.1d). Turn your hand, bringing it back to the starting point.
3. Repeat the movement a few times, then suggest to your patient that you do the other hand to keep the body in balance.

Once you are confident and the patient is happy about being touched (and for those who already know about the benefits of massage), the following sequences can then be carried out, taking the essential oils efficiently into the blood stream, to give the desired benefits.

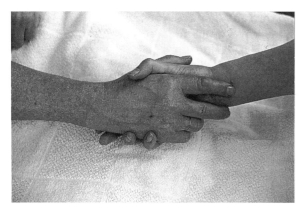

Fig. 6.1a

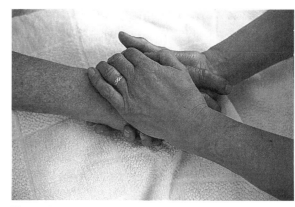

Fig. 6.1b

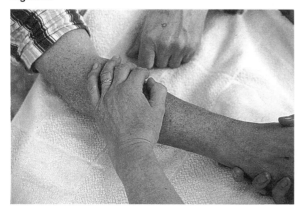

Fig. 6.1c

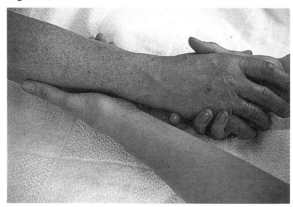

Fig. 6.1d

Hand and arm massage

1. Start with movements 1, 2 and 3 above, 3 or 4 times. Where possible, take this stroke right up to and around the deltoid and 'cradle' the whole shoulder, returning via the inner side of the arm, to finish at the wrist.
2. Still holding the patient's hand as in Fig. 6.1a, make large friction circles with the left thumb from wrist to elbow on the upper side of the arm, returning with a single superficial stroke as in 1. Repeat 3 or 4 times.
3. Turn the arm over, leaving the left hand holding the medial side of the patient's hand and placing the fingers of the right hand on the lateral side of the forearm make friction circles with the right thumb between the radius and ulna as far as the medial epicondyle, returning gently via the lateral side of the forearm to the wrist, with fingers underneath (Fig. 6.2a). Repeat 3 or 4 times.
4. Leaving the fingers of both hands over the extensor retinaculum, push the thumbs across the inside wrist firmly in a zig-zag movement, back and forth several times with one thumb in front of the other (Fig. 6.2b).
5. Slide the fingers down until they cover the back of the hand and stroke up the palmar interosseous muscles firmly, using the whole length of each thumb alternately, from finger level to wrist, several times (Fig. 6.2c).

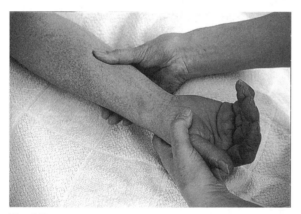

Fig. 6.2a

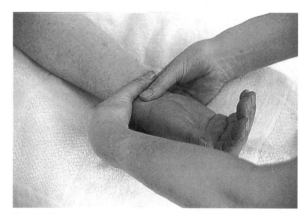

Fig. 6.2b

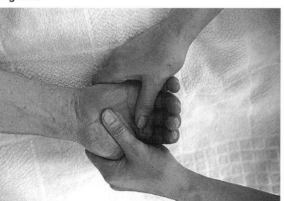

Fig. 6.2c

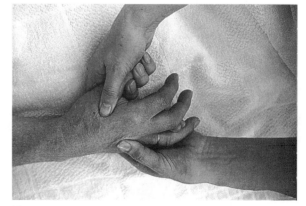

Fig. 6.2d

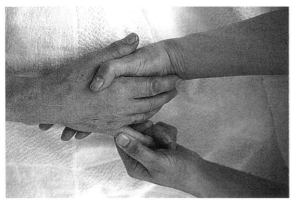

Fig. 6.2e

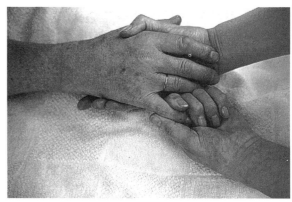

Fig. 6.2f

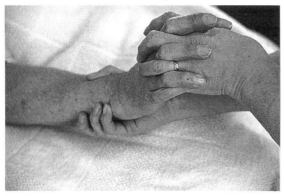

Fig. 6.2g

6. Turn the hand over and repeat wrist zig-zags as in 4, on dorsal side of arm.
7. Move fingers down until they cover the patient's palm and stroke firmly between the metacarpals for their full length; right thumb between patient's thumb and first finger (returning via the radial side of the hand) and left thumb between 3rd and 4th fingers (returning via the ulnar border of the hand). Repeat strokes, this time with right thumb between 1st and 2nd fingers, left between 4th and 5th fingers (Fig. 6.2d).
8. With fingers of right hand still supporting the palm of the patient, make friction circles with your left thumb up the little finger; at the base, turn your own palm uppermost and using your first finger and thumb, slide down the sides of the finger to the tip (Figs 6.2e and 6.2f). Move to ring finger and repeat frictions and return movement. Repeat on the other two fingers, using your right thumb to massage the patient's thumb.
9. Push the fingers of your left hand through your patient's fingers (Fig. 6.2g) and, holding the patient's forearm with your right hand, rotate the wrist slowly and firmly anti-clockwise, then clockwise.
10. Smoothly change to the handshake hold and repeat number 1 several times.

To treat the patient's left hand, reverse directions for 'right' and 'left' in the text.

Foot and lower leg massage

When learning to massage the feet, one very important factor has to borne in mind. The foot must be touched or held *firmly*. Many people have a dread of someone touching their feet and in the majority of cases it can be traced to someone once having held their feet so lightly it tickled or felt insecure and therefore unpleasant.

1. Place your hands across the dorsum of the right foot at toe level (Fig. 6.3a) and move them firmly up the lower leg to the patella. Separate them towards the lateral and medial sides of the leg, returning gently via these to the ankle (Fig. 6.3b), turning the hands again as you reach the toes, ready to repeat the movement 3 or 4 times.
2. When you have mastered this, incorporate the following sandwich into the last part of the movement. As you approach the foot on the return journey, let the fingers of the right hand slide across the instep onto the sole of the foot, meanwhile turning the fingers of the left hand across the dorsum of the foot towards the wrist of your right hand (Figs 6.3c, 6.3d), squeezing both hands together as they move towards the toes. Lift off the right hand only, replacing it in front or behind the left hand, ready to repeat the whole of movement 1 (with the sandwich) several times.
3. On the last journey hold the foot firmly in the sandwich for a moment or two, before progressing to the next movement.
4. Turn your hands so that the fingers are underneath the foot and with your thumbs carry out gentle frictions on the metatarsals—as in hand massage (Fig. 6.3e). The frictions need to be gentle because this reflex area of the foot is often tender, due to poor lymphatic circulation or bronchial conditions (which the movement can help if done regularly).

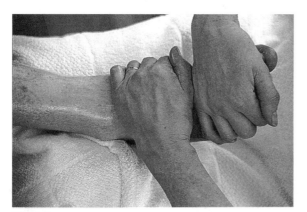

Fig. 6.3a

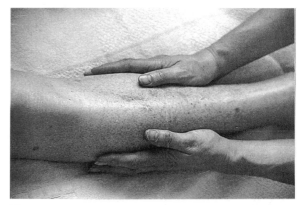

Fig. 6.3b

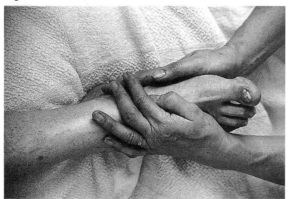

Fig. 6.3c

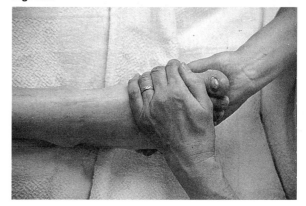

Fig. 6.3d

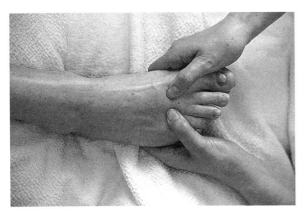
Fig. 6.3e

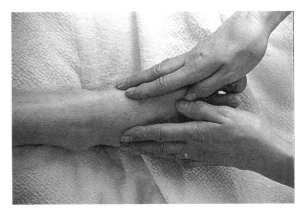
Fig. 6.3f

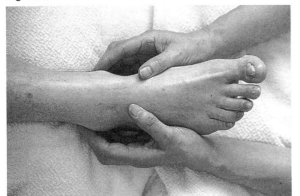
Fig. 6.3g

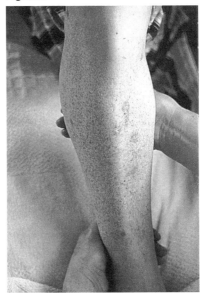
Fig. 6.3h

5. Bring your fingers back to the anterior surface of the foot and move them towards each malleolus (Fig. 6.3f). Take the first and second fingers, pressing firmly, in a circle behind each malleolus (Fig. 6.3g), relaxing the pressure as you come to the front of the foot. Repeat these circles several times. This movement covers the foot reflex point for the groin lymph and is ideal for relieving lymphatic congestion in the groin and increasing circulation in the legs generally.

6. Turn your hands into the position for movement 1 and repeat this movement (together with the sandwich, as in movement 2) several times, finishing by continuing the squeezing movement until you are no longer in contact with the foot.

   For the left foot, reverse directions for right and left in the text.

Should you wish to increase leg circulation further, ask the patient to bend his/her knee, placing the foot flat on the bed. Sit on the toes (place a towel over them to protect your clothes from the oil if necessary) and continue as follows:

7. Carry out movement 1 several times, but only from and to the ankle.

8. Slide one hand onto the tendo calcaneus and move it with pressure up the gastrocnemius muscle, following with the other hand, then the first hand again, etc.—about 12 alternate strokes in all (Fig. 6.3h).

9. Repeat movement 5 around the ankle bones.

10. Finish with movement 1.

Swiss reflex massage

This technique was devised by Shirley Price when in Switzerland in 1987, and is based on reflexology while differing from it. Reflexology is 'an ancient technique which makes use of somewhat mysterious connecting pathways or energy flow lines in the body' (Price 1983). These culminate in various areas of the body and occur mainly in the feet, hands, ears and tongue, where reflexes representing every part of the body can be found. These reflexes are valuable as a diagnostic aid and the body can also be treated effectively using these points. As in professional aromatherapy, it is necessary to undertake an accredited training in order to be able to understand thoroughly the position, significance and interpretation of each bodily system and each reflex point.

In a Swiss reflex treatment, these same reflexes are massaged, together with a specific dialogue between therapist and client. A bland cream base is used with the addition of essential oils selected by the same method as for an aromatherapy massage treatment. The ratio of oil to cream is 30 drops to 30 ml. The treatment is simpler to learn than the techniques involved in reflexology, but knowledge of the location of the representative reflexes is of primary importance before the treatment can be carried out successfully. As with all practical subjects, attending a practical course is the best way to learn. However, the basic principles are described below.

Swiss reflex treatment involves special client participation, including daily practice by the client at home. Without daily participation by the client, the results are approximately the same as they are using reflexology or normal massage; with daily participation, positive results are gained much more quickly than by reflexology. Therapists trained in this method at the Shirley Price International College of Aromatherapy have had extraordinarily positive results (see Cases 6.1, 6.2).

N.B. Always begin with the solar plexus reflex area (Fig. 6.4a) and finish on the kidney–bladder area (Fig. 6.4b).

1. Apply a very small amount of cream all over the dorsum and sole of the right foot.

Case 6.1   Therapist: Shirley Price

Mrs A, who had just recovered from a second attempt on a hip replacement (the healing of the second was helped considerably by aromatherapy), was to undergo an operation in six months time to fuse her cervical vertebrae on account of the severe arthritic pain there. She was reluctant to undergo this, as due to the death of her husband she needed to be able to drive. She wore a surgical collar, which she hated.

On the first visit, Mrs A received Swiss reflex treatment on her feet and was shown how she could carry it out herself at home. The following essential oils were added to a 30 ml pot of bland, nongreasy Swiss reflex cream base:

- 10 drops *Rosmarinus officinalis* [ROSEMARY] for its antiinflammatory action
- 4 drops *Origanum majorana* [SWEET MARJORAM] for its antiinflammatory and analgesic properties
- 8 drops *Juniperus communis* [JUNIPER BERRY], properties as above
- 8 drops *Lavandula angustifolia* [LAVENDER], properties as above.

The client was given the pot of cream to take home for her daily use.

At the second visit 2 weeks later, the therapist was disappointed that no improvement had been made. However, she discovered her 58-year-old client had faithfully been massaging the wrong reflex! This experience indicated to the therapist the importance of giving the client a marked chart, illustrating exactly not only the sequence of the treatment but also the reflex points to be massaged.

2 weeks later, Mrs A was experiencing somewhat less pain and a slight improvement in neck mobility. The improvement continued over the next 2 weeks and at the fourth appointment Mrs A arrived smiling and wearing a collar homemade from firm foam sponge wrapped in a pretty scarf.

6 weeks after this, with no further clinic treatments, but a visit every 2 weeks to confirm all was progressing well, she had her appointment with the consultant prior to the operation. He was amazed at the change in her mobility and the lack of pain. He asked her what she had been doing, and unfortunately Mrs. A was too embarrassed to say she had been rubbing her big toe—as it was early in the history of complementary therapies in Britain, her reluctance was probably understandable.

---

2. Carry out foot movements 1 (but up to the ankle only) and 2 (see above), several times to warm the foot, then wrap in a towel.
3. Repeat the two movements on the left foot and wrap in a towel.
4. Holding the right foot by placing the palm of the left hand over the phalanges and metatarsal of the big toe, begin by massaging the whole of

---

Case 6.2 Therapists: Shirley Price and Debbie Moore

The second case concerns a gentleman who had been in a mining accident 19 years previously. One of the beams had fallen on his shoulder, which was damaged; a rib was broken, which had pierced his lung, so apart from being unable to move his arm away from his side, and walking by moving his feet only 6 or 7 inches at a time, he was having breathing difficulties.

He had been under a consultant for the whole 19 years and was becoming progressively worse, rather than better. His wife had heard the therapist speaking on the radio about aromatherapy and decided to try this treatment for Frank. When they arrived, it was obvious that administering essential oils by a body massage would not be the best for Frank. The answer was the Swiss reflex treatment, which was given to him twice a week for the first 2 weeks, once a week for 2 further weeks, once a fortnight for the next month, then once a month and eventually once every 2 or 3 months. The oils selected for Frank, in 30 ml of the bland reflex cream base were:

- *Piper nigrum* [BLACK PEPPER] for its expectorant, antispasmodic and analgesic properties
- *Juniperus communis* [JUNIPER BERRY], properties as above
- *Boswellia carteri* [FRANKINCENSE] for its immunostimulant and expectorant properties
- *Lavandula officinalis* [LAVENDER] for its antispasmodic, analgesic and general tonic properties.

Frank's wife was taught how to do the daily treatment and it was obvious she never missed a day; after 6 weeks Frank could raise his right arm about 10 cm; after another 2 months this was increased to 30 cm, his shoulders and head were half-way to being erect and his feet were able to take steps as long as his foot.

6 months later, not having seen him for 3 months, I saw him leaving our centre with his head erect and an almost normal, albeit slow, step. When I went up to him, he proudly showed me how he could lift his arm almost up to his shoulder and was looking forward to the day he could comb his own hair.

---

the solar plexus reflex area with the whole of the length of your right thumb (Fig. 6.4a) in a circular motion as firmly as the tolerance of the individual patient will allow (if the patient is highly stressed even a gentle stroking will seem painful). Maintain just enough pressure to give the patient slight discomfort until the client is able to tell you that discomfort is no longer evident. If the discomfort is still present after 1 minute, the original pressure was too strong and the movement should be repeated with just enough pressure to take the patient to his/her lowest pain threshold.

5. Massage (as described above) any reflex areas whose representative organs are presenting a problem to the patient—e.g. lung area for bronchial problems, digestive system area for constipation (concentrating on the large intestine reflex area, in a clockwise direction), spinal areas for rheumatism or arthritis. Change your hand positions when necessary.

6. Placing your right hand across your body and placing it over the patient's toes, massage in a firm circle, following the kidney-ureter-bladder line (Fig. 6.4b) and relaxing the pressure on the return half of the circle.

7. Repeat movements 2 and 3 and rewrap in the towel.

8. Repeat movements 2-7 on the left foot, reversing right and left in the text.

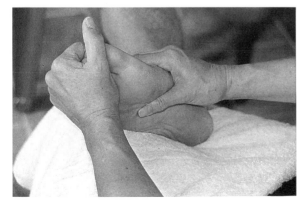

Fig. 6.4a

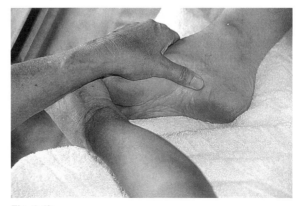

Fig. 6.4b

Shoulder massage

As a general rule the tensions and anxieties we feel manifest themselves first of all as tension nodules in the trapezius muscle. It is not always apparent as continual pain, but can be experienced immediately when someone presses firmly on the exact area of taut muscular fibres we call nodules.

The best time to give a shoulder massage (unless needed at any time to dissipate a headache) is just before retiring; this not only hastens sleep itself, but ensures a more relaxed body during slumber, which in turn puts the body into healing mode (see Ch. 7).

If a special back and shoulder massage stool is not available, the best position for the patient to receive a shoulder massage is sitting straddled on a chair with not too high a back. There should be a pillow over the chairback, on which the arms and head can rest. This position is not always possible, and depends on the age and health of the patient. If it is impractical, the patient may sit normally on a stool or low backed chair. Then proceed as follows:

1. One foot should be in front of the other, the front foot pointing towards the chair, with the rear foot at right angles to it and about 30 cm behind it. Shake your own hands to ensure that they are completely relaxed, before placing them gently over each clavicle (Fig. 6.5a).

2. Take your relaxed hands (you should see spaces between each finger) across the clavicles, cradling each deltoid and across the latissimus dorsii to the base of each scapula—when wrists will be pointing towards the spine; turn your hands until the fingers almost face one another (Fig. 6.5b) and move firmly with pressure up the back—one hand on either side of the spinal column—until you reach the clavicles again, with your fingers curving (draped) over the shoulders as at the start. Repeat 3 or 4 times.

3. Keeping your fingers on each clavicle, make friction movements with your thumbs across the upper trapezius from the neck to the acromion process (Fig. 6.5c) and repeat several times.

4. Still keeping fingers in same position, stretch the thumbs down the spine as far as they will go without undue effort. Place them in the spinal channels and make friction circles up the channels as far as you can go without exertion (Fig. 6.5d). Repeat several times, circling several times on any spot where you feel there is tension before continuing.

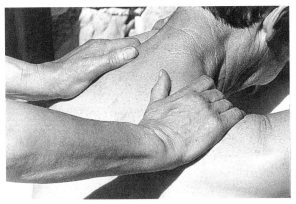

Fig. 6.5a

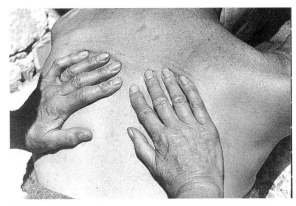

Fig. 6.5b

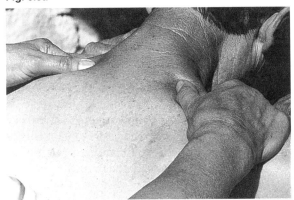

Fig. 6.5c

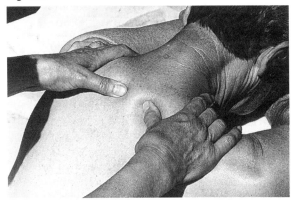

Fig. 6.5d

5. Move round to the left side of the chair (keeping your hands in contact with the patient), so that the patient's shoulder is directly facing the centre of your body. For this movement your feet should be about 45 cm apart, so that you can bend your knees in order to carry out the movement effectively, without strain.

   Open your hands as shown in Fig. 6.5e and, as you place the v of the left hand at the head of the humerus (level with the acromion process), bend your right knee (swinging the body to the right) and stroke up the deltoid to the hair line—your fingers will be in front of the shoulder and your thumb behind. As you reach the hair line, swing your body over to the left, bending your left knee, and stroke up the same area with your right hand as your left hand slides off the back of the neck (Fig. 6.5f). This time your thumb is in front of the shoulder and your fingers behind. Continue this alternate effleurage for a moment or two.

6. With your thumb, feel for painful tension nodules in the deltoid muscle. Firmly make friction circles over the knotty tissue with your thumb cushion (Fig. 6.5g). Use the full length of both thumbs in single alternate strokes if the thumb tires too quickly.

7. Repeat the shoulder effleurage described in movement 5.

8. Leaving your right hand on the shoulder, place your left hand on the patient's forehead and, keeping the fingers of your right hand apart from your thumb (as in movement 5), place it at the base of the neck (Fig. 6.5h); squeeze your thumb and fingers together as you move firmly up the rotator muscles of the neck (sternocleidomastoid and upper trapezius) to the hairline. Without lifting your hand from the patient, relax down to the base of the neck and repeat several times.

9. Keeping your hands on the patient, walk round to the back of the chair and repeat movement 2.

10. Without lifting your hands, walk round to the right hand side of the chair and repeat movements 4, 5, 6 and 7 on the other shoulder.

11. Keeping contact with the patient, walk round to the back of the chair and repeat movement 2, finishing at the base of the scapula with wrists together, and gradually and gently bring your fingertips to the centre and lift off.

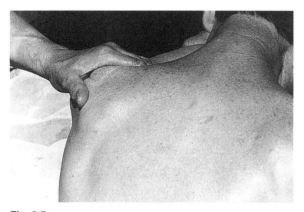

Fig. 6.5e

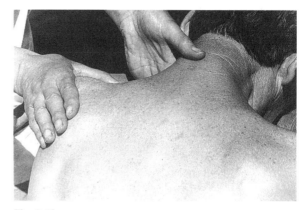

Fig. 6.5f

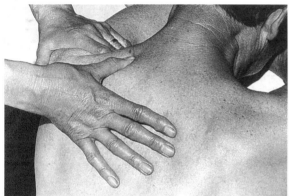

Fig. 6.5g

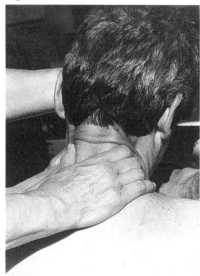

Fig. 6.5h

Forehead massage

Starting with the fingertips of the left hand on the right temporalis (the length of the hand lying along the frontalis as in Fig. 6.6a); move the hand slowly and gently across to the left temporalis (Fig. 6.6b), keeping contact as long as possible until the fingertips are almost on the hair; before lifting off, place the fingertips of the right hand onto the left temporalis, laying the length of the hand across the frontalis and moving across to the right temporalis (Fig. 6.6c); keeping the continuity and rhythm, repeat the two strokes with alternate hands for a few minutes. This stroke can also be done in an upward direction, but teaching may be needed to master this (Figs 6.6d-f).

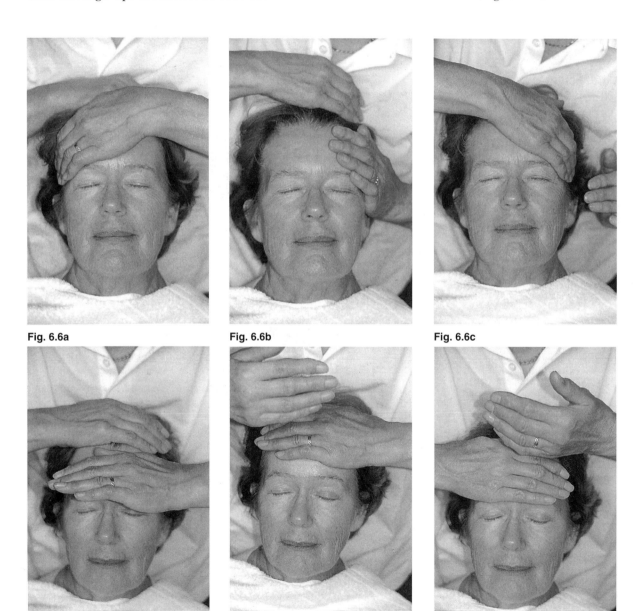

Fig. 6.6a

Fig. 6.6b

Fig. 6.6c

Fig. 6.6d

Fig. 6.6e

Fig. 6.6f

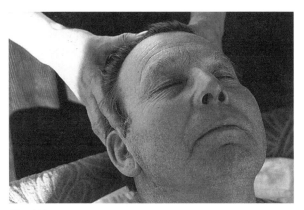

Fig. 6.7a

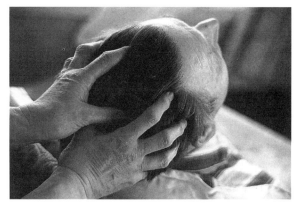

Fig. 6.7b

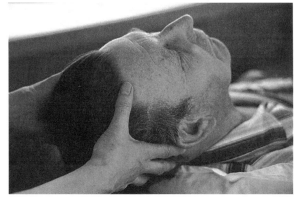

Fig. 6.7c

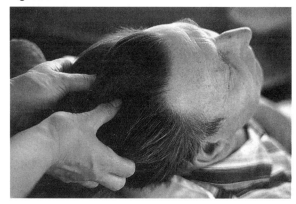

Fig. 6.7d

Scalp massage

If you have been giving a forehead massage, scalp massage follows naturally. No further oil is needed because your hands will still be lubricated from stroking the forehead. When executed gently and firmly, massage of the scalp is exceedingly relaxing. If a client wishes to receive a scalp massage only, gently place onto the face a small amount of the diluted oil you would have selected had you been massaging part of the body. Then proceed as follows:

1. Place the hands on the scalp as shown in Fig. 6.7a and, without moving the fingers through the hair, move the scalp firmly and slowly over the bone beneath.
2. Place the hands as shown in Fig. 6.7b and, once again, firmly and slowly move the scalp over the bone beneath.
3. Move the hands to another position and repeat.
4. Repeat movements 1, 2, and 3 several times.
5. Place the hands as shown in Fig. 6.7c and bring the thumbs and fingers (stroking the scalp all the way) to meet each other at the centre of the scalp (Fig. 6.7d), then gently draw the fingers and thumbs through the hair to the ends.
6. Repeat this movement several times.

Simple back massage

In a hospital situation this should be kept reasonably brief unless it can be carried out on a massage bed of the right height, to ensure the correct posture of the therapist, and prevent backache. Where possible, the feet should be approximately 45 cm apart, the rear foot facing in towards the bed, the front foot pointing towards the patient's head. Your hip should be level with the patient's gluteus maximus, enabling you to reach the shoulders without strain. To follow the directions given here, it is necessary to stand on the patient's right side.

1. Check hands are relaxed and use the whole hand, starting with hands on either side of the spine at sacrum level, fingers pointing towards the opposite shoulder (Fig. 6.8a). Effleurage up the latissimus dorsi (covering as much of the back as possible with your relaxed hands), pushing both hands up either side of the back and around the deltoid (Fig. 6.8b). Return with a superficial stroke right down the lateral sides of the body before bringing the hands back to the starting point. Turn the hands and repeat the movement several times.
2. Repeat the same movement, but only around the scapula, several times, finishing with fingers over shoulders.
3. Lift up your palms only, leaving fingers anchored at the clavicle and, using thumbs, make friction circles on the deltoid across the shoulders (Fig. 6.8c).
4. Place the thumbs into the hollow channels on either side of the spine at the hairline, and make small circles with the pressure on the upward half of each circle. The return journey should be extended downwards so that the circular movement will be accomplished a little lower down the back each time, until the thumbs are just above the coccyx. Repeat movement 1 several times, then turn to face patient, with feet 45 cm apart and centre of body opposite waist line of patient.
5. Place both hands on the gluteus maximus farthest from you (Fig. 6.8d). Move the left hand towards you, to the right gluteus maximus with pressure (Fig. 6.8e) on the initial lift. As the left hand returns to the left side of the body, the right hand moves towards you to the right side of the body (Figs 6.8f and 6.8g). As

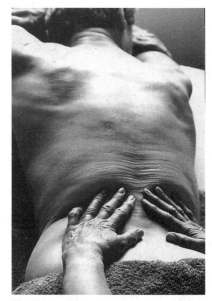

Fig. 6.8a

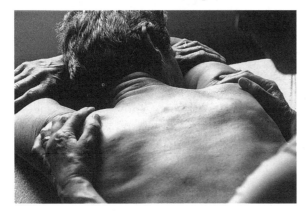

Fig. 6.8b

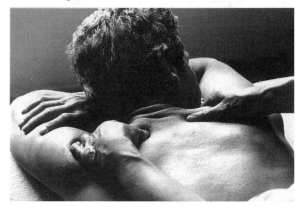

Fig. 6.8c

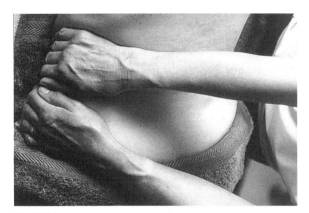

Fig. 6.8d

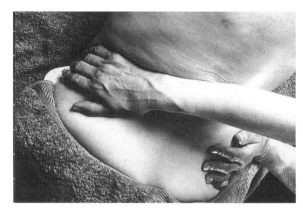

Fig. 6.8e

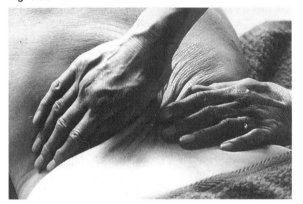

Fig. 6.8f

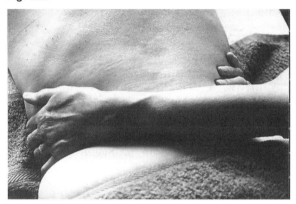

Fig. 6.8g

the right hand returns to the left side of the body, the left hand moves towards you again—to the right side. At every move, each hand is directed slightly higher up the body. Continue this two-way movement up to the top of the latissimus dorsi, sliding both hands in a superficial movement down the lateral sides of the back, ready to repeat the whole movement several times.

6. Return to the position required for movement 1 and repeat that movement several times.

7. Using the whole of the length of the thumb and thenar muscle (Fig. 6.8h) push up firmly from the sacrum past waist level until the thenar muscle is lying in the waist itself. Take the thumb over to the fingers, then turn hands towards sides of body until fingertips touch the bed. Do not take fingers around body, but when the fingertips make contact with the bed, allow them to bend as the thenar muscle comes to meet them, making a fist on the bed.

8. Repeat movement 1 several times.

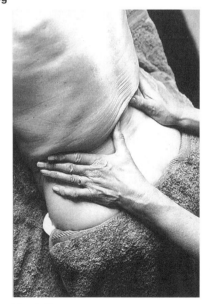

Fig. 6.8h

Abdominal massage

Abdominal massage has been well documented since the beginning of the 20th century as a natural method of relieving constipation (Hertz 1909). It is also used on people hospitalized for differing reasons such as the elderly, cerebral palsy, Parkinson's Disease, HIV+ etc. (Emly 1993). Movements which follow the peristaltic action of the colon are particularly important.

Stand at side of bed and place one hand on top of the other at the top of the diaphragmatic arch (Fig. 6.9a). Check your hands are relaxed and think about your palm when directing the movement. Then proceed as follows:

1. Bring the hands gently down the centre of the body until you can see the navel at the tips of your fingers (Fig. 6.9b). Turn your fingers outwards (Fig. 6.9c) and take them to just under the waist. Lift both hands, keeping full contact and bringing them towards each other downwards (keeping palms down) to the pelvic bone. With fingers in the original over-lapped position, gently slide up the centre of the body to the sternum. Repeat the whole movement several times.
2. Taking both hands (overlapped) to the right iliac fossa (Fig. 6.9d), move them slowly and gently in a clockwise circle up the ascending colon, across the transverse colon and down the descending colon several times, finishing where you began.
3. Keeping hands reinforced and fingers relaxed, make small clockwise circles, in one big circle, with your palms, following the colon as in movement 2 (Fig. 6.9e).
4. Place both hands on the far, lateral side of the abdomen (Fig. 6.9f) and do movement 5 from the back massage above but gently, with less pressure.
5. Repeat movement 3. For severe constipation, the fingers of the underneath hand may be made into a fist in order give a slow, more determined stimulus to the colon.
6. Repeat movement 2.

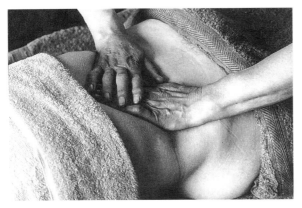

Fig. 6.9a

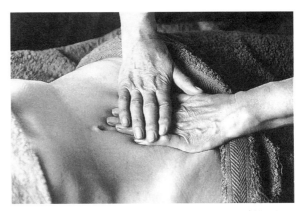

Fig. 6.9b

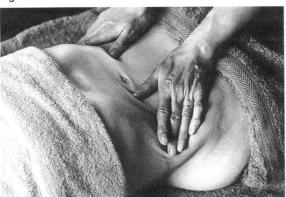

Fig. 6.9c

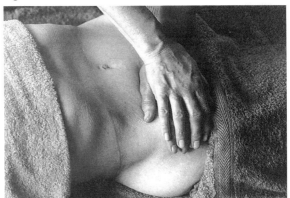

Fig. 6.9d

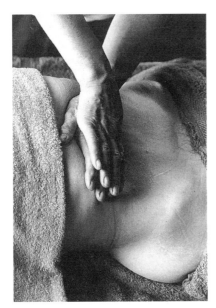

Fig. 6.9e

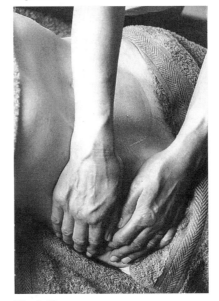

Fig. 6.9f

Pregnancy and labour

During pregnancy normal massage is encouraged up to the 5th month. As the pregnancy develops, the mother-to-be cannot lie comfortably on her tummy, and the following special techniques show how the massage sequences above can be adapted at this stage:

- Back massage is possible if the mother-to-be can be in any of the following positions— whichever she finds most comfortable:
  —semi-prone, often referred to as Sim's position; on the left (or right) side and chest, the opposite knee and thigh drawn up so that it can rest on the bed, the trailing arm along the back (Fig. 6.10a)
  —sitting on the bed with legs in a squatting position, resting the top half of the body on the backrest plus pillows (Fig. 6.10b)
  —sitting straddled on a chair as suggested for shoulder massage above
  —sitting on a stool facing the side of the bed, resting arms and head on a pillow on the bed (Fig. 6.10c).
- Leg massage can take place with the patient in a sitting position on the bed, supported by a backrest and pillows.
- Abdominal massage should be very gentle and is excellent for calming the baby and relaxing the mother. Raise the upper half of the body with pillows. Movement 1 has been found to be very effective during a contraction (Fern 1992).

Summary

Massage has profound benefits, not only for the recipient; and its recent neglect in official healthcare is slowly beginning to be remedied. This chapter has identified the main benefits, as well as the most important contraindications. It has also provided a basic grounding in simple massage techniques, and suggested some of the more useful massage sequences.

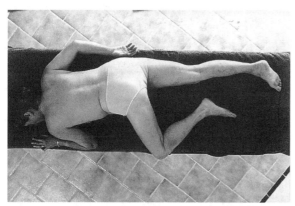

Fig. 6.10a

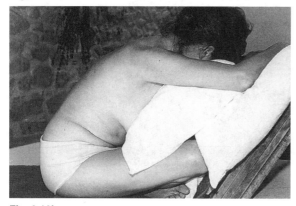

Fig. 6.10b

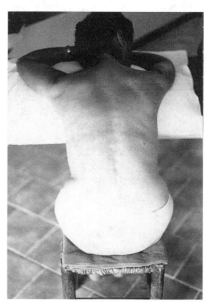

Fig. 6.10c

REFERENCES

Anckett A 1979 Baby massage alternative to drugs. Australian Nursing Journal 9(5): 24–27

Beard G, Wood E C 1964 Massage—principles and techniques. Saunders, Philadelphia, p. 1

Breakey B 1982 An overlooked therapy you can use ad lib. Registered Nurse July: 50–54

Burnside I 1973 Touching in talking. American Journal of Nursing 73(12): 2060–2063

Emly M 1993 Abdominal massage. Nursing Times 89(3): 34–36

Fern E 1992 Directorate of Maternity & Gynaecology. Practice Group (Midwifery, Gynaecology & Neonatal Care) Aromatherapy. Midwifery Procedure no. 23. Ipswich Hospital

Hertz A F 1909 Constipation and internal disorders. Oxford University Press, Oxford

Horrigan C 1991 Complementing cancer care. International Journal of Aromatherapy 3(4): 15–17

MacNish S 1991 The soothing touch. International Journal of Aromatherapy 3(1): 17–19

Mennell J B 1945 Physical treatment, 5th edn. Blakiston, Philadelphia

Montagu A 1986 Touching—the human significance of the skin. Harper & Row, New York

Price S 1993 The aromatherapy workbook. Thorsons, London

Rouse J 1993 Touch for health. Spirit of the Age. Spring: 18–20

Sanderson H, Harrison J, Price S 1991 Aromatherapy and massage for people with learning difficulties. Hands On, Birmingham

Tattam A 1992 The gentle touch. Nursing Times 88(32): 16–17

Waller M 1991 The healing touch in an age of technology. The Independent. October

Wise R 1993 Flower power. Nursing Times 85(22): 45–47

Worrell J 1977 Touch: attitudes and practice. Nursing Forum 18(1): 1–17

7

Aromas, mind and body

Introduction

This chapter explores the connections between a person's thoughts, feelings and immune status, and suggests that the ability of essential oils to affect all these states makes aromatherapy worth considering as a truly holistic therapy.

THE IMPACT OF THE MIND AND EMOTIONS ON THE BODY

Throughout the ages, whatever their culture, tradition and background, whether surgeon-barber or medicine man, people concerned with healing have always been aware that there is a connection between thoughts, emotions and the state of health of the physical body. The following quotation, from an article in the *British Medical Journal* of 1884, shows accurate observation of the connection between the state of the emotions and physical well-being: 'the depression of the spirits at these melancholy occasions (funerals) ... disposes them to some of the worst effects of the chills' (Wood 1990a). In modern times this has been recognized not only by psychotherapists and those in psychosomatic medicine, but also in general medicine.

Can a pessimistic outlook influence our immune system directly? The answer must be yes. The way that we assess situations determines our emotional responses to them. Emotions release hormones and hormones can influence immunity. But it is important to realise that this process doesn't happen (or *needn't* happen) automatically, without our knowing about it. In the last analysis it is the way we think and feel that triggers the immune change.

(Wood 1990b)

These effects can be real, and changes in blood chemistry have been recorded even when the emotions are conjured up artificially, as in the case of superstition. There is a superstition in the theatre, for example, that playing the part of Macbeth will bring bad luck of some sort, such as ill health. 3000 years ago the impact and influence of the intangible human mind on the material body had been observed and recorded in the Bible: 'A merry heart doeth good like a medicine; but a broken spirit drieth the bones' (Proverbs 17: 22).

Psychoneuroimmunology

Since the mid 1980s there has been a significant advance in the study and understanding of the connections between mind and body. Previously, the psyche, the nervous system and the immune system were studied more or less as independent systems functioning alongside each other but without direct connections. However, a new scientific discipline, known as psychoneuro-immunology (PNI), has appeared, and a partial understanding of how the brain and the immune system communicate with each other is developing. They are being looked at now in terms of their intercommunicational system of chemical messengers, their interconnections via nerve tissue and their effects and interactions one with another.

The immune system

Neuropeptide messengers produced by the immune system and nerve cells, including those of the brain, provide two-way communication between the emotional brain and bodily systems via hormonal feedback loops. The limbic system (hypothalamus and pituitary), the spleen, the adrenal and thymus glands all have nerve interconnections. Thus emotions are capable not only of directing the body but also of receiving and being modified by information feedback from cells in the body.

Adrenalin and cortisol are two of the many chemical messengers whose release can be triggered by negative emotion associated with sudden or long-term stress: these two hormones influence the immune system directly to switch it

off (Borysenko 1988 p. 14). ATCH (adrenocortical trophic hormone) suppresses pituitary action by stimulation of the adrenal gland to produce adrenalin which is a stimulator of the autonomic nervous system (ANS).

In the wake of research like this, the idea has gradually gained ground that emotional states can translate into altered responses in the immune system: negative thoughts and sad emotions, perhaps resulting from such occasions as bereavement or because of other types of stress, can sometimes lessen the effectiveness of the immune system temporarily. Hence the body puts into physical effect nonmaterial thoughts and emotions—to produce a beneficial healing effect or to inflict self-damage. This idea is echoed by many writers.

The effect of the emotions on health

It has not been possible up to the present for anyone to show a link between any particular emotion and any specific physical disease— 'Pessimism is not linked to any particular disease' (Wood 1990b)—although pessimism or depression amplifies symptoms of pain. It can probably be said though, that the course and eventual conclusion of nearly all disease is affected by nonphysical thoughts, feelings, emotions and attitudes, in turn influenced by personality.

Studies have confirmed the power of the mind to bring about dramatic changes in the physiology of the body as evidenced in the fight-or-flight response.

Fight-or-flight response

Many thousands of years ago people developed a response to dangerous situations designed to protect the body. This is known as the automatic primary stress response and the arousal system is located in the brain stem. When a person is presented with a threatening set of circumstances, the median hemisphere of the hypothalamus instantly puts into the bloodstream chemical messengers (catecholamines). These, in conjunction with the sympathetic nervous system, trigger a whole array of interconnected reactions— release of steroids, glycogen and adrenalin, faster breathing, increased heart rate, raised blood pressure, dilated pupils, and so on—all designed to prepare the body for instant action resulting from the awareness of danger.

Today, in modern society, this ancient inbuilt fight-or-flight response is evoked many times, not only in response to short-term acute physical risk (e.g. war, traffic, mugging, etc.) but also to threats such as job security, divorce and money problems. Long-term stress conditions like these make the traditional response inappropriate: not only does it not do any good, it can actually be harmful to the body it is supposed to protect. The high-tech high-pressure lifestyle lived by so many people is responsible for many threatening situations, both chronic and acute, and it is now generally recognized that some, if not most, physical problems in our society have a non-physical component in their aetiology. Helen Flanders Dunbar, one of the first researchers in this area, wrote: 'It is not a question of whether an illness is physical or emotional, but how much of each' (Dunbar 1954).

Anticipation stress

Some life events cast a shadow before them. It is known that students are prone to catch colds at examination times and it has also been shown that such times of stress for candidates reduce the efficiency of the immune system. This is due to lowered production of interferon leading to decreased function of natural killer cells. The effects of stress of this kind are popularly recognized in the case of brides-to-be who may catch a 'bride's cold'. Why stress should have the effect of decreasing the body's defences is not clear, and as yet unexplained. It is noteworthy that some of the more ambitious students suffer a greater reduction in the immune system defences, perhaps because the examination represents a bigger threat to them (Borysenko 1988 pp. 12-16).

Grief

The effect of emotions on health is recognized by the insurance industry. Statistics exist for various stressful situations which make people more prone to accidents and poor health, e.g. divorce,

marriage, holidays, death, etc. They show for instance that there are 50% more deaths than would normally be expected in widowers during the first year after the loss of a wife (even though the suicide rate amongst single men is very high to begin with). The depression following the death of a wife is likely to have an adverse effect on the protective immune system and so on the health of the survivor.

Voluntary stress

While repeated stressful situations may produce ill effects and people may suffer chronic illness as a result, many people joyfully expose themselves to repeated stress with no apparent ill effect, e.g. in sports such as mountaineering, car racing and skiing. This can be explained in the following way. On the one hand, if repeated stress is unwanted and creates unhappiness, then it will have unwanted effects. On the other hand, if the repeated stressful situations are sought and enjoyed, the resultant happiness will bring beneficial effects to the person as a whole. In sporting contexts the euphoria resulting from release of endorphins is recognized as 'runner's high'.

Thinking and healing

Using the mind to control pulse rate and breathing, and to bring about general relaxation of the body, has long been practised in many different cultures. A few have mastered the technique to such a degree that they have almost reached a state of suspended animation. This has been documented in people practising transcendental meditation (Benson 1979). In the meditative state the brain waves drop from the beta rhythm to the slower alpha rhythm and the blood circulation is diverted more to the brain and vital organs, with less going to the muscles; the heart rate is slower, blood pressure is lower and little oxygen is used.

All this is initiated by thought alone, effected via the hypothalamus. Hesse, experimenting on cats in the 1950s, found that when the hypothalamus was stimulated, increased activity or relaxation was produced (Hesse & Akerl 1955).

Sometimes, as in the case of people suffering a terminal illness, this mind-to-body effect means that healing is possible even though a cure is not.

Today there is a realization that for optimum healing the sufferer must be fully involved in all stages of the treatment from diagnosis to final cure, and it is generally recognized that all true healing comes from within (as demonstrated by the effectiveness of the placebo). Healing is accomplished by mental and physical routes, with primary roles played by the patient, doctor and nurse, while family and friends take secondary supportive parts. As Plato wrote in the 3rd century BCE:

The curing of the part should not be attempted without treatment of the whole. No attempt should be made to cure the body without the soul, and, if the head and the body are to be healthy, you must begin by curing the mind. ... For this is the great error of our day in the treatment of the human body, that physicians first separate the soul from the body.

Trust and placebo

Another well-known example of the effect of thought on the physical body is the placebo effect. This happens when the cure or amelioration of an illness is due to the patient's trust and belief either in a prescribed substance (whether or not the substance in question is passive), faith in the healer or, frequently, a combination of both. For instance, it has been shown that dummy painkillers are 56% as effective as morphine in the treatment of severe chronic pain (Chaitow 1991). This remarkable and much used placebo effect is important in all healing. When people are made to feel better, positive healing thoughts are generated which encourage the healing process. If an aromatherapy treatment does no more than make people feel better in themselves, it is at least a move in the right direction, for such feelings put the whole person into a healing mode. Positive healing thoughts in the mind can induce healing reactions in the bodily healing processes.

Similarly the efficiency of the immune system is reduced by negative belief and thought. It is not unreasonable to draw the conclusion that we are, in some measure, potentially masters of our own fate as far as our health is concerned, in the sense that immunity from disease appears to be enhanced or diminished by beliefs, and by the environment insofar as it affects our emotions. 'Immunity is to some degree under mental control' (Wood 1990a). Fortunately the human race is intrinsically optimistic, with a will to survive.

Relaxation response

When we are safe, in a calm atmosphere, we have the opposite of the stress response—tension, blood pressure, oxygen use and so on are all reduced. This highly desirable and very important state has been termed the relaxation response (Benson 1975). It can be brought about by many means including reading, listening to favourite music, contemplating nature and, indeed, aromatherapy.

WHERE DOES AROMATHERAPY FIT IN?

We must now consider how aromatherapy can play an effective and worthwhile part in the mental-physical sphere of healing. It is established beyond doubt that essential oils can have physical impact in that they are bactericidal, antiinflammatory, antifungal, an appetite stimulant, hyperaemic, expectorant, etc. (see Ch. 4 and Table 7.1) and that at the same time they possess properties which can affect the mind and emotions, to sedate, calm and uplift.

Table 7.1 Effects of essential oils used internally and externally (from Schilcher 1984)

External application	Internal application
hyperaemic	expectorant
antiinflammatory	appetite stimulating
antiseptic/disinfectant	choleric, cholekinetic
granulation stimulating	carminative
deodorizing	antiseptic/disinfectant
insecticide/insect repellent	sedative
	circulation stimulating

Case 7.1 Midwife/aromatherapist: Elizabeth Kell SRN, SCN, FP, UK

J came to the antenatal clinic at the Southern General Hospital in the early weeks of pregnancy and was extremely anxious and agitated. She was suffering from phobias, unable to enter a lift at any time and preferred rooms which were light and had windows with very open aspects. It became extremely difficult for J to attend for care because of her anxiety state due to her phobias.

I was asked by her consultant to use aromatherapy with her and the first consultation took place in the antenatal clinic in a quiet bright room. After an initial chat J relaxed slightly, when she felt she could relate to me and trust me. I offered her a hand-massage, which I thought would be less threatening for her at the outset and would allow her to feel more confident with me. She relaxed very well, enjoying the hand-massage (using neroli and lavender in a base oil of sweet almond). We then progressed to shoulder- and back-massage with J sitting astride a chair, relaxing her arms on a pillow placed on the back of the chair. The oils used were lavender and Moroccan chamomile in a base oil of peach kernel.

After this she felt much more able to discuss her fears and worries and counselling was able to take place. I was then more able to decide what J's problem was and we discussed how her partner K could help her to cope with her fears. I gave her a tape of simple relaxation techniques, such as breathing and visualization, which J used daily until her next visit. One of her main fears was coming into the labour suite in labour. We decided it would be beneficial to try and use aromatherapy with J in a suitable labour room which we would hopefully use when she did eventually arrive in labour. This enabled her to become very familiar with her surroundings and with the midwives.

In the early stages J often cancelled visits to the clinic because of her anxiety state. I therefore visited her at home and occasionally when necessary would accompany her to the antenatal clinic. J was referred to a psychiatrist at one point during her pregnancy, but she did not wish to take the medication prescribed at that point. It was decided to continue with aromatherapy treatments and her pregnancy progressed well, although her anxiety state fluctuated considerably. Aromatherapy was used to calm and reassure her.

When she was admitted to the labour suite, I administered back- and leg-massage (using jasmine, lavender and Moroccan chamomile in a base oil of peach kernel) and inhalation of jasmine oil. She progressed well and surprised everyone, including herself, by remaining very calm throughout. Unfortunately, she did need to have a forceps delivery, but coped extremely well with this. J's feelings were that aromatherapy had a great deal to offer her during her pregnancy and labour. She was delivered of a beautiful baby boy and both mother and baby did extremely well.

They are therefore ideal tools for tackling not only physical problems but at the same time mental and emotional states, especially if the essential oils are carefully selected on a holistic basis.

Aromas affect emotions

Odours are important in everyday life though notoriously difficult to describe. We are surrounded—sometimes almost suffocated—by aromas, some natural but many synthetic. Fragrances are added to almost everything from floor polishes to foods and buildings, inflicted on us whether we want it or not—like background music—and who knows how we are being affected, since the emotions produced can be very strong and unforgettable. This psychosomatic effect of smell is experienced by many people. The unfamiliar mixture of odours encountered in hospitals, for example, can produce feelings of fear with physical manifestations such as sweating, nausea, and fainting in visitors as well as patients, and the memory of the smell of school cabbage can spoil meals throughout life.

The chain of events involving aroma, emotion and physical change, for so long a mystery, is now beginning to be explained scientifically in psychoneuroimmunology as are the special benefits to be derived from the use of aromatherapy (Table 7.2). Essential oils consist of natural molecules and are to be welcomed at the very least as a means of introducing a little bit of nature into the mainly synthetic hospital environment. The use of carefully selected essential oils makes good sense therapeutically and financially, for they are simple and inexpensive in use and no costly equipment is required.

Olfactory physiology: new developments

Speaking at the 12ième Journées Internationales Huiles Essentielles (1993), Professor André Holley of Lyons reported that changes in thinking have occurred concerning odour reception, following identification of a very large family of genes responsible for coding olfactory receptors (Buck & Axel 1991). Like receptors are grouped

Table 7.2   Mental and nervous system effects of essential oils mentioned by various authors. The figures indicate the number of mentions

	Anguish	Breathlessness (nervous)	Calming, relaxing	Depression (nervous)	Fatigue (nervous)	Hypochondria	Hysteria	Insomnia	Irritability	Melancholy	Memory loss	Migraine
Aniba rosaeodora (lig.) [ROSEWOOD]	1			2								
Boswellia carteri [FRANKINCENSE]	1		1	4					1	1	1	
Cananga odorata (flos) [YLANG YLANG]	2		1	1				1	1	1	1	
Carum carvi (fruct.) [CARAWAY]												
Cedrus atlantica (lig.) [ATLAS CEDARWOOD]	1		1						1	1	1	
Chamaemelum nobile (flos) [ROMAN CHAMOMILE]	2		1	2			1	1	1			1
Chamomilla recutita (flos) [GERMAN CHAMOMILE]												1
Cinnamomum zeylanicum (cort.) [CINNAMON BARK]			2	3								
Cinnamomum zeylanicum (fol.) [CINNAMON LEAF]												
Citrus aurantium var. *amara* (flos) [NEROLI BIGARADE]	1		1	2				1	1		1	
Citrus aurantium var. *amara* (fol.) [PETITGRAIN BIGARADE]	2		2	1				1	1		1	
Citrus aurantium var. *amara* (per.) [ORANGE BIGARADE]	2			2				2	1			
Citrus aurantium var. *sinensis* (per.) [ORANGE SWEET]	2		2					1				
Citrus bergamia (per.) [BERGAMOT]	1		1	1				2	1			
Citrus limon (per.) [LEMON]	2		2					2	1	1		2
Citrus reticulata (per.) [MANDARIN]	3		2	1				2	1	1	1	
Commiphora myrrha [MYRRH]	1			1					1			
Coriandrum sativum (fruct.) [CORIANDER]	1			1				1				
Cupressus sempervirens [CYPRESS]			2	2				1	3			
Eucalyptus globulus (fol.) [TASMANIAN BLUE GUM]	1	1										2
Foeniculum vulgare var. *dulce* [FENNEL]												
Hyssopus officinalis [HYSSOP]	1			1								
Juniperus communis (fruct.) [JUNIPER BERRY]				2				1	1		1	
Lavandula angustifolia [LAVENDER]	4	1	2	3		1	2	2	2			2
Lavandula × *intermedia* 'Super' [LAVANDIN]	1							1				1
Lippia citriodora [VERBENA]	2		1	1								
Melaleuca alternifolia (fol.) [TEA TREE]												
Melaleuca leucadendron (fol.) [CAJUPUT]				1			1					
Melaleuca viridiflora (fol.) [NAIOULI]	1			3					1		1	
Melissa officinalis [MELISSA]	2		1	1		1	2	2	1	2		2
Mentha × *piperita* [PEPPERMINT]	1	1		1					2		1	4
Myristica fragrans (sem.) [NUTMEG]												
Ocimum basilicum [BASIL]	4			2				1	1	1	1	3
Origanum majorana [MARJORAM]	5		1	2			1	3	2	1	1	4
Pelargonium graveolens [GERANIUM]	2		1	1				1	1	1	1	
Pimpinella anisum (fruct.) [ANISEED]												2
Pinus sylvestris (fol.) [PINE]				2								
Pogostemon patchouli [PATCHOULI]												
Ravensara aromatica [RAVENSARA]				1				1				
Rosa damascena, Rosa centifolia [ROSE OTTO]	1			1				1	1		1	
Rosmarinus officinalis [ROSEMARY]				2			2			1	2	3
Salvia officinalis [SAGE]			1	1		1						
Salvia sclarea [CLARY]	1		1	1	1			1	1			
Santalum album (lig.) [SANDALWOOD]	1		1	1				1	1	1	1	
Satureia hortensis, S. montana [SUMMER AND WINTER SAVORY]	1			3	1							
Syzygium aromaticum (flos) [CLOVE BUD]											1	
Thymus serpyllum [WILD THYME]				2	1							
Thymus vulgaris ct. alcohol [SWEET THYME]	2			1	1				1	1	1	
Thymus vulgaris ct. phenol [RED THYME]	1			3								
Valeriana officinalis [VALERIAN]	1		1				1	2				
Vetiveria zizanioides [VETIVER]	1			1								
Zingiber officinale [GINGER]				1					1		1	

Table 7.2 *(continued)*

	Nervous breakdown	Nervous system balancer	Nervous debility	Nervousness (excitability)	Nightmares	Sedative	Sleep problems	Sorrow, sadness	Stress	Tinnitus	Vertigo
Aniba rosaeodora (lig.) [ROSEWOOD]				1	1			1			
Boswellia carteri [FRANKINCENSE]				1	1			1			
Cananga odorata (flos) [YLANG YLANG]				2	1						
Carum carvi (fruct.) [CARAWAY]											1
Cedrus atlantica (lig.) [ATLAS CEDARWOOD]				1	1						
Chamaemelum nobile (flos) [ROMAN CHAMOMILE]	1					1		1			1
Chamomilla recutita (flos) [GERMAN CHAMOMILE]											
Cinnamomum zeylanicum (cort.) [CINNAMON BARK]											
Cinnamomum zeylanicum (fol.) [CINNAMON LEAF]											
Citrus aurantium var. *amara* (flos) [NEROLI BIGARADE]				2	1		1				
Citrus aurantium var. *amara* (fol.) [PETITGRAIN BIGARADE]					1			1			
Citrus aurantium var. *amara* (per.) [ORANGE BIGARADE]				2	1	1	1	1			1
Citrus aurantium var. *sinensis* (per.) [ORANGE SWEET]				1							
Citrus bergamia (per.) [BERGAMOT]				2	1	1					
Citrus limon (per.) [LEMON]					2	1					1
Citrus reticulata (per.) [MANDARIN]				2		1	1	1	2		
Commiphora myrrha [MYRRH]				1	1						
Coriandrum sativum (fruct.) [CORIANDER]	1		1		1				2		1
Cupressus sempervirens [CYPRESS]		1		2						1	
Eucalyptus globulus (fol.) [TASMANIAN BLUE GUM]								1			
Foeniculum vulgare var. *dulce* [FENNEL]											1
Hyssopus officinalis [HYSSOP]											
Juniperus communis (fruct.) [JUNIPER BERRY]	1			1							
Lavandula angustifolia [LAVENDER]	1	1	1	4		2	2				2
Lavandula × *intermedia* 'Super' [LAVANDIN]	1			1			1				
Lippia citriodora [VERBENA]				1		2	1		1		
Melaleuca alternifolia (fol.) [TEA TREE]	1										
Melaleuca leucadendron (fol.) [CAJUPUT]											
Melaleuca viridiflora (fol.) [NAIOULI]						1	1				
Melissa officinalis [MELISSA]	1			2	1	2	1	1			1
Mentha × *piperita* [PEPPERMINT]											1
Myristica fragrans (sem.) [NUTMEG]						1					
Ocimum basilicum [BASIL]	1		1	1						1	1
Origanum majorana [MARJORAM]			1	4	1	2	1		1		2
Pelargonium graveolens [GERANIUM]	1			3	1		1				
Pimpinella anisum (fruct.) [ANISEED]											1
Pinus sylvestris (fol.) [PINE]								1			
Pogostemon patchouli [PATCHOULI]											
Ravensara aromatica [RAVENSARA]				1			1				
Rosa damascena, Rosa centifolia [ROSE OTTO]				1				1			
Rosmarinus officinalis [ROSEMARY]		1				1					1
Salvia officinalis [SAGE]		1	1								1
Salvia sclarea [CLARY]	1			1	1			1			
Santalum album (lig.) [SANDALWOOD]				1	1						
Satureia hortensis, S. montana [SUMMER AND WINTER SAVORY]	1										
Syzygium aromaticum (flos) [CLOVE BUD]	1										
Thymus serpyllum [WILD THYME]											
Thymus vulgaris ct. alcohol [SWEET THYME]	1			1				1			
Thymus vulgaris ct. phenol [RED THYME]	1		1				1				1
Valeriana officinalis [VALERIAN]				2	1	3					
Vetiveria zizanioides [VETIVER]											
Zingiber officinale [GINGER]				1							

together, some specialized for one type of molecule, others more general but with weaker reactions. Considerable advances have also been made in the description of the transduction steps leading from receptor activation by odour molecules to ionic currents generating the peripheral message. Behind this peripheral activity there is a mass of intensely active neurones, involved in such things as memory of odours. Memory is distributed all over the brain, not just in one area, but studies on olfactory memory have revealed new properties of the olfactory bulb in the process of memory storage and it is thought that odour memories probably reside in the olfactory bulb and are modified by other information. Olfactive sensitivity could be dependent on environment.

Inducing the relaxation response

When, during a massage, the touch of the therapist is combined with the mental and physical effects of the essential oils, the client is helped to achieve a temporary separation from worldly worries, somewhat akin to a meditative state. This induces the relaxation response, which activates the body's healing mode, and is outstanding for the relief of tension and anxiety, both physical and mental.

Whatever the method of application, it is our feeling that most of the healing effect of true essential oils takes place primarily through inhalation (see Ch. 5) via the mind and emotional pathways, and that a lesser part of the healing effect takes place via the physical body. There is no doubt that smelling the herb volatile oils can affect the mood and general feeling of well-being in the individual. This is especially true when the essential oils are applied with whole-body-massage: the physical and mental relaxation achieved over a period of 90 minutes has to be experienced to be appreciated fully. To select essential oils to address the mental, emotional and physical needs of the client it is necessary to take time to identify the cause(s) of the health problem. It is probable that all essential oils have an effect on the mind as well as the body, although much research needs to be done in this respect—natural unadulterated essential oils have undeniably powerful effects which need to be properly researched and directed.

The influence of aromas on the mind

Consider that aromatics, such as incense, were used first as calming agents to induce a state of contentment. Sounds like one of our modern day tranquilizers, however the aromatic—unlike the pills—is completely safe. As far back as ancient Greece, the physician Galen recommended the use of aromatic herbs against hysterical convulsions. Burning bay leaves were inhaled by the Oracle at Delphi to induce a trancelike state enabling communication with the gods. Aromatic woods were later burned to drive out 'evil spirits'. Even then, aroma was known to have an effect on the psyche.

(Lee & Lee 1992)

Over 70 years ago a series of experiments on rats provided confirmation of the anecdotal sedative effects of some oils: when the oils were dispersed in the air the rats took longer to perform tasks (Macht & Ting 1921). The oils used included lavender, rose and valerian. This method is effective (Jirovetz et al 1992) because of the huge area in the lungs available for absorption of airborne oils into the blood stream.

Also in the 1920s three papers were published by Gatti & Cayola which looked at the action of essences on the nervous system (1923a), the therapeutic effects of essential oils (1923b) and the use of valerian oil as a cure for nervous complaints (1929) (see also Ch. 4). They noted that the physical effects of the sedative/stimulant action of the oils were achieved more quickly by inhalation than by ingestion, and that opposite reactions could be obtained depending on whether the dose was small or large. Our experience confirms, for instance, that a low dose of lavender is calming and helpful for sleep, but a high dose makes sleep difficult.

Since the 1920s further experiments have been carried out and knowledge of the psychotherapeutic effects of essential oils has grown. Nevertheless, much more research is needed before aromatherapy can take its rightful place. Aromatherapy works but further investigation is needed to discover how and why.

Work by Professor Ammen at Tübingen University has shown that rosemary containing 39% 1,8-cineole was refreshing and improved locomotor activity in mice (Buchbauer 1988). According to Dember and Warm of the University of Cincinnati, people do much better in a task that requires sustained attention if they receive regular puffs of an aroma (New Scientist 1991). The test of concentration involved staring for 40 minutes at a pattern on a computer screen and hitting a key whenever the pattern changed very slightly. People generally did well to begin with, but performance eventually fell off and the fragrance effect was likened to a mild dose of caffein. Peppermint was found to be stimulating, lily of the valley relaxing. The effects of peppermint have also been investigated at the Catholic University of America in Washington DC, where changes were found in brainwave patterns associated with alertness. It was also shown that the aroma enhanced the sensory pathway for visual detection, which allowed the subjects more control over their allocation of attention (Parasuraman 1991).

Researchers at the Rensselaer Polytechnic Institute in Troy NY State, looked at how fragrances alter the way people think and behave. It was found that subjects set themselves higher goals when placed in a room intermittently blasted with air-freshener and that they were more willing to negotiate in a friendly manner, and were able to resolve conflicts more successfully (Baron 1990). At the Memorial Sloan-Kettering Hospital in New York, 'applespice' fragrance (constituents unknown) is used to calm patients receiving whole-body scans in an attempt to prevent waste of money if they panic and press the eject button.

Research carried out in the early 1990s at the Middlesex Hospital Intensive Therapy Unit (ITU) assessed the effects of aromatherapy and massage on post-cardiac surgery patients (see Ch. 11). Foot massage for 20 minutes with and without the use of neroli essential oil on day 1 (post-operative) showed that significant psychological benefit was limited to respiratory rate as an immediate effect of massage. A further follow-up questionnaire on day 5 (post-operative), showing a marked reduction in anxiety compared with a control group using a bland vegetable oil, indicated a trend towards greater and more lasting psychological benefit (Stevenson 1994).

Summary

Great advances have been made in our knowledge of the interactions of the mind, emotions, nervous system and immune system, and there is growing recognition of their combined impact on general health. Essential oils have an important role to play in bringing about a state of relaxation which can favour healing.

REFERENCES

Baron R A 1990 Environmentally induced positive affect: its impact on self efficacy, task performance, negotiation and conflict. Journal of Applied Social Psychology 20: 368–384

Benson H 1975 The relaxation response. Morrow, New York

Benson H 1979 The mind/body effect. Simon & Schuster, New York

Booth A L 1988 Less stress, more success. Severn House, London

Borysenko J 1988 Mending the mind, mending the body. Bantam, Toronto

Buchbauer G 1988 Aromatherapy: do essential oils have therapeutic properties? Proceedings of the Beijing International Conference on Essential Oils, Flavours, Fragrances and Cosmetics. International Federation of Essential Oils and Aroma Trades, London

Buck L, Axel R 1991 A novel multigene family may encode odorant receptors: a molecular basis for odor recognition. Cell 65: 175–187

Chaitow L 1991 Mind your immunity. Here's Health October: 19–20

Dunbar H F 1954 Emotions and bodily changes, 4th edn. Columbia University Press, New York

Gatti G, Cayola R 1923a L'azione delle essenze sul sistema nervoso. Rivista Italiana delle Essenze e Profumi 5(12): 133–135

Gatti G, Cayola R 1923b Azione terapeutica degli olii essenziali. Rivista Italiana delle Essenze e Profumi 5: 30–33

Gatti G, Cayola R 1929 L'essenza di valeriana nella cura delle malattie nervose. Rivista Italiana delle Essenze e Profumi 2: 260–262

Hesse W R, Akerl K 1955 Experimental data on the role of the hypothalamus in mechanisms of emotional behaviour. American Medical Association Archives of Neurology and Psychiatry 73: 127–129

Jirovetz L, Buchbauer G, Jäger W, Woidich A, Nikiforov A 1992 Analysis of fragrance compounds in blood samples of mice by gas chromatography, mass spectrometry, GC/FTIR and GC/AES after inhalation of sandalwood oil. Biomedical Chromatography May/June 6(3): 133–134

Lee W H, Lee L 1992 The book of practical aromatherapy. Keats, New Canaan, Connecticut, p. 125

Macht D I, Ting G C 1921 Experimental inquiry into the sedative properties of some aromatic drugs and fumes. Journal of Pharmacology and Experimental Therapy 18: 361–372

New Scientist 1991 On the scent of a better day at work. 2 March: 18

Parasuraman R 1991 Effects of fragrances on behavior, mood and physiology. Presented at the annual meeting of the American Association for the Advancement of Science, Washington DC

Plato The Republic. (trans. Lee D) Penguin, Harmondsworth

Rovesti P 1973 Aromatherapy and aerosols. Soap, Perfumery & Cosmetics 46: 475–477

Schilcher H 1984 Ätherische Öle—Wirkungen und Nebenwirkungen. Deutsche Apotheker Zeitung 124: 1433

Stevenson C J 1994 The psychophysiological effects of aromatherapy massage following cardiac surgery. Complementary Therapies in Medicine 2: 27–35

Wood C 1990a Sad cells. Journal of Alternative & Complementary Medicine, October: 15

Wood C 1990b Say yes to life. Dent, London, p. 60

Aromatherapy in context

8

Pregnancy and childbirth

Introduction

A wide range of conditions occuring from the onset of puberty to beyond the menopause respond well to the use of essential oils. There is little published scientific research regarding the use of essential oils in any hormonal context apart from pregnancy, but many aromatherapists in private practice have used them to good effect with their female clients' (or their own) problems.

This chapter concentrates on aromatherapy with regard to pregnancy and childbirth. In these contexts essential oils can be very powerful and must be used with great care. At one extreme, gross misuse has lead to documented cases of abortion and death. At the other extreme, as is shown in Reed and Norfolk's pilot study (see p. 146), correct use of oils in labour can reduce a woman's need for drugs such as pethidine. This chapter aims to identify which oils are safe to use with women in various stages of pregnancy and which should be avoided. It also explains which oils can be used safely by the lay-person, and which only by qualified professionals. For ease of access, oils of the following types are listed: those which are emmenagogic, abortifacient, hormonal or uterotonic. Additionally, oils to be used for specific conditions arising during pregnancy are given.

Clearly the use of essential oils during pregnancy requires great expertise, and in a midwifery setting only those qualified in aromatherapy should use such oils, always in strict adherence to existing protocols and guidelines.

POWERFUL OILS IN PREGNANCY

There are several essential oils which have therapeutic effects not required during the first trimester of pregnancy, e.g. they may be emmenagogic and are therefore best avoided then. However, some of these oils may be used correctly and safely later on in the pregnancy, and it is our wish to try and clarify this potentially confusing situation. Many books on aromatherapy are derivative and consequently few authors are able to explain their recommendations of particular oils. This lack of firm information has led many aromatherapists to avoid using any allegedly unsafe oils during the whole gestation period, even though some of the proscribed oils are not necessarily unsafe in relation to pregnancy.

For example, essential oils which appear on a general 'never to be used' list are sometimes conflated with those oils which may need to be used during pregnancy, but with care. Also, many lists of oils to be avoided during pregnancy include those containing aldehydes and phenols (such as *Cymbopogon citratus* [LEMONGRASS] and *Syzygium aromaticum* [CLOVE BUD], whose toxicity is mainly a potential irritant effect on the skin), and contraindications bear no specific relation to the actual pregnancy (see App. B.6). Some oils listed contain coumarins and are therefore photosensitizers (App. B.7), but again, this does not affect their use with particular regard to pregnancy. The essential oils in Appendices B.6 and B.7 should be treated with caution by everyone, not just those who are pregnant.

Balacs (1992) began the clarification of this area by giving reasons for his list of oils to be avoided in pregnancy. His article and *The Aromatherapy Workbook* (Price 1993) are intended to be more informative and to put back into perspective the use of powerful and extremely useful essential oils.

To save confusion and misuse, members of the general public are best advised to stop using an essential oil appearing on *any* restrictive list until the pregnancy is well advanced, and to avoid *entirely* the use of certain oils (see Apps B.4 and B.5). There are plenty of essential oils which can be used by them with safety during this 9-month period.

Importance of appropriate training

Restrictions directed at the general public should not be used as the blueprint for qualified aromatherapists. Pharmacists and doctors are trained to prescribe powerful drugs, unlike the lay person who is simply told how much or how many to take. Likewise, it is crucial that aromatherapists learn how and why some of the powerful essential oils may be used, in specific circumstances. They should also be aware of the difference between those essential oils which are neurotoxic and abortive, those which stimulate the uterus to contract or are emmenagogic, and those which affect the hormone balance in the body.

Proficient aromatherapists (nurses, midwives or otherwise) should know about all possible toxic effects and *pertinent* contraindications, so that they can select the most beneficial essential oils with discrimination and confidence. This means that if a potentially hazardous oil is required during the early gestation period for a one-off administration (e.g. a 50% dilution of *Hyssopus officinalis* on a bruise, or the inhalation of *Mentha × piperita* for nausea) it can be used without fear of adverse effects.

Effects of gross misuse of essential oils

Because of the complexity of essential oil chemistry, a number of essential oils are labelled as toxic without any evidence of their causing harm to human beings, *except by gross misuse*. Toxicity of the main component of an essential oil does not always constitute proof that the whole essential oil is toxic to humans, whatever the results of research on rats and mice (which are injected with or made to ingest essential oils—see Ch. 3). Other research has shown 'that the results of animal testing cannot be directly extrapolated to humans ... The amounts used in aromatherapy massage would be 100 000 times less ... hazardous than the doses used in animal testing' (Tisserand & Balacs 1991).

Empirical evidence accumulated over thousands of years would seem to be a truer test than animal research. Such evidence illustrates that when used in small doses (and for a restricted length of time), even the so-called toxic oils on the lists referred to do not normally present a hazard. However, the dangers of gross misuse of essential oils—whether generally considered to be safe or toxic—are also amply documented. Take *Mentha pulegium* [PENNYROYAL], which is reputed to be a strong abortifacient and a much maligned oil so far as pregnancy is concerned. The following cases of women who took large doses of pennyroyal deliberately are all recorded in medical journals.

- To induce menstruation, one woman took about 15 ml of pennyroyal and suffered acute gastritis, recovering fully (Allen 1987).
- Another made herself an infusion with about 15 ml of pennyroyal and 'threepennyworth of rum'. She felt sick after 10 minutes and later became unconscious; she vomited when roused shortly afterwards and recovered by the next day (Braithwaite 1906). No doubt the rum exacerbated the effects of the pennyroyal.
- To induce abortion, a 22-year-old American took approximately 10 ml of pennyroyal and felt dizzy within an hour, recovering the same day. Tests showed her liver and renal functions to be normal and she was discharged 2 days after admission (Sullivan 1979).
- A 24-year-old mother of two, taking an unknown amount of pennyroyal in two separate doses (evening and the following morning) succeeded in aborting on the second day but was admitted to hospital seriously ill. Towards the end of 10 days her general condition was recorded as being satisfactory—all damaged tissues seemed to have recovered fully, except the kidneys. However, she developed pneumonia and died 3 days later (Vallance 1955).
- An 18-year-old American girl took about 30 ml of pennyroyal, thinking she was pregnant. After severe vomiting and vaginal bleeding, she suffered a cardiopulmonary arrest 4 days after ingestion. She died 2 days later following a second cardiopulmonary arrest (Sullivan 1979).

Mentha pulegium can contain anything from 26.8–92.6% of the powerful ketone pulegone (see Potential toxicity below) depending on the country of origin and whether it is cultivated or wild. Lawrence (1989) quotes the pulegone content found in *Mentha pulegium* from the following countries:

- Uruguay (1985)   26.8%
- Angola (1976)   42%
- Greece (1972)   61.9%
- Chile (1986)   92.6%.

The average content is normally around 65%, but it is not known what percentage of pulegone was in the oils the women quoted above used. It is difficult therefore to be certain about what dosage level is safe and when the amount begins to pose a danger. What is clear is that swallowing large quantities (15–25 ml) of any essential oil, even one considered to be safe, constitutes gross misuse, and may cause significant side-effects (see Ch. 3).

Potential toxicity

Oils which are generally regarded as neurotoxic and abortive contain a high percentage of certain ketones (e.g. d-pulegone), oxides (e.g. 1,8-cineole—synonym eucalyptol, also regarded as a bicyclic ether) or phenolic ethers (e.g. myristicin) (see Ch. 3). Whilst not all of these are emmenagogic it is nevertheless thought prudent to be cautious during the whole of pregnancy with all oils which have a high content of these powerful constituents (see App. B.5). They should be used only by professionals and with extreme care—possibly in emergencies only. Such professionals should become familiar with the quantity and effect of each specific component in the oils needing caution. For example, the very toxic *Artemisia absinthum* [WORMWOOD] contains only 35–45% of ketones (thujones); the less toxic *Foeniculum vulgare* var. *dulce* [SWEET FENNEL] by contrast has an approximate 65% phenolic ether content (trans-anethole). Another example is *Eucalyptus smithii* [GULLY GUM], one of the gentlest and safest essential oils, yet it contains 70–80% 1,8-cineole.

In order to establish definitively the toxicity of specific essential oils, reliable and replicable research is needed. In all such research the proportions as well as the names of the ketones or phenolic ethers responsible for the neurotoxicity (and hence the abortifacient effect) should be given for each essential oil tested. For example, the ketones in *Salvia officinalis* [SAGE] can vary with each harvest from 15–70% but did the oil used to label it as abortive and neurotoxic contain 50–60% thujone or 15–20% thujone? Suppliers of this oil to aromatherapy users should ask the distiller to make a test run on 1 kg of plant to check the ketone content before harvesting. The ketone content, as well as the yield of oil, varies throughout the season, becoming higher as the season progresses. (Most farmers naturally prefer to harvest their plants when the yield is at its highest, which explains why an essential oil with a low ketone content may be more expensive.) It will be seen therefore that the properties of an essential oil depend on its total make-up, i.e. the quantities and types of ketones, oxides and phenolic ethers it contains. Even then, synergy within the plant can alter the oil's effects: 'Although sage has more thujone than wormwood, it seems a far safer plant' (Mabey 1988).

CAUTIONS FOR PREGNANT WOMEN

Emmenagogue or abortifacient

Before discussing which essential oils should or should not be used in pregnancy, the terms emmenagogue and abortifacient need to be differentiated. Valnet (1980 p. 268) defines an emmenagogue as 'a substance which induces or regularises menstruation' and an abortifacient as a substance 'capable of inducing an abortion'. It follows that an emmenagogue stimulates an occurrence which is natural in a woman, but which, perhaps through emotional upset or other causes is delayed (Wingate & Wingate 1988 p. 21), whereas an abortifacient is a toxic substance, necessarily powerful, because it has to *fight* nature, not gently help it.

This is a difficult area to clarify, but there is a definite difference between the condition of the uterus in secondary amenorrhoea and its condition during pregnancy. In the former, progesterone is produced by the ovary in order to stimulate the thickening of the uterus lining and when the supply of progesterone ceases because of non-fertilization, the lining is shed. In pregnancy, the placenta, which is completely formed and functioning 10 weeks after fertilization (Myles 1993), takes over the production of progesterone and also secretes hormones into the mother's circulation to maintain the pregnancy (Wingate & Wingate 1988 p. 376). 'Even if an essential oil is proven to have an emmenagogic action, this does not necessarily mean it is a potential abortifacient' (Balacs 1992). Although there is insufficient research yet to confirm this, the experience of many aromatherapists (including the authors') would seem to indicate its truth.

Cautions

Notwithstanding the above, there are cautions which should be strictly observed with pregnant women, even when using very dilute essential oils for short periods of time (N.B. very dilute = high dilution = a low percentage of essential oils in the mix; low dilution = a higher percentage of essential oils in the mix). These cautions are listed below.

- In the case of women with poor obstetric history it is advisable to avoid using all emmenagogic or abortive oils—even if only because, should an abortion threaten, the mother (and perhaps the nurse/midwife, aromatherapist or aromatologist) may feel psychologically that an essential oil used, however sparingly or dilute (and however unlikely), may have been the cause.
- The patient's medical history should always be referred to in case of possible further contraindications, e.g. epilepsy, significant rise in BP, kidney damage, etc.
- Nurses not adequately qualified in aromatherapy or aromatology should only work with essential oils under the direction of a qualified aromatherapist or aromatologist (see Ch. 14). Midwives should follow the United Kingdom Central Council (UKCC) rules for midwives (see paras 40.2, 41.1), the Standards for the Administration of Medicines (paras 38 and 39)

and the Code of Practice (Introduction and para. 3.3.3), where they are applicable to aromatherapy and aromatology. They should also abide by any locally agreed policies, protocols or guidelines, many of which have already been drawn up by various Midwifery and Gynaecological Services (e.g. the Ipswich Hospital).

- Essential oils should always be used on pregnant women at 50% normal strength, both in the bath and for application or massage, e.g. 8 drops in 50 ml carrier oil or lotion (this is barely one drop in 5 ml, which is about a teaspoonful), i.e. just under 1% dilution. Half strength is used for two reasons:
  — pregnant women often have a heightened sense of smell
  — normal strength could be too potent for a fetus.
- If a breastfeeding mother uses essential oils on the breasts to stimulate lactation or clear mastitis, the oils should be used immediately *after* feeding; the nipples should be cleaned with a bland oil before putting baby to the breast at the next feed. (N.B. Half normal dilution should also be used when breastfeeding.)

For a list of neurotoxic and abortive oils which may *not* be used during pregnancy or in general aromatherapy use, see Appendix B.4. (N.B. Some oils listed there may be used by aromatologists and herbalists who have received the appropriate training.)

Emmenagogic essential oils

Emmenagogic essential oils are recommended to promote menstrual flow in non-pregnant women suffering from amenorrhoea, or irregular or scanty menstruation. The oils listed below are considered by the majority of writers to be emmenagogic. Such oils should not be used in the first trimester of pregnancy, unless needed in an emergency or for a short period of time. In such instances they should be used exclusively under the direction of an aromatherapist or aromatologist. Where there is a history of miscarriage, they should not be used at all.

- *Achillea millefolium* [YARROW] contains little or no thujone as opposed to sage oil which may contain 50% (Leung 1980) but the plant has been used as an abortive in the past (Chandler et al 1982) and so the essential oil must be regarded as emmenagogic until proven otherwise. There is also a taxonomic problem with yarrow and Lawrence (1984) speaks of yarrow being a complex of hardly separable species, which is another reason for caution.
- *Foeniculum vulgare* var. *dulce*—also hormone-like, diuretic and galactogogic; facilitates delivery—(average phenolic ether content 60%).
- *Myristica fragrans* [NUTMEG]—also facilitates delivery; is hallucinogenic in overdose—(average phenolic ether content 6%).
- *Petroselinum sativum* [PARSLEY SEED] (average phenolic ether content 55%).
- *Pimpinella anisum* [ANISEED]—also hormone-like; facilitates delivery—(average phenolic ether content 83%).
- *Salvia officinalis*—also hormone-like—(average ketone content 35%).

The following essential oils are those which some books, but not all, suggest are emmenagogic and should be used with caution during pregnancy. No evidence has yet been produced to support or refute these suggestions and, under the guidance of adequately trained aromatherapists, it would appear from the facts below that their use may not be detrimental to the well-being of a pregnant woman. However, this does not necessarily mean that all of them should automatically be regarded as safe oils, because even safe oils can be used wrongly, and far from safely.

- *Chamaemelum nobile* syn. *Anthemis nobilis* [ROMAN CHAMOMILE] (contains around 13% of a ketone). The link to amenorrhoea is due to nervous problems (Valnet 1980 pp. 104–5).
- *Chamomilla recutita* syn. *Matricaria recutita* [GERMAN CHAMOMILE]—hormone-like (Franchomme & Pénoël 1994)—(contains around 20–30% oxides).

These two essential oils are recommended for amenorrhoea, but their emmenagogic properties are generally considered to be very mild.

- *Commiphora myrrha, C. molmol* [MYRRH]. Myrrh is thought to be an emmenagogue perhaps because it is hormonal; in Grieve (1991 p. 572) it is not made clear whether the plant or the essential oil is responsible for the therapeutic action (see *Levisticum officinale* below). As a result it appears in many British aromatherapy books as a proven emmenagogue. None of the French books cites it as such and Balacs (1992) considers it to have 'doubtful toxicity'.

- *Juniperus communis* (fruct. ram. fol.) [JUNIPER BERRY, TWIG, LEAF)—diuretic. Formacek & Kubeczka (1982) found *Juniperus communis* to contain approximately 87% terpenes, with a small percentage of alcohols and no ketones, yet a *Juniperus communis* cited in Franchomme & Pénoël (1990 p. 361) is given as containing two ketones (percentages not given). It is cited occasionally as an essential oil to be avoided in pregnancy, yet Franchomme cites no contraindications for this oil. Valnet (1980) gives it as an emmenagogue, though he does not cite amenorrhoea as an indication for its use—only painful menstruation, and it is not clear whether he means the essential oil or a decoction of the berries. This is crucial, as larger plant molecules can have different effects from the smaller volatile molecules. Franchomme makes no reference to the reproductive system whatsoever, nor do four other French aromatherapy books. The property of *Juniperus communis* upon which all are agreed is its diuretic effect. This is sometimes suggested as the reason to avoid its use during early pregnancy, though it is an accepted fact that the baby draws all its needs from the mother, sometimes at her expense.

- *Levisticum officinale* [LOVAGE]—diuretic (contains around 50% phthallides, about which not much is known). The essential oil is distilled from the roots. The leaves were once used as an emmenagogue (Grieve 1991 p. 500), which may be the reason why the essential oil has been assumed to be emmenagogic also.

- *Melaleuca cajuputi* [CAJUPUT]—hormone-like—(contains around 30–40% oxides). Franchomme (Franchomme & Pénoël 1990 p. 369) is the only person to advocate this essential oil needing

care in use during pregnancy. He does not give it as emmenagogic.

- *Mentha × piperita* [PEPPERMINT]—hormone-like—(contains 20–50% alcohols, 15–40% ketones). Like several essential oils, the main constituents in peppermint essential oil are variable, making decisions regarding its emmenagogic properties difficult. The pulegone content is usually between 0.3–0.6%, though American peppermint may be just under 3% (Gilly et al 1986). Peppermint is sometimes distilled after drying the plant, when the ratio of menthone (16–36.1%) to menthol (46.2–30.8%) is radically different (Fehr & Stenzhorn 1979). Valnet (1980 p. 173) and Tisserand (1977 p. 269) list it as an emmenagogue, though Franchomme (Franchomme & Pénoël 1990 p. 374) lists it as a hormone-like oil which regulates the ovaries; he does not contraindicate it for pregnant women. Bardeau (1976 p. 216) states that it calms painful periods.

- *Ocimum basilicum* [EUROPEAN BASIL]. Because of its phenolic ether content (methyl chavicol), which varies within wide limits, depending on the species, the origin and the time of harvesting, basil is often cited as an emmenagogue. Valnet (1980) cites it as such, though Franchomme (Franchomme & Pénoël 1990) gives no mention of its use for any gynaecological condition and states that regardless of the percentage of methyl chavicol there are no known contraindications. Most of the basil oils available to aromatherapists contain a high percentage of methyl chavicol, the lowest being around 50% (and often as high as 75–80%). The plants from which the authors obtain their European basil oil have a very low methyl chavicol content, usually around 12%.

- *Origanum majorana* [SWEET MARJORAM] (contains around 40% terpenes and 50% alcohols). When this essential oil is contraindicated for pregnancy it is no doubt being confused, by the use of the common name, with *Thymus mastichina* [SPANISH MARJORAM]. This essential oil is a species of thyme and has totally different constituents, with an oxide content of 55–75%. There is no mention of any emmenagogic effect or of having to treat *Origanum majorana* with caution in any of the French aromatherapy literature (including Franchomme & Pénoël 1990, Valnet 1980) and no evidence has yet been produced to support the contraindication of *Thymus mastichina*, despite its high oxide content. Until there is, it may be prudent to use this latter oil with care. 'Marjoram' essential oil should not be purchased without knowing its botanical name.

- *Rosa damascena, R. centifolia* [ROSE OTTO]—hormone-like—(contains over 60% alcohols). Rose otto is cited several times as being antihaemorrhagic (Bardeau 1976 p. 268, Franchomme & Pénoël 1990 p. 392, Roulier 1990 p. 298), but no sources mention its having any emmenagogic properties. Wabner (1992 personal communication) states that it regulates menstruation because of its hormonal influence, but that it is not emmenagogic.

- *Rosmarinus officinalis* [ROSEMARY]—different chemotypes (ketone content 14–35%, oxide content 18–40%). The chemotype labelled by Franchomme (Franchomme & Pénoël 1990 p. 393) as an emmenagogue is the camphoraceous rosemary. He cites the verbenone chemotype as neurotoxic and abortive (which would indicate care when used with pregnant women), but gives no contraindications regarding the reproductive system for the cineole chemotype. Roulier (1990 p. 298) on the other hand, gives no contraindications regarding the verbenone chemotype, yet warns against use of both the cineole and the camphoraceous type on pregnant women. He gives neither of them as an emmenagogue. The rosemary quoted in Valnet (Valnet 1980 p. 177), which is not given as a specific chemotype and does not appear to contain verbenone is given as an emmenagogue.

- *Salvia sclarea* [CLARY]—hormone-like—(contains 60–70% esters). The French authors mentioned above cite clary, referring only to its hormonal properties (Roulier 1990 p. 302) specifically in regard to amenorrhoea, but with no mention of its being emmenagogic. It is considered emmenagogic by Holmes (1993), although no references are given. According to Culpeper (1983), the juice of the herb (not the essential oil), drunk in beer, accelerates menstruation. This could be due to its hormonal properties, as sclareol (the diterpenol responsible for the hormone-like property of clary) is present in the juice in a much higher quantity than in the essential oil, due to the size of the molecule (see Ch. 1).

- *Vetiveria zizanioides* [VETIVER] (average ketone content 22%). Only one source has been found to cite *Vetiveria zizanioides* as an emmenagogue, i.e. Franchomme & Pénoël 1990 p. 405.

Hormonal essential oils

A few essential oils which are hormonal but not neurotoxic or abortive are sometimes contraindicated during the first half of pregnancy, e.g. *Salvia sclarea, Rosa damascena* and *R. centifolia* (see above) but it is our belief and that of Balacs (1992) that this is not necessary. Indeed, many of my (S. Price) clients before 1985 used these and other now contraindicated oils such as *Juniperus communis* in an informed manner during their pregnancies with positive results only.

This is undeniably a complex and perplexing area, and books on aromatherapy and essential oils do not always agree with each other. For example, *Commiphora myrrha, C. molmol* is a hormone-like essential oil, high in terpenes—all are agreed on that. Its phenol content, when mentioned, is extremely low—some authors give ketones present and no phenols and some vice-versa. In no book does it appear to contain anything untoward in the way of toxic chemicals, yet it is cited as toxic in Opdyke (1979). (Acute oral LD_{50} is equivalent to 1.65 g per kg of subject's weight; in tests, no irritation or sensitization was noted.)

Hormone-regulating oils do not necessarily affect the uterus in the same way as an emmenagogue. Instead they are oils which stimulate the endocrine system, some being effective for many women's hormone-related problems such as primary or secondary amenorrhoea, irregular or scanty menstruation, PMS, pregnancy and menopausal difficulties (Price 1993 pp. 220–235). However, several of the hormonal oils contain not only emmenagogic properties but also a ketone or phenolic ether (marked * below). These oils should be used with prudence during pregnancy.

Essential oils with hormonal properties come into their own not only to assist uterine contractions (see Uterotonic essential oils in labour below) but also after the birth, to support the production of prolactin. *Foeniculum vulgare*, for example, is known to promote lactation (Franchomme & Pénoël 1990 p. 354, Valnet 1980 p. 125).

The following are hormone-like, hormone-regulating essential oils (see Table 4.8):

* *Chamomilla recutita*
* *Commiphora myrrha, C. molmol*
* *Foeniculum vulgare* var. *dulce**
* *Melaleuca cajuputi*
* *Melaleuca viridiflora* [NIAOULI]
* *Mentha × piperita*
* *Pimpinella anisum**
* *Pinus sylvestris* [PINE]
* *Rosa damascena, R. centifolia*
* *Salvia officinalis**
* *Salvia sclarea*.

MIDWIFERY AND ESSENTIAL OILS

Many conditions occurring during pregnancy and childbirth, from backache and heartburn to oedema, stretch marks and uterine inertia, can be relieved or prevented by the use of various essential oils. This is being increasingly recognized by midwives. According to Sue Lundie, a midwife and aromatherapist working for Derby City General Hospital Trust, midwives working with both hospital and home deliveries are 'finding aromatherapy a useful adjunct to the range of options they are able to offer their clients to assist them in their efforts to make pregnancy, labour and the puerperium a natural and enjoyable experience' (Lundie 1993a).

With this welcome entry of aromatherapy into midwifery, it is imperative that essential oils be administered by properly trained staff, working to well thought-out guidelines and protocols (see Ch. 14). This is not always the case, however. Many nurses and midwives (not qualified in aromatherapy or aromatology) are using essential oils on their own initiative, occasionally with unfavourable results.

Health Care Professionals working in areas where no policies or guidelines exist on the use of essential oils, and who are approached by women requiring advice on their use in pregnancy, should direct them to a qualified aromatherapist.

(Lundie 1993b)

This is a view shared by many aromatherapists in the nursing profession, whether or not they are practising midwives. It is reassuring to know that Community Health Sheffield (NHS Trust), which was the first UK health authority to appoint a clinical aromatologist, does not allow any nurse unqualified in the use of essential oils to administer these except under the direction of the aromatherapist, and only he/she can be responsible for making up the essential oil prescriptions.

A good example of a practice guide for the use of aromatherapy in midwifery is provided by the Ipswich Hospital Practice Group in midwifery, gynaecology and neonatal care. It begins by quoting the following from the Handbook of Midwives Rules (UKCC 1993 41.1):

A practising midwife shall not on her own responsibility administer any medicine, including analgesics, unless in the course of her training, whether before or after registration as a midwife, she has been thoroughly instructed in its use and is familiar with its dosage and methods of administration or application.

The Ipswich midwifery guide specifies dilutions and lists essential oils which may be used with safety and those with possible hazards. These last contain essential oils with skin irritation risk, the restricted use of which would apply to all users of these oils and which may be contraindicated for other than pregnant women (see App. B.6). It then sets out the possible uses for lavender oil (type not specified) as a sedative, in labour and postnatally, in baths and by inhalation. It gives the aims of using essential oils in labour as being to:

* ease tension
* induce relaxation by relaxing the muscles
* improve the circulation
* lower the blood pressure
* provide the therapeutic benefits of touch
* strengthen the rapport between client and midwife
* give the birthing partner (if participating) a positive role to play.

There then follows a list of precautions and local contraindications plus procedures for treating four common occurrences during labour and breast-feeding (included in the lists in the next section).

GENERAL INDICATIONS FOR USE DURING PREGNANCY

The lists below show which essential oils have been used to date to alleviate which pregnancy-related condition. For ease of access, the conditions have been organized in four sections: antenatal, preparation for labour, labour and postnatal. The oils in each list are referred to by their common names, as they appeared in the literature from which they have been collected, viz: Burns (1992), Fawcett (1993), Guenier (1992), Cornwall & Dale (1988), Lundie (1993a), MacInnes (1993), Norfolk & Reed (1994 personal communication), Parr (1994 personal communication).

Appendix B.1 lists further essential oils which can facilitate delivery, suggested in sources other than those included here.

For methods of use of all the oils listed below, see Chapter 5.

Antenatal

Backache

- lavender, ginger, Roman chamomile—bath, massage
- Roman chamomile, lavender, rosemary—bath, application
- sweet marjoram, rosemary—bath, application in a carrier
- black pepper, sweet marjoram, Roman chamomile—bath, massage
- chamomile (type not specified), rosemary—massage, compress
- lavender, chamomile (type not specified), frankincense, eucalyptus.

Constipation

- lavender
- black pepper, sweet orange—abdomen massage, Swiss reflex

- orange (type not specified), Roman chamomile, black pepper.

Cramp

- marjoram (type not specified)
- sweet marjoram, cypress—massage, bath.

Emotional upsets

- Douglas pine, juniper, geranium, rose otto, cedarwood, clary
- clary, rosewood—inhalation from tissue.

Fatigue

- coriander, grapefruit, lavender, neroli, rosemary
- lemon, rosemary—inhalation
- grapefruit, bergamot, geranium.

Haemorrhoids

- cypress—bath, compress
- cypress, geranium—bath, compress
- cypress, geranium and sandalwood—application
- cypress, frankincense—application in a lotion
- cypress, lavender, frankincense, myrrh.

Headaches

- lavender 1 drop neat—massaged into temples or in cold compress
- basil—inhaled.

Heartburn and indigestion

- Roman chamomile, mandarin, orange, peppermint, petitgrain, sandalwood—application
- Roman chamomile, ginger—5 drops each coriander, cardamom, dill in 50 ml carrier lotion—application
- coriander, ginger, lavender, lemongrass
- sandalwood, fennel—application in a lotion
- ginger 1 drop, in a teaspoonful carrier oil
- peppermint.

Hormone balancing

- geranium (see Table 4.8 on p. 71).

Hypertension

before 36 weeks

- rosewood, sandalwood, ylang ylang.

after 36 weeks

- lavender, sweet marjoram, ylang ylang—5 drops in total in bath.

pregnancy induced

- stress relieving oils in general
- ylang ylang—bath; lemon 1 drop—tea (see Ch. 5)
- ylang ylang, marjoram (type not specified), lavender.

Insomnia

- lavender 1–2 drops—pillow/nightclothes
- Roman chamomile, lavender, sweet marjoram, mandarin, patchouli, sandalwood, ylang ylang—bath, inhalation (pillow, vaporizer)
- sandalwood, ylang ylang—on nightclothes during whole 9 months
- lavender, sandalwood, ylang ylang.

Nausea/vomiting (morning sickness)

- peppermint 1–2 drops—inhalation (tissue)
- petitgrain, orange, (lavender), ginger, lemon—inhalation
- ginger, rosewood, petitgrain—inhalation
- lavender, ginger
- petitgrain, rosewood—inhalation, ginger—ingestion (1 drop in a teaspoonful vegetable oil). [N.B. Unrefined hazelnut oil has a pleasant taste.]

Oedema

- lemon, orange (high dilution), geranium, lavender—upward massage only
- patchouli, petitgrain—upward massage only.

Perineal tears (prevention)

- lavender, geranium—daily massage of the perineum and posterior vaginal wall with two fingers
- lavender, tea tree 6–8 drops—bath or cold compress

- frankincense, German chamomile (in wheatgerm oil)—daily massage.

A study was carried out which looked at 29 first time mums who performed 6 weeks of daily massage of the perineum against a control group of 26 women who did not. Episiotomy and second degree tear occurred in 48% of those massaging compared with 77% in the control group (van Arsdale & Avery 1987).

Pregnancy rashes

- Roman chamomile 6 drops, rose otto 1 drop, in 50 ml carrier lotion (more quickly absorbed than oil)—application
- peppermint 1 drop, Roman chamomile 4 drops, sandalwood 2 drops, in 50 ml carrier oil or lotion
- chamomile (type not specified).

Stress and tension

- lavender
- ylang ylang, rose, neroli, rosewood, sandalwood, cedarwood
- bergamot, frankincense, geranium.

I have found frankincense of great use … for anxiety and stress in women hospitalised with antepartum haemorrhage or threatened premature labour.

(Lundie 1993a)

Stretch marks

- lavender, Roman chamomile, mandarin—application
- geranium, frankincense, lavender
- rosewood, carrot seed, rose otto
- frankincense, German chamomile, neroli—massage.

Urinary tract infections

- bergamot, Roman chamomile, sandalwood—sitz baths, washes (bath)
- juniper berry, sandalwood, cedarwood—bath.

Vaginal infections

- bergamot, lavender, tea tree—sitz bath, washes
- tagetes, tea tree, rose otto 1 drop each—bath.

Varicose veins
- cypress, lemon—gentle massage upwards only, compress
- cypress, lavender, lemon—bath, careful massage.

Labour preparation
- clary, rose otto, sage—last 2–3 weeks
- clary—massage twice daily
- sage and fennel (to strengthen womb and Braxton Hicks Contractions—bath, application, sage tea (1 teaspoonful fresh, or 1/2 teaspoonful dried, sage to 1 cup boiling water).

Uterine tonic
See Uterotonic essential oils in labour (p. 144).

Induction
- Any essential oil with relaxing properties.

Labour

Contractions
- lavender
- clary, geranium
- clary—inhalation.

See also Uterotonic essential oils in labour.

Discomfort, pain
- lavender 5 drops—bath
- bergamot, geranium, lavender, palmarosa, rose otto
- black pepper, sweet marjoram—massage.

Hypertonic uterine action
- geranium, lavender.

Puerperal depression
- bergamot, clary, grapefruit, mandarin, neroli, rose otto, vetiver
- clary, frankincense, neroli—inhalation, massage.

Ruptured membranes
- lavender 3 drops—bath.

Stress and anxiety
- clary, lavender, rose otto, ylang ylang
- lavender
- clary, rose otto, ylang ylang—inhalation, massage
- lavender, petitgrain, ylang ylang
- benzoin, frankincense, rose
- clary, chamomile (type not specified), lavender.

Uterine inertia
- clary, lavender.

See Uterotonic essential oils in labour.

Postnatal

Anxiety
- lavender—bath/tissue.

Blood loss minimization
- cypress, lavender —baths.

Breast engorgement
- geranium 6 drops—in bath or warm compress.

Caesarean section wounds
- lavender, tea tree—baths/compress
- frankincense, neroli, rose otto—bath.

Cracked nipples
- lavender, Roman chamomile, rose otto
- frankincense, myrrh, patchouli—lotion.

Despondency
- bergamot, clary, neroli, ylang ylang
- clary, geranium, juniper.

Emotional imbalance
- geranium, Roman chamomile, rose otto— inhalation, bath.

Fatigue
- bergamot, geranium, lavender, mandarin, petitgrain, rosemary, rose otto.

Grief following stillbirth

- frankincense, melissa, rose otto—inhalation, massage, bath.

Haemorrhage

- cypress, sweet marjoram—compress
- cypress, lavender.

Lactation

increase

- fennel tea—1 teaspoonful crushed seeds to 1 cup boiling water; fennel 7 drops, geranium 2 drops in 30 ml carrier—massage
- 7 drops fennel in 50 ml carrier—massage
- aniseed and lemongrass—massage.

decrease

- geranium—bath or compress
- peppermint—bath or compress
- geranium, lavender—compress
- geranium, lavender, peppermint—compress
- peppermint and sage—bath, compress.

Mastitis

- lavender, geranium (decongestant), peppermint (cooling)—compress.

Perineum

bruised

- cypress 2 drops, lavender 2 drops, sweet marjoram 3 drops, in 50 ml wheatgerm oil.

infected

- lavender, tea tree 4 drops each—baths or compress
- cajuput, pine, sandalwood 2 drops each—bath, compress.

painful

- lavender 6–8 drops—bath
- juniper, lavender, marjoram
- neroli, tea tree 4–6 drops—bath
- cypress, frankincense, lavender, myrrh.

trauma

- lavender 8 drops in 50 ml cold water—compress.

Swollen ankles following delivery

- geranium—massage
- geranium, patchouli, petitgrain—massage.

Baby

Colic

- fennel—tea for mother if breast feeding; ginger, Roman chamomile 1 drop each in 25 ml carrier oil—massage baby
- dill, mandarin, Roman chamomile.

Cradle cap

- cedarwood 1 drop in 10 ml carrier oil
- eucalyptus, geranium, lavender.

Crying unduly

- sandalwood, ylang ylang—on a tissue
- chamomile (type not specified), lavender.

Uterotonic essential oils in labour

Oxytocin, the hormone which stimulates the uterus to contract, can be supported by a few essential oils which are uterotonic, even though these may be neurotoxic/abortive. By virtue of their ability to stimulate the uterus to contract, they are recommended for use in the last stages of labour, to facilitate the birth. Essential oils containing ketones and phenols are also useful during this time because of their analgesic properties—the analgesic effect of the terpenes is not as strong (Price 1993 p. 53). For oils with analgesic properties see Analgesic oils below and Appendix B.9.

Franchomme (Franchomme & Pénoël 1990 pp. 354, 387) suggests the essential oils listed below. Their stimulating action on the uterus can facilitate the birth better than simple 'relaxing' oils such as 'lavender' (unspecified) or *Salvia sclarea*. That is not to say that an essential oil from one of the *Lavandula* species (or *Salvia sclarea*) would not be supportive: enabling the mother to relax is of prime importance, and results not only in less pain being felt during labour (Reed & Norfolk 1993—see Trial below), but also allows the mother to maintain awareness and enjoy the last unique and precious moments of birth. However, it would make sense to include a little of one of the following more strongly uterotonic oils in a mix in order to add to the benefits.

The following are essential oils which facilitate delivery (i.e. are uterotonic):

- *Cymbopogon martinii* [PALMAROSA]
- *Syzygium aromaticum* (flos) (difficult deliveries)
- *Foeniculum vulgare* var. *dulce*
- *Mentha × piperita*
- *Myristica fragrans*
- *Pimenta dioica, P. racemosa* [BAY] (difficult deliveries)
- *Pimpinella anisum*
- *Thymus vulgaris* ct. geraniol [SWEET THYME].

These oils should be employed during the last 2–3 weeks of pregnancy, massaged into the abdomen and the lower back twice daily. They may also be useful during labour itself.

Aromatherapists who can prescribe essential oils for internal use may recommend a weak tea made with *Salvia officinalis* 2 drops, one tea bag (preferably tannin-free China tea) and 0.75 l water. The tea bag should be removed after a short, quick stir. 1 cup, three times a day is recommended during the last 3 weeks, and each cup will contain less than 1 drop of essential oil. Bernadet (1983 p. 120) recommends a tea made with the leaves of *Salvia officinalis* for the same purpose, and peppermint tea may also be helpful. Other essential oils mentioned above may also be administered in this way, but always under the careful direction of an aromatologist or consultant.

PILOT STUDIES

The use of essential oils to assist labour has been well documented. In a hospital in New South Wales, Australia, for instance, clove and lavender are used to intensify contractions. 'Feedback indicates that these oils (clove oil with lavender) are particularly valuable in strengthening and enhancing contractions, whilst at the same time, easing the pain and discomfort of labour' (Cutter 1992). At the onset of labour, a warm bath is taken with 1 or 2 drops of clove oil added; for massage 1 drop of clove oil is added, together with lavender, to make a 1% concentration and used 1 week before labour is expected.

The two pilot studies presented here were carried out in British hospitals, and their results are very encouraging.

PILOT STUDY USING ESSENTIAL OILS DURING LABOUR

Midwives in the John Radcliffe Maternity Hospital under the care of Ethel Burns (lecturer practitioner delivery suite) undertook a pilot study in 1990 to find a way of relieving pain and keeping mothers calm during labour and delivery (Burns & Blamey 1994). In this 6-month study 585 women took part (91% had full data recorded), and 10 different essential oils were used. It is important to bear in mind, when considering the data below, that this hospital is a regional referral unit, with a significant number of women with complicated pregnancies.

The oils were chosen according to the qualities attributed to each of them in aromatherapy literature, e.g. relaxing, sedating, antispasmodic, uterotonic, oestrogen-like, cooling, refreshing, antiinflammatory, antidepressant. The oils were:

- chamomile (unspecified)
- clary
- eucalyptus (unspecified)
- frankincense
- jasmine absolute (not a distilled oil)
- lavender (unspecified)
- lemon
- mandarin
- peppermint
- rose absolute.

Different oils were chosen and used for specific purposes:

- the reduction of maternal anxiety—used 321 times (predominantly lavender)
- to relieve nausea—used 130 times (predominantly peppermint)
- to increase contractions—used 111 times (predominantly clary)
- pain relief—used 88 times.

An evaluation sheet was devised to record the following data: parity, fetal distress, labour onset; analgesia before and after oils, which oils were used, how often, for what reasons and at what stage in labour, and type of delivery. Both the mother's and the midwife's evaluation of the effectiveness (and side-effects if any) were recorded.

Methods of use

The following range of methods of use was used:
- 2 drops essential oil in 100 ml water, sprayed onto a face flannel, pillow or bean bag
- 4–6 drops in a bath
- 2–3 drops in a footbath
- 1 drop onto absorbent card for inhaling
- 2 drops in 50 ml almond oil for massage
- 1 drop peppermint directly on the forehead
- 1 drop frankincense directly on the palm.

All women had given their consent and were defined as being 'in labour' when contracting regularly and painfully, with a cervical dilation of at least 3 cm.

Results

Labour

80% of the women started with essential oils without any form of analgesia and of these:
- 13% used no other form of analgesia
- 67% were given essential oils first, before any other analgesia.

Delivery

The percentages of different types of deliveries were:
- 71% spontaneous vaginal delivery
- 20% instrumental delivery
- 8% Caesarean section
- 7% emergencies
- 1% elective
- 1% unrecorded.

Effectiveness

The number of essential oils employed in different combinations in this study makes it impossible to arrive at any definite conclusions about the effectiveness of any one particular essential oil. However, the overall effects of essential oils recorded by the women themselves are given below.
- 62% found them effective
- 12% did not
- 17% were unsure
- 9% did not record a decision, but 27% of these made positive comments.

Side-effects

3% (16 people) recorded transient side-effects and of these:
- 8 comments were about peppermint—5 said the drop placed on their forehead had had a burning effect. [Authors' comment: peppermint is an essential oil best not used neat, especially near the eyes. In dilution (even 20%) this oil may retain its cooling qualities, but in concentration it often has the opposite effect to that desired. For example, it is antiirritant in low concentration (1% or less) but can be irritant if used in high concentration (above 10–20%, depending on the individual).]
- 2 comments were about lavender—it had exacerbated the nausea of 1 woman and made the husband of another feel sick.
- 6 comments were regarding clary: 2 did not like the aroma, 2 felt nauseated and 2 did not feel it worked.

Conclusions

Burns & Blamey (1994) concluded that 'The results indicate a high degree of overall satisfaction in using aromatherapy during labour/delivery, on the part of women and midwives. ... A relaxed woman in labour is empowered to have greater control over what happens to her'. It is now the hope of the John Radcliffe hospital to run a randomized controlled trial in the future should funds become available.

TRIAL USING LAVENDER (UNSPECIFIED) DURING LABOUR

A survey using lavender baths during labour was carried out by Lynne Norfolk and Lynne Reed, aromatherapist/midwives at Ipswich Hospital in 1992 (Reed & Norfolk 1993), with the support of their Director of Midwifery Services (E Fern) and using the practical procedure written by her (Ipswich Directorate of Maternity and Gynaecology) to protect both clients and midwives from any possible misuse of oils. All midwives worked under the direction of Norfolk and Reed. The aims of the survey were:
- to determine if there was any pain relief and relaxation to be gained from lavender baths
- to ensure there were no adverse side-effects from them.

Clients taking lavender baths (using 5 drops lavender oil) and their midwives were asked to complete a questionnaire. The questionnaire covered five areas: Apgar score; type of delivery; length of labour; additional pain relief; midwife and client perception of the effects of lavender baths. A total of 38 questionnaires were handed in (19 primigravidae and 19 multigravidae clients).

Results

Apgar scores

On this assessment of neonatal condition:

- 3 women scored 10
- 30 women scored 8 or 9
- 2 women scored 7—(1 had a total of 250 mg pethidine and 1 had 150 mg shortly before delivery)
- 1 woman scored 6 (stale meconium was present)
- 2 women did not have the score recorded on the questionnaire.

N.B. Those scoring 7 or below had other associated contributing factors.

Types of delivery

The deliveries were as follows:

- 34 normal
- 2 forceps
- 1 LSCS (failure to progress)
- 1 ventouse extraction (suction cup).

Length of labour

The length of labour of each of the 38 women in the trial is shown in Table 8.1. The shortest primigravidae labour was 3 h 10 min, the longest 22 h 37 min. The shortest multigravidae labour was 40 min, the longest 12 h 47 min.

Table 8.1 Length of labour (in hours) of 38 women taking lavender baths (after Reed & Norfolk 1993)

	Primigravidae*	Multigravidae
Up to 4 hrs	—	8
Up to 5 hrs	—	5
Up to 6 hrs	8	2
7–13 hrs	4†	4
14–22 hrs	5	—

* 2 primigravidae replies not received
† all under 10 hours

Table 8.2 Additional pain relief required during labour by 38 women taking lavender baths (after Reed & Norfolk 1993)

	Primigravidae	Multigravidae
Entonox	3	6 (1 plus massage)
Pethidine 100 mg	5	3
Pethidine 150 mg	8 (7 one dose)	3 (1 plus massage)
Epidural	2	0
TENS	0	0
Massage only	1	0

Additional pain relief

Altogether, 18 out of the 19 primigravidae clients required additional pain relief during labour, contrasting with 12 of the 19 multigravidae clients. The amount and type of additional pain relief required by these clients is shown in Table 8.2.

Perceived benefits

Table 8.3 shows the benefits the midwives and their clients felt they gained from taking lavender baths.

Table 8.3 Results of questionnaires given to 38 midwives and their clients assessing effects of taking baths, with 5 drops unspecified lavender oil added, during labour (after Reed & Norfolk 1993)

	Midwives			Clients		
	Helped	Did not help	No reply	Helped	Did not help	No reply
Relaxation	36	0	2	31	2	5
Pain Relief	30	4	4	23	7	8
Enjoyment	34	1	3	30	1	7

Conclusions

Fetal wellbeing

The good Apgar scores would suggest that 5 drops of lavender in baths present no risks to the baby.

Type of delivery

34 of the 38 clients achieved a normal delivery.

Length of labour

It is not possible to assess whether or not labour was shortened by having lavender baths, but some appeared to progress very rapidly. However, two facts became obvious. Progress was better:

- in those who used the lavender bath when a 2+ dilation or more was established
- in those who spent more than 30 minutes in the bath (this may be due in part to the hydrotherapy effect).

Relaxation and pain relief

The majority of clients found the baths helpful and enjoyable. Over half felt that the baths helped with pain relief.

Analgesic oils

It would be interesting to carry out a study similar to the one described above using analgesic essential oils (high in terpenes, ketones or phenols—perhaps phenolic ethers also), to determine the pain relief and relaxation benefits for women in labour, since the relief of pain would automatically induce relaxation (Franchomme & Pénoël 1990). The following list shows the percentage of these components present in analgesic essential oils (all figures are approximate):

- *Lavandula angustifolia* [LAVENDER]—8% terpenes, 6% ketones
- *Coriandrum sativum* [CORIANDER]—25% terpenes, 12% ketones
- *Juniperus communis* (fruct, ram)—60% terpenes
- *Syzygium aromaticum*—15% terpenes, 70% phenols
- *Melaleuca alternifolia* [TEA TREE]—55% terpenes
- *Mentha × piperita*—25% terpenes, 25% ketones (rectified oil can contain 60% ketones)

- *Myristica fragrans*—70% terpenes, 3% phenolic ethers
- *Origanum majorana*—40% terpenes, 0.5% phenolic ethers
- *Piper nigrum* [BLACK PEPPER]—85% terpenes
- *Zingiber officinale* [GINGER]—75% terpenes.

Case 8.1 Aromatherapist: Beryl MacInnes MISPA, ITEC, SPDA, SPCD, UK

T is aged 39—fit and healthy, with two other children aged 6 and 2. She was disappointed with her lack of control over the induced birth of the elder. The younger was born naturally, with the help of aromatherapy. Drugs were not used, resulting in T being fully alert and in control throughout her labour and delivery.

She came to see me 8 weeks into her third pregnancy, feeling nauseous and very tired. I gave her a full treatment, using 2 drops *Citrus aurantium* var. *amara* (fol.) (balances and uplifts the nervous system), and 1 drop *Citrus paradisi* (per.) (for debility) and 2 drops *Citrus sinensis* (per.) (digestive stimulant, relieves nausea). I gave her the same mix of essential oils to use in the bath.

12 weeks. She had felt less fatigued after the first treatment and had slept well that night. She was still feeling a certain amount of nausea. I again carried out a full treatment, adding *Zingiber officinale* to the mix to help the nausea, and gave her some ginger to use as an inhalation for home use. After this, she was not so tired, slept well and her nausea was much improved.

17 weeks. She had haemorrhoids, for which I made up a lotion for daily application containing *Cupressus sempervirens* (vasoconstrictive), *Pelargonium graveolens* (decongestive, cicatrizant) and *Santalum album* (soothing). I also gave her a mixture of sweet almond and avocado, with essential oils of *Chamaemelum nobile*, *Citrus reticulata* (per.) and *Lavandula angustifolia* to apply daily to her abdomen, breasts and thighs to help avoid stretch marks. I would have liked to add *Boswellia carteri* but she did not like the aroma of this particular oil.

22 weeks. Feeling well, quite energetic, no sickness. Haemorrhoids still a slight problem, but had improved. No digestive problems, and her pregnancy was progressing well. Her treatment oils were 2 drops *Citrus aurantium* var. *amara* (per.) (uplifting and relaxing), 1 drop *Pelargonium graveolens* (hormonal balancing), 1 drop *Rosmarinus officinalis* (stimulates nervous system). She responded to this treatment with increased energy and a sense of well-being.

35 weeks. Still feeling well, but rather tired and a little emotional. No evidence of oedema or heartburn, blood pressure normal. Relaxed and positive approach towards the birth. Treatment: 1 drop *Chamaemelum nobile*, 1 drop *Melissa officinalis* (relaxing), 1 drop *Lavandula angustifolia* (backache), 1 drop of *Salvia sclarea* (uterotonic in preparation for the birth). Felt 'wonderful' following her treatment; was not tired, despite a restless night. I mixed a combination of cold-pressed sweet almond and wheatgerm oils for her to massage her perineum daily to encourage elasticity, prevent tearing, to nourish any previously damaged tissue and to prepare this area for the impending birth.

37 weeks. Feeling rather uncomfortable: the baby's head had engaged, causing some pressure on her bladder, and there was flatulence and some lower backache. Despite this, still optimistic, no anxiety. I massaged her back and legs using 1 drop *Chamaemelum nobile*, 1 drop *Lavandula angustifolia*, 1 drop *Zingiber officinale* (these three to soothe the digestive system, relieve flatulence and backache) and 1 drop *Pelargonium graveolens* (stimulates digestion and circulation). Following the massage, she felt relaxed with renewed energy—the backache eased.

During this period I massaged her back, legs and abdomen each week. The selection of oils included *Salvia sclarea* (uterotonic, imparts optimism and euphoria). The main consideration was in keeping her as relaxed and comfortable as possible, considering the increasing size and pressure of the fetus.

41 weeks. The consultant confirmed that T and baby were still well, and told her that if the baby had not arrived at 42 weeks, she would be admitted to hospital to be induced. She had been assured that this method would only be used as a last resort. As the baby was a week late, T was feeling quite agitated and worried about the prospect of a further week's wait. To help allay her fears, I massaged her back, legs and abdomen, using 2 drops *Melissa officinalis* (uplifting, balancing), 1 drop *Cupressus sempervirens*, 1 drop *Pelargonium graveolens* (circulatory system, leg cramps and haemorrhoids, which T was worried would recur, due to pressure in the bowel area). T became noticeably calmer and more relaxed with the pressure in her back eased. The baby seemed so familiar with my hands and oils that as I worked on the abdomen, I could feel it moving and responding to the calming oils and the gentleness of the massage, reacting in the same way as T does.

42 weeks. T was admitted to hospital, where she had a Prostin pessary inserted in the vagina. Fetus heartbeat and uterine action were monitored for the first 30 minutes and registered a strong and steady foetal heartbeat and some uterine activity. She was feeling rather anxious and a little nauseous, so I massaged her feet and back with *Lavandula angustifolia* (nausea, relaxation). Although this Maternity Unit does not use aromatherapy, they were quite happy for us to proceed as we wished, using the oils. The Prostin pessary resulted in T getting irregular contractions and backache. After 6 hours she had only dilated to 2–3 cm. I again massaged her back, applying hot compresses and using a mixture of *Jasminum officinale* and *Salvia sclarea*.

T's progress was slow but natural. She chose not to have her membranes ruptured or to be induced intravenously. At 22:00, some 13 hours following admission, she was still making very slow progress. Her contractions were not very strong, but enough to prevent her from sleeping and she was beginning to feel tired and despondent. Throughout this period her blood pressure, pulse and fetal heartbeat were good. She was offered temazepam to help her sleep or pethidine to ease the pain, but she declined both. I then massaged her feet with a mixture containing 3 drops *Salvia sclarea*, paying special attention to massaging very firmly the repro-

ductive area reflexes. The massage and oils were used to help speed up and regulate contractions.

She began to progress more quickly and at 01:00 she had an extremely strong contraction: her membranes ruptured and she continued having strong and regular contractions. She remained totally focused and committed, breathing deeply, inhaling *Lavandula angustifolia* on a tissue and having the same oil in cold compresses applied to her forehead and back of neck.

By 03:30 she had fully dilated to the amazement of the nursing staff who had predicted that she would not give birth until the following day and would almost certainly need further medical intervention. T was taken to the delivery suite, still very much in control over her own labour. She spent 2 hours in the final stages, using only gas and air and still totally focused on what she had to do. The delivery midwife gave her freedom of choice in the position she wished to deliver. T's beautiful baby boy eventually emerged at 05:45, weighing in at 8 lb 12 oz (well over 2 lb heavier than her previous two children). She delivered in the squatting position, immediately cradling her baby and even cutting her own umbilical cord. She had only experienced a superficial tear, which needed a few stitches.

Case 8.2 Aromatherapist: Katie Watts, UK

Mrs E, who was at that time 36 weeks pregnant, had been admitted to hospital due to bleeding from a low-lying placenta, a large baby and polyhydramnios (an excess of amniotic fluid surrounding the baby).

24 November. At her request, I gave her a relaxing full body massage on the ward using jasmine, lavender and rose otto in grapeseed with calendula and wheatgerm carrier oils. She reported feelings of 'floating' for 4 hours post-massage.

29 November. Due to the complications of her pregnancy she was to be induced on the following Tuesday so we arranged for a more stimulating massage. I used a blend of lavender, geranium, rose and clary.

30 November. She informed me that although the massage was relaxing, 2 hours later she had noticed the Braxton-Hicks contractions becoming more regular and more intense. This tailed off 2 hours later.

1 December. Mrs E's labour was induced for artificial rupture of the membranes. I joined her at 16:30 when she was in early labour. She was connected up to a monitor which shows a variation in the fetal heartbeat and muscular tension in the uterus (demonstrating contractions).

One indication of fetal well-being is the presence of beat-to-beat variability on the heart trace. (Beat-to-beat variability means the alteration of speed of the baby's heart rate, which should be greater than 5 beats per minute; a reduction is an indication of low oxygen supply.) This was the case prior to the massage and the baby's condition started to cause some concern.

Permission from the hospital was obtained and the massage was begun at 17:11 to the delight of the attending hospital staff who commented on the wonderful aroma. I gave Mrs E a full-body-massage (suited to pregnancy) using jasmine, lavender and rose otto

Mrs E was turned to her right side at 17:23. The final part of the abdominal massage finished at 17:40. It was interesting to note that the beat-to-beat variability improved to a point of acceptability at 17:47, and was subsequently maintained for a further 20 minutes until 18:05 when Mrs E used a bed pan (possibly the stimulating effect of the massage caused the bladder to fill). Gravity acted on the weight of the uterus, then suppressed the blood supply to the placenta and in conjunction with the contractions led to a marked deceleration in fetal heart beat, a result of an even lower level of oxygen getting to the placenta, a more severe indicator of fetal distress.

Mrs E also had an epidural which was only effective on one side despite adjustment. In advanced labour there was increased pain which progressed round the back and into the pelvis with contractions. This area was massaged further and with increased pressure during the contractions when the pain intensified. Mrs E felt great relief from this and benefitted from the physical and moral support.

At 22:58 a baby boy was assisted (due to fetal distress) into the world, weighing 9 lb 4 oz.

Since the birth Mrs E has used an essential oil mix of cypress, jasmine and lavender in the bath to help tighten up the perineum and heal the episiotomy, which has been consistently clean and dry.

Retrospectively, Mrs E felt she had benefited enormously from my attendance and on discussion with the hospital practitioner it was felt that the blend of aromatherapy and midwifery practice was to the patient's benefit.

Case 8.3 Aromatherapist: Lynne Reed, UK

Antenatal

a. Gravida 5 Para 3 with hyperemesis gravidarum. This lady had suffered with hyperemesis during all of her previous four pregnancies and had even undergone a termination previously because of this condition. She was admitted to hospital for intravenous therapy to correct her electrolyte balance and after several days was discharged. She was re-admitted a few days later still unable to keep any food down. It was at this time that I was asked if I thought aromatherapy could help her.

She was offered various oils to smell to ascertain how well they would be tolerated. The ones she felt most happy with were *Citrus aurantium* var. *amara* (per), *Citrus paradisi* (per), *Citrus sinensis* (per) and *Mentha × piperita*. Lemon was not well-tolerated as she associated it with the lemon squash that she had been drinking, which had made her sick. I gave her a drop of peppermint oil in a glass of water to sip occasionally when she felt queasy, to settle her stomach. The orange and grapefruit oils were inhaled from a tissue.

The following morning she said that she felt a bit better and that she had remembered that in the past citrus fruits were the one thing that she could eat without feeling or being sick. We decided therefore that as soon as she felt able, these were the foods she should try to begin with.

I arranged to see her 2 days later, only to find that she had been discharged, requiring no further admissions.

Labour

b. Primigravida. This lady made good use of *Lavandula angustifolia* baths in early labour to aid relaxation. She had 1 dose of pethidine 100 mg when the contractions became too much for her. She wanted a water birth (contraindicated within 3 hours of having pethidine) so was anxious not to have more.

05:00 6 cm dilated and an ARM (artificial rupture of membranes) was performed. She commenced on Entonox and back-massage was given. We made use of a long footstool which she could sit astride with myself behind her, her upper body being supported with a beanbag on the bed.
05:30 Fully dilated.
05:45 Entered the bath for delivery (no lavender because of the baby's eyes) and the vertex was visible.
05:55 She had a normal water birth.

Essential oils used: 2 drops *Lavandula angustifolia*, 2 drops *Chamaemelum nobile*, 1 drop *Salvia sclarea*.

c. Primigravida in early labour.

16:15 2 cm dilated.
20:05 3 cm dilated.
21:30 Coping quite well.
23:15 Persuaded to take a bath with 5 drops *Lavandula angustifolia*. This was enjoyed but she could not get really comfortable in the bath.
23:45 5 cm dilated. Pethidine requested and 100 mg given.
00:45 6 cm dilated; spontaneous rupture of membranes occurred.
01:00 A back- and gentle abdominal massage were given using 1 drop each of *Chamaemelum nobile*, *Chamomilla recutita* and 2 drops each of *Cananga odorata* and *Lavandula angustifolia*.
01:30 Fully dilated
02:54 Normal delivery

d. Primigravida. 36 week gestation with spontaneous rupture of membranes due for induction because of prolonged rupture of membranes.

04:00 1 cm dilated, with weak to fair contractions every 5–10 minutes. She was offered a relaxing bath with essential oils of *Lavandula angustifolia* and *Salvia sclarea*. She stayed in the bath for 1 hour.
06:00 Contracting fairly strongly, once every 5 minutes.
07:00 Fully dilated, with an urge to push.
07:15 Confirmation of full dilation was made and good progress was continued.
07:40 Normal delivery.

Total length of labour: 3 hours 45 minutes.

e. Primigravida. Had made use of TENS machine at home. Admitted to hospital for delivery.

23:30 2 cm dilated with intact membranes.
00:30 Given bath with 5 drops *Lavandula angustifolia*.
02:30 9 cm dilated; requested additional pain relief. Reluctant to leave the bath, so vaginal examination carried out in the bath. An ARM was performed and entonox commenced.
03:30 Vertex was visible, but progress in the second stage was slow. Advised to get out of the bath.
04:30 Transferred to a delivery bed. A gentle abdominal massage was given using 2 drops each of *Chamaemelum nobile*, *Lavandula angustifolia*, 1 drop of *Salvia sclarea*.
05:00 Normal delivery. No other form of pain relief.

f. Primigravida

01:00 5 cm dilated. ARM performed.
01:45 Bath with 5 drops *Lavandula angustifolia*.
02:15 Full dilation confirmed. Urge to push.
03:00 Vertex visible on the perineum.
03:10 Normal water birth.

The delivery took place in the same bathwater containing lavender because it would have had time to either evaporate or blend well in the water.

Various combinations of essential oils were used for massage in labour. In 50 ml of carrier oil were blended (number of drops of each oil in brackets):

- *Chamaemelum nobile* (3), *Lavandula angustifolia* (1), *Salvia sclarea* (3) in 50 ml carrier oil
- *Cananga odorata* (3), *Lavandula angustifolia* (1), *Pelargonium graveolens* (3) in 50 ml carrier oil
- *Cananga odorata* (2), *Jasminum officinale* var. *grandiflorum* (1), *Lavandula angustifolia* (2) in 25 ml carrier oil.

The main aim was:

- To stimulate the pituitary and thalamus to encourage the secretion of endorphins and encephalins to reduce pain.
- To utilize the sedative properties of lavender and Roman chamomile to aid relaxation.

Summary

The majority of female admissions to hospital are connected with pregnancy and birth, which are not health problems unless there are complications. Pregnancy is an area of great interest to aromatherapists, nurses and midwives and consequently a great deal of experience has been accumulated in maternity wards and by visiting midwives all over Britain. Small-scale trials of essential oils used in labour have given encouraging results. It is hoped that larger controlled studies will endorse these findings, and that the use of aromatherapy (including some of the more powerful oils) by qualified professionals in antenatal, maternity and postnatal settings will increase accordingly.

REFERENCES

Allen W T 1897 Note on a case of supposed poisoning by pennyroyal. The Lancet 1: 1022–1023
Balacs M Á 1992 Safety in pregnancy. International Journal of Aromatherapy 4(1): 12–15
Bardeau F 1976 La médecine aromatique. Laffont, Paris
Bernadet M 1983 La phyto-aromathérapie pratique. Dangles, St-Jean-de-Braye
Braithwaite P F 1906 A case of poisoning by pennyroyal: recovery. The British Medical Journal 2: 865
Burns E, Blamey D 1994 Using aromatherapy in childbirth. Nursing Times 90(9): 54–60
Burns E 1992 Dedicated to better birth. International Journal of Aromatherapy 4(1): 9–11
Chandler R F, Hooper S N, Harvey M J 1982 Ethnobotany and phytochemistry of yarrow, *Achillea millefolium*, Compositae. Economic Botany 36(2): 203
Cornwall S, Dale A 1988 Aromatherapy in Midwifery Practice. Hinchingbrooke Hospital, Huntingdon
Culpeper N 1983 Culpeper's colour herbal. Foulsham, London p. 47
Cutter K 1992 Dedicated to better birth. International Journal of Aromatherapy 4(1): 11

Fawcett M 1993 Aromatherapy for pregnancy and childbirth. Element Books, Shaftesbury
Fehr D, Stenzhorn G 1979 Untersuchungen zur Lagerstabilität von Pfefferminzblättern, Rosmarinblättern und Thymian. Pharmazeutische Zeitung 124: 2342–2349
Fern E 1992 The Ipswich Hospital Directorate of Maternity & Gynaecological Practice Group (Midwifery, Gynaecology & Neonatal Care). Aromatherapy, Midwifery Procedures Nos 23A, 23C, 23D, 23E
Formacek K, Kubeczka K H 1982 Essential oils analysis by capillary chromatography and carbon-13 NMR spectroscopy. Wiley, New York
Franchomme P, Pénoël D 1990 L'aromathérapie exactement. Jollois, Limoges
Gilly G, Garnero J, Racine P 1986 Menthes poivrées— composition chimique analyse chromatographie. Parfumerie Cosmétiques Aromates 71: 79–86
Grieve M 1991 A modern herbal. Penguin, London
Guernier J 1992 Essential obstetrics. International Journal of Aromatherapy 4(1): 9–11
Holder R 1995 Aromatherapy in hospitals—a study in acceptance. The Aromatherapist 2(2) April

Holmes P 1993 Clary sage. International Journal of Aromatherapy 5(1): 15–17

Lawrence 1984 Progress in essential oils: Yarrow oil. Perfumer & Flavorist 9(4): 37

Lawrence B M 1989 Progress in essential oils: Pennyroyal. Perfumer & Flavorist 14(3): 71

Leung A Y 1980 Encyclopedia of common natural ingredients used in food, drugs and cosmetics. Wiley, New York p. 409

Lundie S 1993a Aromatherapy in maternity care. Unpublished paper

Lundie S 1993b Introducing and applying aromatherapy within the NHS. The Aromatherapist 1 (2): 30–35; (3): 32–37; 2(1)

MacInnes B 1993 The use of aromatherapy in pregnancy and childbirth. Unpublished dissertation, Shirley Price International College of Aromatherapy, Hinckley

Mabey R 1988 The complete new herbal. Elm Tree Books, London p. 72

Myles M 1993 Textbook for midwives 12th edn. Churchill Livingstone, Edinburgh p. 43

Opdyke D L J (ed) 1979 Monographs on fragrance raw materials. In: Food and Cosmetics Toxicology. Research Institute for Fragrance Materials, Pergamon Press, New York

Price S 1993 The aromatherapy workbook. Thorsons, London

Reed L, Norfolk L 1993 Aromatherapy in midwifery. Aromatherapy World, Nurturing Issue, Summer: 12–15

Roulier G 1990 Les huiles essentielles pour votre santé. Dangles, St-Jean-de-Braye

Sullivan J B, Peterson R G 1979 Pennyroyal poisoning and hepatoxicity. Journal of the American Medical Association 242(26): 2873–2874

Tisserand R 1977 The art of aromatherapy. Daniel, Saffron Walden

Tisserand R, Balacs M A 1991 Research reports. International Journal of Aromatherapy 3(1): 6

United Kingdom Central Council 1993 Handbook of midwives' rules. UKCC, 23 Portland Place, London

Vallance W B 1955 Pennyroyal poisoning: a fatal case. The Lancet 2: 850–851

Valnet J 1980 The practice of aromatherapy. Daniel, Saffron Walden

van Arsdale L, Avery M 1987 Unpublished paper

Wingate P, Wingate R 1988 The Penguin medical encyclopaedia. Penguin, London

9

People with learning difficulties

Introduction

Therapy using essential oils with massage has had some surprising successes in one of the least responsive therapeutic areas—the treatment of people with learning difficulties. Several case histories will be presented, along with advice about the need for particular caution in the selection and presentation of oils in this context.

SPECIAL NEEDS

Since the 1970s there has been a markedly positive change in understanding and attitudes towards adults and children whose mental or physical attributes are retarded in some way. Treated as outcasts from society before then, there was little regard for their needs as individuals, nor much attempt to improve their happiness and well-being. They were rarely touched, except possibly to receive rough treatment, and it is believed that the lack of positive tactile stimulation could lead to the rocking, hand-wringing and head-banging that play such a large part in the behaviour pattern of many people with learning difficulties.

Touch is a basic behavioural need in much the same way as breathing is a basic physical need. When the need for touch remains unsatisfied, abnormal behaviour will result.

(Montagu 1986)

Fortunately, such people are now being recognized in their own right:

Mentally disordered people should be treated with the same respect for their dignity, personal needs, religious and philosophical beliefs, and accorded the same choices, as other people. Special consideration should be given to those with particular cultural and communication needs.

(Mental Health Act 1983)

153

Case study 9.1 Aromatherapist: Mary Anna Hanse SPDipA, UK

I was asked if I would visit a busy ward of a hospital for mentally handicapped people in the Midlands, to see if my work had any relevance to the severely disturbed, deaf and blind residents there with severe mental handicaps, and with whom nurses wanted to improve communication. The visit was a most rewarding experience, because it really did show the value of touch. I spent about 4 hours in a ward and worked with three patients.

The first person is a man call M, who goes around on all fours and likes to bash his head on the tiled floor. The staff said that when they intervened and tried to stop the bashing it made matters worse: M accelerated the behaviour and they had to leave him to work through the self-mutilation. When I saw him rhythmically hitting his forehead on the floor until the sores he had accumulated on his forehead bled onto the tiles, I suggested that I try to massage his back to see what would happen. I used a carrier oil with relaxing essential oils and started first to introduce the aroma near his face for him to inhale. I talked to him as I worked, in case some vibration could be picked up, or something communicated. I worked in large circles on his back, first very gently, and as his response was immediate and positive, I used a firmer stroke. The instant I started, M straightened up and stopped the head-banging. He sat on his knees, fully absorbed and not moving an eyelash, for the 10 minutes or so that I worked on his back. M remained peaceful for the rest of the afternoon.

The second person I worked with was a young man with severe nasal congestion who refuses to be touched by anyone apart from two or three staff he knows well. Staff had been using the usual drugs, which did not seem to clear the congestion, and G was keeping others as well as himself awake at night. Recently he had been taken to see a specialist in another hospital because the congestion was so troublesome, but G would not let the consultant near him and they had to bring him back unhelped. I put some essential oils for sinusitis and catarrh on a tissue and, while a nurse held them near his face, I worked on his feet, using a Swiss reflex cream containing the same essential oils. Before starting on his feet I chatted to him and very gently first touched and stroked his hands and face. On his feet I worked on the sinus reflex points. After a while his sinuses started running and he was needing to spit, etc. The staff were surprised not only at the blockage moving, but at G allowing touch from a stranger.

Finally, the most moving and surprising, was the response of a 19-year-old girl called F. This young woman is very disturbed. When I saw her, the word that came to my mind was torment. She was continually thrashing backwards and forwards, punching her head with her fists, slapping her head and face, sticking her fingers into her eyes, pushing away hands that tried to touch her. She ceaselessly thrashed around. I was told that she refused to let people touch her. Her carers and parents, who show so much concern for her, never have the satisfaction of knowing whether she appreciates it. She does not communicate this.

I stayed with her for about 2 hours. At first with total rejection, and then ever so slowly, there was a gradual acceptance of my presence and then of my touch. The last half hour or so, F was relaxed and lying back on the bean bag, sometimes with her arms behind her back with a little smile and sometimes giving a gurgling laugh of pleasure. I held her on the solar plexus area between rib-cage and stomach, with the other hand on the adrenals at the back. It seemed that there was a healing calm produced by hands placed on the body, combined with the effect of the relaxing essential oils and the total effect was dramatic. The nurses were wishing that it could have been photographed or better still, videoed, as they had never seen F like that. There was a concentration on what was going on in the ward; a focus and a quiet calmness—the nurses said that all the residents seemed more calm than usual.

I believe that there is much useful work that could be done in the area of profound handicaps, using essential oils and having the confidence to use hands for communication and healing.

People with learning difficulties require the same (and probably more) care, love, touch and attention as a person whose illness or disability takes a different form. Terms like 'challenging behaviour' and 'learning difficulties' have replaced words like 'mentally deficient' and 'backward', and instead of keeping patients/ clients away from contact with the outside world, every effort is made to help them to achieve as normal an everyday life as possible. This is brought about primarily by using and developing the sense of touch (and also, it is believed, the sense of smell):

Touch is central to our work with people who have severe learning difficulties ... addressed by considering the quality of touch which people receive in everyday interactions. ... Gently holding a hand, a kind touch on the arm, a pat on the back or holding someone who is crying can often convey silently but more clearly and easily than words how people really feel.

(Sanderson et al 1991 p. 11)

The child or adult needs to feel loved and to be completely accepted, including the acceptance of any particular physical impairment or negative emotional behaviour. A feeling of being loved will help to increase the person's feeling of self-worth, as will praise when something positive is achieved or the person's hair or other grooming features are pleasing to the eye. Also, 'it is important that tasks which are given should be attainable with short term goals, so that there is early reward, for nothing breeds success more than success itself' (Bischoff 1992) and success will boost a person's self-belief.

TREATMENT

Massage, as discussed in Chapter 6, is merely an extension of touch, which relaxes the muscles and 'encourages the mind to take a break from its usual frenetic activity' (Bischoff 1992). The addition of essential oils to a bland massage oil extends massage into a therapy which can have profound effects on the mind, thus beneficially affecting the emotional and physical behaviour of the person with learning difficulties.

The fact that aromas can trigger the memory (van Toller & Dodd 1988 p. 153) suggests that on the second and subsequent occasions when the same oil is used, memories of the first occasion are aroused. If these memories are happy ones, treatment will be enhanced each time, building on any therapeutic benefit generated by the first treatment and this has, indeed, been found to be the case (Price 1987).

It is believed that, as with most health problems for which essential oils are used, stimulation and/or relaxation are prime factors in the initiation of the healing process—whatever the health problem. This is remarkably evident in the case of those with learning difficulties: their power of communication is considerably increased, and challenging behaviour is decreased. The use of essential oils accelerates any progress being made—and a positive constructive circle is begun, resulting in the person becoming independent in small personal tasks previously attended to by a carer (Sanderson et al 1991 pp. 80–81).

Essential oil range and selection

The range of oils from which selection is made is very important in the case of people with learning difficulties and should not include those containing aldehydes, ketones, oxides, phenols or phenolic ethers as principal constituents. The oils to avoid are listed in Appendices B.4–8 and it is

---

Case study 9.2 Aromatherapist: Lucile Bischoff SPDipA, South Africa

R is 21 years old, with mild to borderline mental retardation and suspected temporal lobe epilepsy, for which he is prescribed Tegretol 200–300 mg. His mother disappeared soon after his birth, and his father is an alcoholic who was battered himself as a child and physically and sexually abused R and his 3 brothers. The children were removed and placed in a home. R can look after himself and works in sheltered employment at the home.

Aromatherapy was introduced to try and help with his erratic mood swings, which fluctuate from sulking, or very aggressive behaviour with self abuse. It is not known to what extent his retardation is related to the emotional factors. He does have a 'girlfriend' at the home but there are frequent arguments, some of them quite physical.

Treatment 1. On my first visit to the home I brought some plants to show the children where the oils came from. R recognised the lavender and said that you could make tea from it, much to the surprise of Mrs S (the helper assigned to help me). I think this boosted R's ego quite a bit as he stated that he was very clever. He showed considerable interest in the oils and enjoyed smelling them. I decided to let him dictate the course of treatment, allowing him to choose his own oils. Any communication was directed at Mrs S and not to me. He was very curious but also nervous about the massage so I first worked on the other children so that he could see exactly what it involved. By the time it was his turn he was very eager and stated that if I did the same on him he might just fall asleep. I gave him a back massage and a gentle foot massage which he enjoyed. Deciding to let him choose his own oils and length of treatment broke the ice and helped to build his confidence and trust. He enjoyed the treatment and said he felt quite sleepy afterwards.

Treatment 2. I was greeted with a smile; he was in a good mood as he had helped on the switchboard that morning, which I think made him feel important. The results from the previous treatment were favourable. He had slept in the afternoon and also been in a good mood with no fighting. This time, our conversation was a bit better and we chattered about a geranium plant I had given him on the previous visit, as I felt that something of his own to look after might help with his moods. Although there was an improvement in our conversation, I felt that most of the time he was being polite. He enjoyed his back massage the most.

Treatment 3. R was waiting for me to arrive this time. He seems to be a happier person, smiling more and seeming to be content. He brought his own music for the session which we played while I was working on him, but he soon realised that it was too fast and asked me to change it as it was making a noise. He is relaxing far more during treatments. I noticed that he was closing his eyes and dozing on and off during the treatment.

Matron and the staff are extremely pleased at the change in his behaviour; he was easier to control and not losing his temper as often. I made up an oil for him to use in his bath or to rub onto his hands and arms if he was feeling cross. I also showed him a few breathing exercises. The essential oils used were *Boswellia carteri*, *Cedrus atlantica* and *Citrus aurantium* var. *amara* (flos).

recommended that these are not even kept on the premises.

The selection of the 2 or 3 oils to be presented to each person or child should not be undertaken at random. The medical details of each case should first be studied, and then oils pre-selected which will influence the symptoms presented. From these, 2–3 oils are chosen for their relaxing or uplifting properties (whichever is felt to be the effect required). This means that although the selection has been made to affect the mental and emotional side of the client primarily, it will also alleviate any symptoms being suffered, such as constipation, insomnia, rheumatic pain, poor circulation, respiratory disorders etc.

For example, someone who cannot sleep well and who suffers from rheumatism could be offered *Citrus limon*, *Origanum majorana* and *Chamaemelum nobile* as their oils from which to choose. (For a full list of oils to help insomnia see the main therapeutic cross-reference chart at the end of the book.)

Having selected the essential oils which would be most helpful to the person concerned, the way in which these are presented is of great importance. The aim is to select an aroma which is acceptable to and appreciated by the person for whom it is intended, so time should be taken when introducing the essential oils. Never offer more than 3 and offer them one at a time, noting the reactions carefully: Did the hand push it away? Was the head averted? Did the person come closer? Did he or she reach out for the hand holding the aroma? The end result will be enhanced when an oil favoured by the person is used, and the preferred one, on its own, should be used first in whatever method of treatment is adopted.

In visualization therapy, if a colour is introduced by the therapist while the subject has already begun to visualize one of his or her own choice, confusion disrupts the relaxation (van Toller & Dodd 1988 p. 152). The same potential for confusion (and reduced benefit) applies to the choice of essential oils for those with learning difficulties: if the therapist decides to mix together two that the person favoured, this is not the same thing as using one which the client has actually smelt.

Presentation of aromas

The essential oils can be presented in two ways:

- 1 drop on a spill or tissue—neat.
- Ready-mixed in a carrier oil on a tissue or on the back of the therapist's hand. Using the hand sometimes enables the therapist to make physical contact with a client who previously has not been enthusiastic about being touched.

If the diluted method is preferred, small bottles of each essential oil diluted in jojoba oil can be kept for this purpose alone. (Jojoba is a liquid wax resistant to oxidation that keeps well.)

Should the person appear to like more than one (or all) of the offered oils equally, this is not necessarily a sign to blend these together (see above): a different aroma will be produced. Simply select one of the favoured single oils for the first few treatments, or offer a mix or blend of

---

Case study 9.3 Clinical Aromatologist: Barbara Payne SPDipA, SPCD Aromatology, UK

During a visit to one of the Mencap homes in Bridlington I was asked if there was anything I could do to help J, a 30-year-old resident of the home, with learning and physical disabilities, and very bad bouts of depression. She had always found communication to be problematic, particularly with visitors. She had hardly ever slept right through the night, which sometimes made her tired and irritable the next day.

J looked continually at the floor. I offered her a choice of 3 oils to smell and she looked intently at the bottle containing sandalwood essential oil. This was taken to be an indication that she liked the smell. I mixed the oil into a foot-balm base and asked her if she would like me to massage her feet. Again, although interest was shown in the massage offered, she looked intently at the jar and reached out to touch it. I gently started to massage her foot and she was clearly delighted. Her gaze at the jar slowly rose until she was looking straight into my eyes while at the same time stretching out her toes for more.

The staff were amazed at the eye contact as they had never seen her do that before. I spoke gently to her and let her hold the sealed jar, whilst massaging the other foot (which she had eagerly pushed into my hands). I demonstrated to staff how to massage the foot slowly and gently and suggested they might use the cream at J's bedtime. The next day I received a phone call from J's carer to say that J had slept well the whole night and was in a very happy frame of mind. Treatments with the foot-balm have continued and so has the improvement in J. She now sleeps through every night and consequently life has improved both for her and everyone around her.

2 or 3 of the oils on the first list as one more possible aroma to be offered to the client.

Should none of the aromas offered gain a positive reaction, rather than change to yet another oil, a drop of *Lavendula angustifolia* can be added to each spill or tissue, and one of these offered again. The blend offered is still a single aroma, but may be more acceptable.

Where there is a large number of patients/ clients, and time permits, it is useful to keep second sets of neat (and diluted) trial bottles which contain *L. angustifolia* together with an equal amount of a single essential oil. A third set using *Santalum album*, *Pelargonium graveolens* or another popular oil, such as *Citrus reticulata*, in place of *L. angustifolia* is another possibility.

Norfolk Park School, Sheffield, uses essential oils together with massage throughout their school on children with severe learning difficulties, and have produced a video and small book designed to assist anyone working with handicapped adults on a one-to-one basis. Also available is *Aromatherapy for People with Learning Difficulties* (Sanderson et al), which is invaluable for those working in this field.

LEARNING DIFFICULTIES TRIAL

Lucile Bischoff, who is principal of an aromatherapy school in South Africa, carried out a trial study on three children with learning difficulties at the San Michelle Home for the mentally and physically handicapped. Because different essential oils were used for each child and there was no placebo, the study does not show any particular essential oils effecting an improvement. Nevertheless, it is of value in showing that essential oils, together with massage, did have a positive effect on the children concerned. Even though the trial was terminated two treatments short of the set number, the six treatments carried out are still useful, as they show definite improvements in the behaviour of the children. It would be worth doing further controlled studies in this area.

The aims of the study were to see how aromatherapy and massage could benefit people with learning difficulties by:
- promoting self awareness and trust
- increasing communication
- providing tactile and sensory stimulation.

Lucile encountered a few obstacles and limitations. Space was a problem at the home and co-operation and feedback from the staff were not very forthcoming. An epidemic of hepatitis unfortunately broke out before the end of the scheduled number of treatments, prematurely ending the study.

Evelyn

Evelyn was 7 years old, blind and mildly mentally retarded, a suspected syphilis baby. She was incontinent, unable to speak, wash, dress or feed herself. The oils selected (no botanical specification given) were: 1 drop each lavender and geranium essential oil in 10 ml grapeseed carrier oil.

Treatment 1. Evelyn's behaviour was very erratic, changing from extreme excitability to crying and refusal to have a massage. Eventually tolerated a back-massage for a full minute while sitting on Lucile's lap.

Treatment 2. Behaviour far better, although still resisting and frequently asking to be taken to the bathroom. A short foot-, hand- and back-massage was managed.

Treatment 3. Evelyn recognized Lucile's voice and was happy to 'see' her. Although resisting lying down, a breakthrough was felt regarding communication and acceptance.

Treatment 4. Evelyn allowed the massage of her feet, legs, arms and hands for a short while, plus a 2-minute back-massage lying down.

Treatment 5. Still resisting a little, but the length of each massage session increased and Evelyn lay down again for her back to be massaged.

Treatment 6. Evelyn beginning to relax more; lavender and geranium have been placed in her room and on her clothes for identification.

Walter

Walter was 7 years old at the time of the study, hyperactive and on medication for severe MR. His IQ is under 40 and he is considered untrainable. His brother (with whom he has a good relationship) is in the same home and his mother is institutionalized. His medication: Catapres and Melleril.

The oils selected were: 1 drop each of chamomile and lavender essential oil in 10 ml grapeseed carrier oil.

Treatment 1. A short foot-massage was managed without resistance (except for asking the helper to hit Lucile if it hurt him). When asked if he would like a back-massage he jumped onto the bed face down and thoroughly enjoyed one. He asked for oils to be put on his face and stomach.

Treatment 2. Very eager and lay still for a 15-minute massage of his feet, legs, stomach and back. At the end of the treatment Lucile asked for a hug, which he allowed, but with no response on his part. There was no eye contact or communication.

Treatment 3. The helper said that Walter had been talking much more, and after treatment 2 had sat down with crayons and scribbled for the first time. While being massaged, Walter smiled often and was quite chatty, but before and after his treatment, he refused to communicate or respond to a hug.

Treatment 4. Walter was very quiet and refused to communicate, though apparently still enjoying the massage.

Rachael

Rachael was 8 years old, with quadriplegia (which presented the biggest problem), cerebral palsy due to birth trauma, profound MR and epilepsy. Rachael comes from a very loving family. Her medication was Epilim, Tegretol, Valium.

The oils selected were: 1 drop each of chamomile and lavender essential oil in 10 ml grapeseed carrier oil.

Treatment 1. Difficulty experienced with handling, but Rachael's legs and feet (perhaps sensitive as she kept pulling them away) were massaged; she enjoyed the head-massage.

Treatment 2. Handling easier this time—and much smiling and laughing.

Treatment 3. Rachael was much more relaxed. There was no feedback from her mother, which was disappointing.

Treatment 4. Still enjoyed the head massage the most. Enjoyed watching Lucile's shadow on the wall.

Treatment 5. Showed a definite response to the music being played, trying to find it with her eyes when it was switched off. Still no feedback from her mother.

Results

Unfortunately, the hepatitis outbreak prevented further treatments for all three children.

Evelyn
- Massage tolerance increased from 1 minute to 15.
- Improvement in relaxation.

- Ready acceptance of sensory stimulation through touch.
- Improvement in communication.

Walter
- Definite improvement in behaviour patterns.
- More cooperation with tasks performed at home.
- Improvement in communication, especially speech.
- Showed an interest in objects around him (previously non-existent).

Rachael

It was difficult to assess any improvement as there was no feedback from her mother and no cooperation from the staff. However, she was progressively easier to handle and Lucile felt it was worth it for the enjoyment Rachael derived from the treatments. Her circulation must have benefited also.

Even though, so far as the authors are aware, there have been no trials or studies carried out on people with learning difficulties in Britain, a tremendous number of individual cases have been recorded. Peg Holden-Peters, who gives aromatherapy treatments (and uses vaporized essential oils) at Grove Park, a school for children with special needs, as well as at a special unit in Wadhurst Primary school (both in East Sussex) says that:

Out of the 26 children that I have massaged regularly, 20 have been able to relax thoroughly (9 of these quite deeply) and the other 6 have achieved relaxation for short spells of from 2–5 minutes. ... Children who spend most of their days in a wheelchair benefit from having their limbs loosened up by gentle aromatherapy massage. The leg and arm muscles of one child were fiercely resistant, but since aromatherapy began, her hands are no longer tightly clenched and she opens them easily.

(Holden-Peters 1993a)

Other benefits noticed include sleeping more soundly on nights after treatment. Within 2 weeks a 12-year-old who used to whimper when touched was tapping his teacher on the shoulder to request a cuddle and his challenging behaviour was considerably reduced.

Other reports from teachers and conversations with parents have shown the benefits possible by using essential oils with massage on children with special needs.

Very physically disabled children have been loosened up by aromatherapy sessions. Since receiving aromatherapy, two girls with cerebral palsy, who always had their fists tightly clenched, now open them and keep them loose most of the time.

(Holden-Peters 1993)

Summary

In spite of the anecdotal nature of aromatherapy's reported successes with people with severe mental and physical handicaps, it is clear from these few studies and case histories that it would be worth holding properly conducted trials. Not only could more be discovered about the benefits of aromatherapy, but much could be learned about the nature of learning difficulties themselves.

REFERENCES

Bischoff L 1995 How aromatherapy can help people with learning difficulties. The Aromatherapist 2(3)
Holden-Peters P 1993a Aromatherapy and special needs children. Dissertation, Clinical Practitioner's Diploma, Leics
Holden-Peters P 1993b Grove Park. The Aromatherapist 1(1): 22–24
Mental Health Act 1983 Draft Code of Practice. General principles of care and treatment: 1

Montagu A 1986 Touching: the human significance of the skin. Harper and Row, New York
Price S 1987 The effect of essential oils on the memory. Aromanews 6: 6–7
Price S 1993 The aromatherapy workbook. Thorsons, London
Sanderson H, Harrison J, Price S 1991 Aromatherapy for people with learning difficulties. Hands On, Birmingham
van Toller S, Dodd G 1988 Perfumery: the psychology and biology of fragrance. Chapman & Hall, London

10

Stress

Introduction

This chapter examines the phenomenon of stress in modern life. It looks at natural therapies used to combat stress in the hospital environment, and explores in depth the role of essential oils. A trial study is cited which demonstrates that massage with essential oils can significantly reduce stress levels in the patients of GPs. There follows a guide to the selection and combination of essential oils for the relief of stress, which is accompanied by illustrative examples.

THE EFFECTS OF STRESS

In the last few years the word stress has almost become synonymous with substandard health, assuming such significance that it is now accepted as a medical term. A current definition of stress is given by Wingate & Wingate (1988) as: 'Any influence which disturbs the natural balance of a person's body or mind', including 'physical injury, disease, deprivation and emotional disturbance'. There is no doubt that much stress today is due to the modern society in which we live—city and motorway driving, environmental pollution, divorce (which completely changes the traditional form of family life), unemployment, the threat of being mugged or burgled, flying, hospitalization—the list is endless. The emotions associated with stress can include deep anxiety, depression, desolation, grief, heartache, pain and mental torment. There are various forms and degrees of stress, defined only by each individual's ability to cope with a specific situation.

These are normally categorized as belonging to one of two groups—positive and negative stress. Both of these involve a response by the body to internal or external demands made upon it (see Ch. 7).

The right amount

Stress is like a violin string: too much tension and the string will snap, too little and it will not produce any music. However, just the right amount of tension produces vibrant energy. Without a certain amount of stress none of us could function positively. The stress before a race or a job interview is a kind of challenge—to win, or be successful—just as the stress of cooking daily for the family can be a challenge to satisfy the family appetite at specific times and to meet their nutritional needs. These are positive stressors without which we cannot function to our best ability. However, stress, which is not merely nervous tension (Selye 1956), can build up to an excess level—one of negative stress or distress—through physical injury, illness, work overload, emotional disturbance and even lack of a challenge.

According to Selye (1956) there are three stages in the development of the body's response to stress:

1. The initial direct effect of the body exposed to a stressor, bringing about the alarm stage, where
   a. a temporary cessation of digestive juices occurs
   b. the respiratory and heart rate increase
   c. extra oxygen is transported to the brain and the muscles (in preparation for strenuous action or emotional strength)
   d. energy is released quickly from stored fats and sugars
   e. extra adrenalin is produced
   f. the immune system shuts down.
2. The resistant stage, where the extra oxygen, energy and adrenalin are brought into action to enable the body to cope with this unacceptable situation (expected to be temporary).

With isolated occurrences the body is able to rid itself of the stress and the body functions return to normal. However, without help or release, the responses in 1 above are continuous and the body tries to adapt itself to the stressor in an effort to reach a balanced state. If the level of stress is prolonged or becomes chronic and is allowed to continue without help, the body reaches the third stage.

3. Exhaustion, with reversion to the alarm stage, resulting inevitably in eventual health problems. These may manifest as headaches, inability to sleep, digestive problems, skin disorders, susceptibility to infections, etc. due to the closing down of the immune responses.

Breakdown

Early on in stage 3, people may become irritable, even aggressive, critical, restless, inefficient, withdrawn, moody and with an uncontrollable urge to cry at the least setback. They may find that coffee, cigarettes or alcohol give temporary relief to their mental stress, or they may take tranquilizing medication, any of which may eventually add to their discomfort.

The combination of several ongoing stressors can result in a nervous breakdown, or what is sometimes termed burnout. The nervous system, influenced so strongly by the mind (see Ch. 7), is unable to cope and lethargy, inactivity, apathy and indifference set in. In this state, almost a 'waking coma', nothing seems possible to the sufferer, i.e. there is a breakdown in nervous energy. As the English philosopher John Locke put it (at the end of the 17th century): 'Though the faculties of the mind are improved by exercise, yet they must not be put to a stress beyond their strength'.

It is important to be able to recognize the danger signals and find a natural method of combating them, so that severe consequences can be avoided. The following diagram illustrates the relationship of stress to performance: when stress goes beyond a certain level, fatigue sets in and the performance level drops (Fig. 10.1).

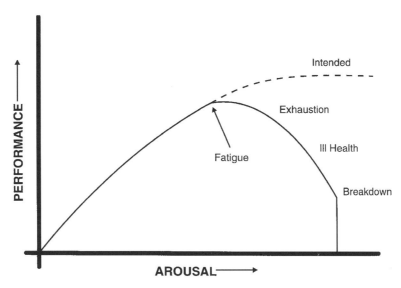

Fig. 10.1   The effect of stress on performance (Dr Kenneth Nixon)

Natural methods of stress-relief

Of the numerous ways of reducing stress, the following are the most frequently practised in hospitals in the UK and USA:

- Relaxation. For instance, the Northern View Day Hospital in Bradford successfully uses muscle relaxation techniques combined with a self-hypnosis tape and relaxing music to reduce levels of stress in the elderly (Harrison & Skinner 1992).

Case 10.1   Aromatherapist: Lynne Reed SPDipA, UK

An antenatal case. Primigravid lady resting in hospital with pregnancy-induced hypertension. The evening that I saw her, her diastolic BP was in the region of 110 mm Hg. Her BP was being recorded at 15-minute intervals using a Dynamap. She was obviously anxious and during the course of our chat, I asked her if she would like me to massage her feet for a little while. This I did, using Swiss reflex cream with 3 drops each of *Cananga odorata* and *Lavandula angustifolia*. We continued this for a little over half an hour, during which time her diastolic BP dropped gradually by 10 mm Hg. The last recording before she settled down to sleep was 95 mm Hg.

- Counselling.
- Reflexology and/or Swiss reflex massage.
- Massage (without oils).
- Therapeutic Touch, or the laying on of hands, is used by nurses belonging to the American Holistic Nurses Association as well as by many nurses in England (Krieger 1979).
- Hydrotherapy (often followed by massage).
- Laughter. Worwood (1990) advises patients to laugh as much as possible since it boosts the endorphin level and makes them feel good. She goes on to say that several hospitals in the United States take the physiological effects of laughter so seriously they have designated 'laughter rooms' where patients can have their prescribed fun. Michigan psychologist Zajonc maintains that even fake smiling triggers a reaction in the brain, making a patient feel better (cited in Price 1993).
- Essential oils. A large number of essential oils are stress reducing and to this end can be used independently on a paper tissue, in the bath and in a vaporizer. Also, the effects of massage are enhanced when essential oils are added to the basic massage oil, as discovered by Passant (1990).

ESSENTIAL OILS IN THE RELIEF OF STRESS

The main function of aromatherapy as introduced in the 1960s, i.e. with obligatory massage, was to relieve stress. The first aromatherapists were taught to concentrate only on relieving the stress, so that the body's own healing mechanism would be brought into play to alleviate symptoms brought on by the stress, such as migraines, problems related to menstruation, eczema, etc. Aromatherapy as practised today combines several aspects of healing which enhance each other's effects. Time is spent observing and listening to the patients, who often unburden themselves of their problems when encouraged by a skilful listener. Simple dietary advice is offered, such as cutting out coffee, tea and caffeinated soft drinks, and relaxing tapes have been introduced by some into their treatments.

A community psychiatric nurse in Leeds remarked to the authors in 1993 that 'therapies such as massage and aromatherapy are being seen more and more in the treatment of depression and anxiety, often being seen as an alternative rather than a complementary therapy'. While many of the drugs used can have a therapeutic part to play, they can also have horrific side effects. Indeed, the anxielitic group of drugs such as Vallium, Librium etc. have such addictive qualities that they are seldom prescribed today except in extreme cases of sudden trauma. And then only with caution and for short periods (Kirk 1993).

Essential oils have not been clinically tested in the same way as drugs but they are potentially less dangerous and far less damaging to the body (see Ch. 3). Their benefits have led to their increasing use by health professionals who have recognized the major role they can play in the reduction of stress.

STRESS PROJECT ON GP REFERRALS

In 1991 a project was carried out over a period of 6 months by Jean Gonella, on 16 women suffering from severe stress (Gonella 1993). The aim was to try and reduce the need for medication such as tranquillizers, antidepressants and hypnotics. Each woman was referred by her GP and fulfilled the following criteria:

- stress level above that acceptable to client/family
- disruption/dysfunction to client/family.

Clients were accepted on project with

- physical symptoms such as backache, headaches, etc.
- subject to panic attacks
- unresolved or prolonged bereavement
- hormone-related problems.

The treatment given was full body massage with the essential oils *Lavandula angustifolia* [LAVENDER], *Pelargonium graveolens* [GERANIUM] and *Santalum album* [SANDALWOOD]. *Salvia sclarea* [CLARY] was added where there were hormonal problems.

Results

The clients had to rate the severity of their problem on a scale of severe, medium, negligible or nonexistent. The results collated from individual questionnaires show the average percentage of problem severity before treatment, with the level after treatment shown in brackets (see Table 10.1).

Although the results are impressive, Gonella would like to see 100 clients given treatment together with an equivalent control group in order to prove that aromatherapy could reduce drug therapy (Gonella 1993).

Table 10.1 Problem severity before and after aromatherapy treatment. Average percentages are given, with the post-treatment level in brackets

	severe		medium		negligible		non-existent
	before	after	before	after	before	after	
anxiety	63%	(0%)	25%	(50%)	12%	(50%)	(0%)
depression	43%	(5%)	30%	(18%)	10%	(52%)	(25%)
insomnia	43%	(5%)	26%	(18%)	5%	(55%)	(25%)
pain	55%	(20%)	38%	(25%)	2%	(50%)	(5%)
tiredness	25%	(10%)	65%	(30%)	5%	(55%)	(5%)
confidence	55%	(12%)	20%	(13%)	25%	(75%)	(0%)
coping skill	50%	(8%)	25%	(22%)	25%	(70%)	(0%)

Selection of essential oils

The essential oils in this section are those recommended by Franchomme & Pénoël (1990), Roulier (1990) and Price (1993). Up to 4 different essential oils may be needed to treat stress holistically. Together they will enhance each other's effects, i.e. a synergy will be created.

Oils are chosen according to the particular stress symptoms presented by the patient. The symptom lists below can be used in the following way to make the appropriate choices. Firstly, decide which if any of the circumstances and symptoms listed in numbers 1–13 apply to the patient. Secondly, decide whether the patient's symptoms are due to deep anxiety or to depression. Then select from the anxiety or depression lists oils also appearing in the more specific lists 1–13. It is important to note that only a selection of the possible essential oils will be given here in order to illustrate the method of selection; for complete lists see Appendix B.9.

Anxiety

- *Cananga odorata* [YLANG YLANG]
- *Chamaemelum nobile* [ROMAN CHAMOMILE]
- *Citrus aurantium* var. *amara* (flos) [NEROLI BIGARADE]
- *Citrus aurantium* var. *amara* (fol.) [PETITGRAIN BIGARADE]
- *Citrus aurantium* var. *amara* (per.) [ORANGE BIGARADE]
- *Citrus bergamia* (per.) [BERGAMOT]
- *Citrus limon* (per.) [LEMON]
- *Citrus reticulata* (per.) [MANDARIN]
- *Coriandrum sativum* [CORIANDER]
- *Cupressus sempervirens* [CYPRESS]
- *Lavandula angustifolia* [LAVENDER]
- *Lavandula × intermedia* 'Super' [LAVANDIN]
- *Melissa officinalis* [LEMON BALM]
- *Ocimum basilicum* var. *album* [EUROPEAN BASIL]
- *Origanum majorana* [SWEET MARJORAM]
- *Pelargonium graveolens* [GERANIUM].

Depression

- *Boswellia carteri* [FRANKINCENSE]
- *Chamaemelum nobile*
- *Citrus aurantium* var. *amara* (flos) [NEROLI BIGARADE]
- *Citrus bergamia* (per.)
- *Juniperus communis* (fruct.)
- *Lavandula angustifolia*
- *Lavandula × intermedia* 'Super'
- *Melaleuca viridiflora*
- *Ocimum basilicum* var. *album*
- *Origanum majorana*
- *Pelargonium graveolens*
- *Thymus vulgaris* ct. geraniol [SWEET THYME]
- *Thymus vulgaris* ct. thymol [RED THYME].

1. Agitation
- *Citrus aurantium* var. *amara* (flos)
- *Citrus aurantium* var. *amara* (per.)
- *Citrus bergamia*
- *Cupressus sempervirens*
- *Lavandula angustifolia*
- *Lavandula × intermedia* 'Super'
- *Melissa officinalis*
- *Origanum majorana*
- *Pelargonium graveolens*
- *Thymus vulgaris* ct. geraniol.

2. Emotional instability
- *Citrus aurantium* var. *amara* (flos)
- *Citrus aurantium* var. *amara* (fol.)
- *Melissa officinalis*
- *Origanum majorana*
- *Pelargonium graveolens*.

3. Fatigue
- *Coriandrum sativum*
- *Cupressus sempervirens*
- *Ocimum basilicum* var. *album*.

4. Headaches and migraines
- *Chamaemelum nobile*
- *Citrus limon* (per.)
- *Lavandula angustifolia*
- *Lavandula × intermedia* 'Super'
- *Melissa officinalis*
- *Mentha × piperita*—digestive
- *Ocimum basilicum* var. *album*—nervous
- *Origanum majorana*—congestive and menstrual
- *Pelargonium graveolens*—congestive.

5. Hypertension
- *Cananga odorata*
- *Citrus limon* (per.)
- *Lavandula angustifolia*

- *Lavandula × intermedia* 'Super'
- *Ocimum basilicum* var. *album*
- *Origanum majorana*
- *Melaleuca viridiflora*.

6. Inability to concentrate, loss of energy (mental and physical)
- *Citrus limon* (per.)
- *Coriandrum sativum*.

7. Indigestion
- *Citrus aurantium* var. *amara* (per.)
- *Citrus reticulata* (per.)
- *Melaleuca viridiflora*
- *Melissa officinalis*.

8. Insomnia
- *Cananga odorata*
- *Chamaemelum nobile*
- *Citrus aurantium* var. *amara* (flos, fol., per.)
- *Citrus bergamia* (per.)
- *Citrus limon* (per.)
- *Citrus reticulata* (per.)
- *Coriandrum sativum*
- *Cupressus sempervirens*
- *Juniperus communis*
- *Lavandula angustifolia*
- *Lavandula × intermedia* 'Super'
- *Melissa officinalis*
- *Ocimum basilicum* var. *album*
- *Origanum majorana*.

9. Irritability
- *Boswellia carteri*
- *Chamaemelum nobile*
- *Citrus aurantium* var. *amara* (fol.)
- *Citrus aurantium* var. *amara* (per.)
- *Citrus bergamia* (per.)
- *Citrus reticulata* (per.)
- *Cupressus sempervirens*
- *Juniperus communis* (fruct.)
- *Lavandula angustifolia*
- *Origanum majorana*
- *Pelargonium graveolens*.

10. Low immunity
- *Boswellia carteri*
- *Melaleuca viridiflora*
- *Origanum majorana*.

11. Muscle tension (mainly neck and shoulders)
- *Chamaemelum nobile*
- *Juniperus communis*
- *Lavandula angustifolia*
- *Lavandula × intermedia* 'Super'
- *Origanum majorana*
- *Eucalyptus smithii* [GULLY GUM] can be added to increase the synergy of any mix (Pénoël 1994).

12. Nightmares
- *Boswellia carteri*
- *Citrus limon*
- *Melissa officinalis*.

13. Sadness
- *Boswellia carteri*
- *Citrus aurantium* var. *amara* (fol.)
- *Citrus reticulata* (per.)
- *Melaleuca viridiflora*.

Combination of essential oils

Although more than four suitable essential oils may be found, the choice should be restricted to three or four. Once chosen, it is advisable and time-saving to to make up a dropper bottle of the essential oils, which should be labelled and used in whichever method is thought most appropriate (see Ch. 5). The relative proportions of each essential oil should be influenced by the aroma preferences of the patient concerned.

Practical examples

The method of selecting and combining essential oils described above is illustrated by the following examples.

Depression due to grief, with nightmares. *Boswellia carteri* is the only common denominator, therefore half the number of drops used should be of this oil. *Melissa officinalis* would be a good second oil, to relieve both the nightmares and the depression.

Depression, with headaches and insomnia. *Chamaemelum nobile, Lavandula officinalis, Origanum majorana.* If the immune system is felt to be low, *Origanum majorana* should be present in the highest proportion in the mix. Should the aroma need adjusting, select any other essential oil from the antidepressive range.

Case 10.2 Aromatherapist: Sandra Agnew, Australia

A 58-year-old male was admitted to hospital on 25 November 1993 in a semi-comatose state after a drinking session, diagnosed as alcoholic cirrhosis of the liver. Clinical signs were disorientation, extreme jaundice, indicated by his eyes (which were bright yellow), distorted and puffy facial features, bloated abdomen and uncontrollable tremors. Biochemical and haematological pathology tests showed grossly impaired liver function, e.g. enzyme 60 times greater than normal values. The family was informed by the Medical Officer that due to the severity of his conditions he was unlikely to survive.

2 days after admittance he was lucid and uncomfortable, apathetic and immobile. His skin was flaky and extremely itchy, especially arms and legs. He was given valium and diuretics to sedate and get rid of excess fluid, and consequently he was drowsy, but aware of his surroundings and recognizing family. The tremors had diminished considerably and he was agitated and worried about his condition.

His daughter, a regular client of mine, approached me to see if aromatherapy was a possibility. I contacted the Medical Officer who confirmed the prognosis and willingly gave permission for an aromatherapy massage, implying that any treatment would be beneficial.

His daughter was shown some basic massage techniques and began massaging daily starting 28 November. After 2 days he commented that he was sleeping soundly because the itchiness was relieved, previously the itch had been waking him. On 10 December the pathology tests were repeated: the liver enzymes, although still elevated, were decreasing and coagulation studies were normal. His mental attitude was greatly improved and he was enthusiastic about the daily massage to the extent that visitors were asked to massage his hands, legs and feet. Mobility and appetite were improving and he wanted to go home.

The following oil blend was used in an almond and avocado oil as a carrier base (for quick penetration and skin healing properties): Roman chamomile (calming to CNS, liver stimulant, relieves pruritus), frankincense (uplifts, soothes, aids digestion), lavender (relieves anxiety, stimulates cell renewal), rosemary (liver decongestant, activates metabolism, stimulates nervous system), clary (calms CNS, panic state, helps withdrawal symptoms of alcohol, strengthens immune system).

He was discharged from hospital on 20 December into the care of his family who continued the daily massage with essential oils. Biochemical test on 5 January 1994 showed liver function to be almost normal. The patient looks and feels well, is in great spirits, eating well and generally enjoying life.

Anxiety, with emotional instability and insomnia. *Citrus aurantium* var. *amara* (flos), *Citrus aurantium* var. *amara* (fol.), *Melissa officinalis*, *Origanum majorana*.

Anxiety with agitation, and high blood pressure. *Cananga odorata*, *Lavandula angustifolia*, *Lavandula* × *intermedia* 'Super', *Origanum majorana*.

Anxiety with agitation, and indigestion. *Citrus aurantium* var. *amara* (per.), *Melissa officinalis*. Should a third oil be desired, one may be selected for whichever symptom is strongest.

Low immunity, with sadness, high blood pressure and indigestion. The only common denominator here is *Melaleuca viridiflora*, which should be present in the mix in the highest proportion. *Origanum majorana* can help to control the hypertension and stimulate the immune system. *Boswellia carteri* uplifts, easing sadness and stimulating the immune system.

Summary

This chapter has examined the phenomenon of stress in modern life, and the role essential oils can play in reducing its effects. Gonella's 1991 trial project clearly demonstrates that massage with essential oils can significantly reduce stress levels in the patients of GPs. The guide presented here to the selection and combination of stress-reducing oils is intended to enable readers to choose and administer appropriate oils for their patients, with a view to achieving similarly beneficial results.

REFERENCES

Franchomme P, Pénoël D 1990 L'aromathérapie exactement. Jollois, Limoges
Gonella J 1993 Stress and aromatherapy trial project. Unpublished paper
Harrison L, Skinner R 1992 Relax for health. Nursing Times 88(49): 46–47
Kirk P 1993 Anxiety, stress and depression. What are the alternatives in the Health Service? Unpublished paper
Krieger D 1979 The therapeutic touch. Simon and Schuster, New York

Passant H 1990 A holistic approach in the ward. Nursing Times 86(4): 26–28
Price S 1993 The aromatherapy workbook. Thorsons, London
Roulier G 1990 Les huiles essentielles pour votre santé. Dangles, St-Jean-de-Braye
Selye H 1956 The stress of life. McGraw Hill, New York
Wingate P, Wingate R 1988 Medical encyclopedia. Penguin, London
Worwood V 1990 Fragrant pharmacy. Macmillan, London p. 109

11

Intensive and coronary care

Introduction

This chapter presents the results of several clinical trials which show the value of essential oils in significantly reducing patient stress-levels in coronary and intensive-care contexts. The treatment of severe burns with essential oils is briefly discussed, illustrated by anecdotal evidence. It is suggested that further studies to corroborate this evidence should be undertaken.

LIFE-THREATENING SITUATIONS

It is difficult to talk generally about the use of aromatherapy in intensive care, because the reasons for needing it are many and often sudden—breathing difficulties, lung viruses (see Case 11.1), strokes, heart attacks, heart surgery, road accidents, etc.

Many factors need to be addressed when looking after the intensive-care patient. These include the possibility of further invasive infections, and the severe stress experienced by patients and relatives. Factors such as these respond to aromatherapy, used now in many intensive- and coronary-care wards throughout Britain.

The overriding concern of the aromatherapist in these environments is patient stress, because 'anxiety can precipitate life threatening arrhythmia and extend infarction areas, if not allayed quickly enough' (Harris 1993). Patients' anxieties have been found to be centred on their personal illness rather than on the hospital surroundings (Rowe 1989), and even though frequent nursing reassurances may prevent intimidation by the

Case 11.1 Aromatherapist: Elizabeth Sonn, UK

Suddenly, my father, normally fit and healthy, was taken seriously ill overnight with an unknown lung virus. He was rushed to hospital, put on a life support machine and the family was told it was only a matter of time!

After 3 days I suddenly awoke to the fact that if the hospital would allow it, I might be able to help. I approached the consultant, who was amazed that I had not spoken up before, and he agreed that I could do whatever was needed.

For the first 2 days I used 2 drops each of eucalyptus and benzoin (in about a teaspoonful of grapeseed oil) for his lung congestion, rubbing it onto his chest wherever the life support equipment would allow! The reflex points on his feet were massaged, using the Swiss reflex method and concentrating mainly on the lung and lymph areas. This was accompanied by gentle music to help relax the mind and balance the emotions. Peace and a wonderful aroma emanated from the room.

Mother did not go unprotected either. She received a massage of lavender and marjoram for her aching legs, emotional exhaustion and stress, and jasmine to give her the courage needed. A mix of Bach Flower remedies were taken also.

I continued to massage my father in the Intensive Therapy Unit at every available time. After 3 days tea tree was added to assist with the viral infection. X-rays taken on the 4th day showed a slight improvement. The doctors and nursing staff were impressed, and such was their interest, that their support increased—along with their curiosity regarding aromatherapy.

2 days later, following a couple of nasty scares, hyssop was added to Father's treatment to help normalize the fluctuating blood pressure. Improvement continued.

1 week later the consultant thought that my father would survive, but that the oxygen level had to be down to 35% before they would remove him from the life-support machine, and this would be a critical phase of his recovery. It could take up to a couple of weeks and at this stage there was a possibility that he would react by panic, fear and irritability. I changed the oils for this point in his recovery: jasmine (confidence booster), rosemary (for clear thinking) and clary (calming). Bach Flower 'Rescue Remedy' was used between his lips.

Within 2 hours of removal from the machine, Father was sitting up. The medical staff remarked with amazement at his speedy recovery. He was removed from the intensive therapy unit within 24 hours and was home within a fortnight, although the prediction had been 8–10 weeks. Once home the massage with essential oils, Swiss reflex treatment and music were gradually stopped. Within 3 months Father was once more to be seen playing golf and swimming a couple of times a week, none the worse for his traumatic experience.

high-tech environment, their state of mind can be calmed further by the use of essential oils. The clinical trials which follow show the effectiveness of aromatherapy in coronary and intensive-care contexts. However, the authors are concerned that only common names are given for the oils used in most studies and trials, especially when there are so many varieties of 'chamomile', 'eucalyptus' and 'lavender', for instance. Full botanical identification is essential if such trials are to be taken seriously.

Trial studies

BATTLE HOSPITAL, READING

Chrissy Dunn, a senior nurse at Battle Hospital, Reading, began to explore massage as a means 'to help patients immobilised by drugs and equipment to relax' (Waller 1991). Under her direction, Patricia Tseng, a nurse trained in aromatherapy, carried out a clinical trial in an intensive-care situation to discover whether essential oils could reduce stress levels of critically-ill patients. It was observed, via the monitors, that the heart and respiration rates of patients slowed down to normal levels, with a similar effect on high blood pressure. It would seem therefore that therapeutic touch with essential oils can sometimes be all that is needed to bring relief from mild pain or discomfort, avoiding the use of chemical analgesia or heavy sedation (Tseng 1991).

ROYAL SUSSEX COUNTY HOSPITAL

Trials were carried out at the Royal Sussex County Hospital early in 1992 (Woolfson & Hewitt 1992) showing that foot massage with essential oil of lavender (botanical name not given) could lower the blood pressure, heart and respiratory rates of people in intensive care. Two treatments a week were given for 5 weeks to patients in both intensive- and coronary-care units. All treatments were given at the same time of day and observations recorded at the beginning, end and 30 minutes after each session.

The trial, carried out by Woolfson and Hewitt, consisted of three groups, each of 12 people, receiving treatment as follows:

- Group 1: 20-minute massage using lavender in a vegetable oil

- Group 2: 20-minute massage using only vegetable oil
- Group 3: 20-minute undisturbed rest period only.

The results showed a consistent decrease in blood pressure, heart rate, pain, respiratory rate and wakefulness in all three groups, with the greatest benefits experienced by patients in Group 1 (see Table 11.1).

Table 11.1 Number and percentage of patients experiencing reductions in physiological stress indicators after: massage with lavender (Group 1); massage alone (Group 2); undisturbed rest (Group 3)

Reduction in:	Group 1 % (No.)	Group 2 % (No.)	Group 3 % (No.)
Heart rate	91.6 (11)	58.3 (7)	41.6 (5)
Pain	50.0 (6)	41.6 (5)	16.6 (2)
Blood pressure	50.0 (6)	41.6 (5)	16.6 (2)
Respiratory rate	75.0 (9)	41.6 (5)	16.6 (2)
Wakefulness	50.0 (6)	33.3 (4)	25.0 (3)

Averaging the totals in Table 11.1, the overall benefits to each group were as follows:

- Group 1: 63.32%
- Group 2: 43.28%
- Group 3: 22.85%.

This trial bears out the theory that although massage alone is beneficial, the greatest benefits in all areas tested here are experienced when essential oils are used as well.

LONDON MIDDLESEX HOSPITAL

A similar trial to the one carried out at the Royal Sussex County Hospital (see above) was undertaken in 1992 (Stevensen 1994) at the London Middlesex Hospital. Intensive-care patients were given foot massage using *Citrus aurantium* var. *aurantium* (flos) [NEROLI BIGARADE]. Neroli was chosen for its calming, antispasmodic, antidepressant and gentle sedative actions. It also has antiseptic qualities and there are no known contraindications to its use in physiological doses.

The trial consisted of four groups of 25 cardiac patients in intensive care. They all fulfilled the following criteria:

- only requiring oxygen through a mask
- no mechanical blood pressure support

- not receiving cardiac pacing during time of procedure
- be English speaking (for speedy communication) and with regard to the feet:
- no pedal arterial line for blood pressure monitoring
- no suppurating or infected skin conditions.

Each patient was given an information sheet and a consent form to sign. The treatment received by each group was as follows:

- Group 1: 20-minute standardized foot massage with 2. 5% neroli in apricot kernel vegetable oil
- Group 2: 20-minute standardized foot massage using only the apricot kernel oil
- Group 3: 20-minute conversation with a nurse, without tactile input or formal counselling
- Group 4: 20-minute period with routine care, but without intervention of any kind.

Each group was assessed physiologically and psychologically 5 times the day after cardiac surgery (referred to as day 1) and again 4 days later (referred to as day 5). The physiological measurements were heart rate, respiratory rate and blood pressure. To assess both positive and negative aspects of the patients' psychological state, a modified Spielberger questionnaire was given, verbally on the day 1, with a written one on day 5. The negative aspects were pain, anxiety, tension; the positive ones, calm, rest, relaxation. The four options for patients' replies were: not at all, slightly, moderately, very.

Additional questions asked the subjects to relate:

- their perception of the massage
- its benefits to date (if any)
- the length of time they perceived the duration of the effects to have lasted, over the 4-day period
- comments on the frequency and timing of the massage
- suggestions regarding future or added treatments
- other comments.

Five assessments took place on day 1 at the following times:

- 1 hour before the intervention period
- immediately before the 20-minute intervention period
- immediately after the intervention period
- 1 hour after the intervention period
- 2 hours after the intervention period.

Results

The physiological results showed statistically significant differences between Groups 1 and 2 and the two control Groups 3 and 4 in the respiratory rates immediately after the intervention. No difference was seen at the next measurement period.

The psychological results were as follows:

- On day 1, Groups 1 and 2 had statistically significantly better psychological results than the control groups, 3 and 4.
- On day 5, there was a significant difference in psychological benefits between Groups 1 & 2. 82% of Groups 1 & 2 remembered having the massage and all of these had found it beneficial. Group 1 had a marked reduction in anxiety compared to Group 2, but the perceived difference in pain reduction between the two groups was minimal. Group 1 found the effects more relaxing, restful and calming than Group 2 and, generally, found the effects to be longer lasting.

This trial shows that touch and massage give positive psychological results to patients in intensive care. It also confirms the findings of the Royal Sussex County Hospital's trials that while massage alone is beneficial, massage *with* essential oils gives enhanced and longer-lasting effects.

ROYAL SHREWSBURY HOSPITAL

Most of the recorded uses of aromatherapy in intensive care are concerned with heart surgery, and another such study was carried out in 1992 at the Royal Shrewsbury Hospital, on the effectiveness of essential oils in reducing the anxiety level of patients admitted to the Coronary Care Unit, and afterwards in the Post-Coronary Care Ward (Harris 1993).

In this study, the method used was inhalation of plant oils from an electric vaporizer. Patients were monitored on admission, 12 hours later, and then prior to discharge to the post-coronary care ward. There were four groups of five people, three groups each being given a single essential oil chosen from lavender, ylang ylang and the absolute of jasmine respectively, the fourth being a control group, inhaling water vapour only. The trial took place over a 4-week period and results were obtained by questionnaire. One person in each of Groups 2 and 4 did not return the questionnaire.

The reduction in anxiety experienced by patients was as follows (number of patients shown in brackets):

- Group 1: 60% (3 out of 5)
- Group 2: 75% (3 out of 4)
- Group 3: 80% (4 out of 5)
- Group 4: 25% (1 out of 4).

Of the 14 people receiving essential oils who returned the questionnaire, 10 (71.4%) experienced a reduction in anxiety. All patients showed a lowering of blood pressure from their initial admission levels and within 12 hours of the study.

Harris contends that 'though a significant drop in blood pressure was noted on the majority of patients, this cannot be wholly attributed to the inhalation of essential oils'. However, even with such small groups, the results appear to show that some benefit was gained.

The Royal Shrewsbury Hospital trial described above shows that positive results can be obtained by inhalation of essential oils without massage. A further trial would determine whether neroli, administered by massage in the London Middlesex Hospital trial, can give 100% reduction in stress levels by inhalation only. Our expectation is that it would. Such a trial would prove interesting, more so if it were to use the three oils employed in the Shrewsbury Hospital and with 20–25 people in each group, as in the Middlesex Hospital trial. A trial of this type would give a fuller picture of the efficacy of essential oils in the reduction of anxiety in an intensive-care situation.

Severe burns

Essential oils can also be used to treat emotional shock and to minimize the risk of infection. This is especially so in the case of severe burns. Damaged tissue is a good incubator for bacteria, and essential oils can play a potentially life-saving role in such cases by sanitizing the micro-environment.

In 1988 essential oils were used in intensive care for a woman with extensive severe burns at the University College Hospital, London (Price 1989). The authors blended oils to be vaporized in her room, to keep the air aseptic. The oils selected were *Pinus sylvestris* [SCOTCH PINE], *Citrus limon* [LEMON], and *Eucalyptus globulus* [BLUE GUM]. *Lavandula angustifolia* [LAVENDER] and *Boswellia carteri* [FRANKINCENSE] were supplied in a base oil for areas of the body which could be touched. Essential oils were put into a regenerative cream base (containing unspecified plant extracts) for use on the patient's face and neck burns. These, although not as seriously affected as other parts of her body, were of great concern for the once-attractive female patient. She not only survived, but the skin on her chest (the worst-affected area) became more elastic and supple than the consultant had thought possible (Parkhouse 1988 personal communication).

Summary

The research studies presented in this chapter clearly demonstrate the efficacy of essential oils in significantly reducing patient stress levels in coronary and intensive-care contexts. It is interesting to note that both the inhalation of oils and different forms of massage with them produce beneficial results. Further studies that directly compared the efficacy of different methods of administration would be welcomed. The evidence regarding the efficacy of essential oils in the treatment of severe burns, though powerful, is still largely anecdotal. Proper clinical studies in this field are needed to corroborate the existing evidence.

REFERENCES

Harris C M 1993 Is there a benefit to patients in using aromatherapy oils in a coronary care unit? Pilot study results. Copies available from The Royal Shrewsbury Hospital

Price S 1989 Essential oils in a burns unit. Aromanews 16: 4

Rowe L 1989 Anxiety in a coronary care unit. Nursing Times 85(45): 61

Stevensen C J 1994 The psychophysical effects of aromatherapy massage following cardiac surgery. Complementary Therapies in Medicine 2: 27–35

Tseng P 1991 Personal profile. International Journal of Aromatherapy 3(2): 10–11

Waller M 1991 The healing touch in an age of technology. The Independent. October

Woolfson A, Hewitt D 1992 Intensive aromacare. The International Journal of Aromatherapy 4(2): 12–13

12

Care of the elderly

Introduction

Some of the greatest benefits to both patient and carers come from the use of essential oils with the elderly, since quality of life is improved for all concerned. Studies are presented which show definite reductions in the need for medication for sleep disturbances in settings where aromatherapy has been tried. Treatments for a variety of conditions often associated with old age are given, with particular reference to rheumatology.

THE EVE OF LIFE

Care of the elderly has always been regarded as one of the least glamorous sides of nursing. It is also one of the richest areas of care, and can make the difference between a winter of discontent or an Indian summer.

Aromatherapy enhances the holistic framework in caring for elderly persons: I find a number of cases where they are not at peace with themselves, the reason being a lot of unfinished business within themselves and their family. The psychological pain this generates, at times causes these physical symptoms to be uncontrolled, despite the use of orthodox medicine. Combine the two, orthodox and complementary, and the outcome is what is termed ideal for patient and carer. Families who sit with loved ones, or not so loved ones, are at a loss what to say and what to do. The three simple words 'I love you' or 'I am sorry' are at times difficult for them to say. At this juncture touch is encouraged as a form of communication and with this communication, essential oils are used.

(Tattam 1992)

Case 12.1   Aromatherapist: Sue Cook, Australia

The nursing home houses 21 residents with varying degrees of senile dementia, as well as the degenerative physical conditions and limited or no mobility that is apparent with many elderly persons. The staff at the home are relaxed in their approach and aim to create an atmosphere of a home environment for all the patients. Medication is kept to a minimum and an activities coordinator is involved with the patients every weekday for group and one-to-one sessions. Family and friends are welcome to participate in the care-giving at any time and as often as possible.

The director of nursing was to choose the patients who would benefit from the type of care Incare offers, and access to medical files and nursing and consultants' notes was given for all patients. Eight were chosen and I would be spending 10–15 minutes with each individual during a 2-hour weekly visit. I decided to use only one essential oil to start with—to prevent confusion, to gather detailed results and acquaint the staff and residents with the benefits of each oil as it was introduced. The blend used was 2.5% dilution of *Lavandula officinalis* in sweet almond oil.

The areas to be worked upon were mutually agreed: hands, feet, shoulders, face etc. Those that were bedridden generally received foot-massage as a means of stimulating circulation there.

The observations after 10 weeks were positive. Lavender was vaporized in a ceramic vaporizer all day and into the evening. The staff enjoy the pleasant fragrance and the oil masked the constant odour of urine. The staff reported back on the pleasant environment the vaporized essential oil creates, both for themselves, the visitors and mainly for the residents.

Of the patients receiving weekly treatment, all have responded to greater or lesser degrees to the aroma, the contact and the one-to-one communication. A reduction in emotional outbursts has been noted for those that are disturbed or disruptive, both during the day and during the night. Recognition of both the oil and the treatment is acknowledged by the majority of the patients. All responded positively to the contact, finding an increase in mobility and decrease in pain. Some individual reactions are reported below.

a   TM: Severe Alzheimer's with emotional disturbances
Had required an increase in night medication due to nocturnal disturbance. TM's partner spends 4 hours per day in physical exercise and social contact, and when the partner was not there, TM exhibited aggressive verbal abuse of other residents. TM showed decreased ability to remember short-term events and seemed to have difficulty recognizing people.

After 10 weeks of aromatherapy, the emotional disturbances had decreased dramatically, nocturnal disruption has ceased after using the lavender on TM's pillow. I was greeted recently by TM using my first name and giving me compliments.

b   JR: Alcohol-induced dementia, blind, reduced mobility
With no family, friends or relatives interested in visiting, JR had regressed to internalization, with little communication or interest in others around. Within 2–3 sessions with JR his severe depression seemed to disappear, with an increase in conversation, attention to surroundings and interaction with other residents.

c   OC: Senile dementia, lives in the past, very confused
Initially OC was reluctant to allow contact or even to converse with a stranger. OC now looks forward to the weekly sessions and jokes about family and events of the past. Conversation is more coherent and recently, through the massage session, OC will massage my hands.

Helen Passant, now retired, was one of the first nurses to introduce massage into a hospital, shortly after she became sister of what was then called the geriatric ward at the Churchill Hospital, Oxford in the 1980s. It soon became apparent to her that with massage the patients' skin became stronger and more resistant to bruising and tissue damage.

Later, essential oils were introduced into the vegetable oil the nurses were using, and it was found that the added benefits of these enabled the conventional sedative drugs to be reduced. Other effects were soon noticed and, through the support of the consultant and the professor of geriatric medicine, herbal and essential oil remedies were included on the drug charts. She found that therapeutic touch and essential oils benefit and can uplift both patients and nurses, giving the latter a more satisfying role. It can open the doors to a closer relationship, 'allowing patients to speak of their dreams and hopes, of their fears and pleasures. To relieve stress and pain on all levels was something I had not thought possible—but it is' (Passant 1990).

Mark Hardy, working with the elderly mentally ill at The Old Manor Hospital, Salisbury, expressed his concern regarding the 'almost habitual way in which night medication is prescribed' (Hardy 1991). Although not every patient experiences side-effects (notably ataxia, confusion and constipation plus other unwanted effects such as dry mouth and incontinence due to abnormally deep sleep), the use of certain essential oils can induce sleep easily. In many cases there is no need for hypnotics, or a reduced dose only. Many of the other side-effects can be alleviated with essential oils.

Dr Park, director of ITU at Addenbrooke Hospital states that aromatherapy has helped to reduce the need for expensive sedation and painkilling drugs on account of the relief obtained from constipation and general aches and pains by the application of this therapy (Macdonald 1993).

Dosage for the elderly

When determining the dosage of essential oils to be used, the weight, age and health (both mental and physical) of the person should always be taken into account (Price 1993b p. 154). With children, and older people whose bodily systems have begun to slow down, only half the normal concentration of essential oils is needed, i.e. 12–15 drops per 100 ml of carrier oil or lotion. The exact number of drops is rarely crucial (except where internal use is concerned) and is usually given as a range. For patients who need to use the oils over a long period of time, it is best to keep to the lower end of the range. *Eucalyptus smithii* [GULLY GUM] is one of the exceptions to this rule as it is extremely gentle in action and should always be used in preference to *E. globulus* [TASMANIAN BLUE GUM] on elderly and children alike (see respiratory section below).

As in all use of essential oils, synergy within and between essential oils is an important consideration (see Ch. 3). Two oils are always more effective than one and up to four oils, when selected with knowledge, can be even more so. Each person is an individual, and one essential oil may not have the required effect on everyone—as with drugs, where one brand is not necessarily appropriate for each person.

TREATMENT OF SPECIFIC CONDITIONS

Circulation

Case 12.2 Aromatherapists: Eleni Hajisava and Mary Ann Gardner, Australia

Hajisava and Gardner visit Lara Lodge in Oakleigh which provides special accommodation for men. The residents are elderly, and a number of them are former alcoholics. They concentrate on foot treatments, using footbaths and massage.

a
A man with a past history of a stroke, had poor circulation to his feet and tended to develop gangrenous spots on his toes. These spots had to be surgically removed when they appeared. He was given footbaths using essential oil of pine, and his feet were massaged with a blend of niaouli for its antiseptic effect. Since starting weekly treatments no further spots have occurred.

b
This man was very immobile and as a result had such poor circulation to his lower extremities that his legs were blue. He was given footbaths using lavender (occasionally with small amounts of rosemary) and mandarin for its antispasmodic effect. As a result the circulation to his legs and feet has been very much improved.

Another benefit to these elderly men who otherwise tend to be isolated, is that these Incare visits give them an opportunity to get together as a group. When Hajisava and Gardner arrive, the residents gravitate to the day room, evidently looking forward to their treatments.

Digestive disorders

Currently, the aromatherapy organizations do not allow their members to give essential oils internally. This is frustrating to many aromatherapists, because complaints involving the digestive system often respond more rapidly to ingestion. In the UK the Aromatology Association (linked to the European body VEROMA) gives insurance for internal use (see Useful Addresses), and studies in aromatology (in addition to an accredited aromatherapy course) need to be taken to qualify for this insurance.

If adequately qualified and suitably insured to prescribe and administer essential oils internally in accordance with the protocol, 8 drops in total of the selected essential oils should be well mixed into 50 ml of vegetable oil or liquid honey and 1 teaspoonful of the mixture administered three times a day, or morning and night depending on the needs of the patient/client. Suppositories for the elderly should contain no more than 2 drops of essential oils.

The essential oils suggested for each digestive condition below may be:

- administered internally, per os diluted as above, or per rectum in a suppository
- applied to the abdomen in a carrier lotion or oil
- massaged into the abdomen.

Should a consultant or doctor disapprove or be wary of using essential oils to treat anything but stress and anxiety, select those essential oils from the suggestions which are recommended also for stress relief (see Ch. 10 and relevant Appendices).

Constipation

Many elderly people suffer from constipation, often as a result of medication taken or a poor, or over-refined diet. Despite the best efforts of the nutritionists even younger people in hospital can become constipated due to a change in environment. As with everything, constipation should be treated in a holistic fashion, endeavouring to discover the cause, and treatment should include regulating the diet.

Essential oils can be effective for constipated patients when used with massage of the abdomen and/or the feet. With the feet, the area to concentrate on is the soft tissue just below the level of the sesamoid bones and above the calcaneus, on the plantar surface of the foot. If not trained in Swiss Reflex treatment (see Ch. 6) or reflexology, start with the right foot and massage in large firm circles directed from the lateral to the medial side; the left foot should then be massaged in firm circles directed from the medial to the lateral side. This directional massage of the colon reflexes, with pressure, helps peristalsis, as does movement 3 of Abdomen massage, carried out firmly and slowly with the heel of the hand (see Ch. 6).

Case 12.3 Aromatherapist: Jeanette Langhamer RGN, UK

This case history took place at a private nursing home in Hull as part of a project to see the difference aromatherapy could make to some of the clients there. It was conducted with the consent and backing of the client's family and the doctor in charge.

K suffers from Alzheimer's disease, which started 3 years ago and she has been blind for 6 years. She also suffered a stroke 5 years ago which left her with a right-sided weakness. Although K has periods of aggression followed by times of normality, she is a delight to care for and has a lot to contribute towards society. She loves music and can recall the words of songs long forgotten by most people. However, she has many problems, for as well as the Alzheimer's disease, she suffers from insomnia, chronic constipation and loss of appetite, among other discomforts.

On my first visit we spent the time in the home's garden as I wanted to give K the opportunity to smell some flowers. Afterwards, over a cup of tea, I introduced her to the essential oils and we had a 'sniffing session'. She instantly recognized the fragrance of rose so we decided, whatever else we would use, rose would be one of the oils in the blend for the massage.

Armed with her favourite music hall tape I gave K her first massage. She loved every minute of the experience and sang all the words to the songs during her massage! I asked for K to be given a nightly bath containing 5 drops of lavender plus 1 or 2 drops of the same oil to be sprinkled on her pillow before going to bed. She enjoyed a tot of whisky, so I suggested that this, together with the bath and pillow use of lavender, be given—eventually instead of her temazepam medication, which was reduced gradually. She was eager to receive this more acceptable nightcap.

I mixed some base cream with a few drops of *Lavandula angustifolia*, to be applied to her forehead when she became aggressive and the nursing staff observed and documented the reactions. The baths and lavender on the pillow were a daily treatment, the massage treatments being conducted on a weekly basis. After 8 weeks she was almost off temazepam; after 12 weeks it was completely stopped with no adverse reactions.

The results up to date are that K's life is much improved and happier. Her right side is stronger now, with more mobility, the constipation problem is under control due to the abdominal massages, the insomnia has been almost eradicated and she responds well to the lavender cream on her forehead.

Each time K heard my voice, she started to get ready for her massage and although blind, she very much enjoyed the oils through her sense of smell, which in turn provoked happy memories from the past. K, her family and all the nursing staff, including the doctor, all feel this has become a worthwhile project.

The most effective oils for constipation are: *Citrus aurantium* var. *amara* (per.) [ORANGE BIGARADE], *Rosmarinus officinalis* [ROSEMARY] (camphor and cineole chemotypes), *Ocimum basilicum* var. *album* [EUROPEAN BASIL], *Piper nigrum* [BLACK PEPPER], *Zingiber officinale* [GINGER].

The last is cited for constipation by Franchomme & Pénoël (1990 p. 406) and for diarrhoea by Valnet (1980 p. 135). Like *Foeniculum vulgare* var. *dulce* [FENNEL], it may be a balancing oil in this direction.

Diarrhoea

This condition can sometimes be just as upsetting to a patient as constipation, and in this case, and where the diarrhoea is of nervous origin, the tranquillizing effect of *Origanum majorana* [SWEET MARJORAM] is effective, together with antiinflammatory oils such as *Melaleuca viridiflora* [NIAOULI], *Mentha × piperita* [PEPPERMINT] (which in addition, will help against nausea) and *Pelargonium graveolens* [GERANIUM]—this last oil is also tranquillizing. These antiinflammatory oils are also useful for colitis and gastro-enteritis, whilst *Syzygium aromaticum* (flos) [CLOVE BUD], *Pimpinella anisum* [ANISEED], *Melaleuca cajuputi* [CAJUPUT] and *Myristica fragrans* [NUTMEG] relieve the spasms (Valnet 1980 pp. 114, 95, 101, 161).

Diverticulitis (diverticulosis)

Diverticulosis, the harmless presence of small bulges in weak points in the large intestine, exists in most elderly people (Wingate & Wingate 1988 p. 147). It is only when one or more of these diverticula becomes inflamed that chronic diverticulitis can set in and constipation, slight abdominal pain and bleeding may manifest. The diet should be changed to one rich in fibre, and massage with the antiinflammatory essential oils (under Diarrhoea above) would be beneficial, with those effective for constipation incorporated where necessary, such as *Citrus aurantium* var. *amara* (per.), which is also antiinflammatory.

Other antiinflammatory oils which act on the digestive system are *Commiphora myrrha* [MYRRH]

Case 12.4 Aromatherapist: Robert Nancarrow, Australia

An elderly woman at the Queen Elizabeth Centre, Ballarat, was unable to open her bowels due to atrophy of the large intestine (colon), and required admission to hospital every 3 weeks for a colonic washout. Doctors were planning to perform a total colectomy (surgical removal of the large intestine), which would have left the woman with a colostomy.

I made a blend of fennel, patchouli, sandalwood and black pepper in vegetable oil, and this blend was massaged gently into the woman's abdomen several times that evening. Next morning she had a normal bowel action. Ongoing care consists of daily abdominal massages and an oral aperient nightly. Other staff members have been taught how to do this massage so that it can be performed daily and not just when I am on duty. Best of all, the woman's bowels are opened regularly, and surgery has been avoided.

(distilled only), *Chamomilla recutita* [GERMAN CHAMOMILE], *Juniperus communis* (fruct.) [JUNIPER] and *Melissa officinalis* [MELISSA].

Indigestion (dyspepsia)

Chronic indigestion can be due to many causes. Common physical reasons, if there is no gastritis or ulcer present, may be eating too quickly, too much or swallowing air with the food. Medication or heavy smoking may also be responsible (Wingate & Wingate 1988 p. 256) In many cases stress can be implicated and this should be treated as well, by abdominal and/or foot massage with relaxing essential oils 30 minutes before a meal.

As a preventive measure and to help those who are eating incorrectly (e.g. too fast, poor diet), 1 teaspoonful from a mix of digestive oils in a vegetable oil (see above for quantities) taken 15 minutes before a meal would be an effective measure. If this is not possible, then the abdomen should be massaged with the same mix 30 minutes before the meal. *Carum carvi* [CARAWAY], *Citrus aurantium* var. *amara* (per), *Foeniculum vulgare* var. *dulce* and *Pimpinella anisum* are the most effective oils. *Ocimum basilicum* var. *album* can be added if the indigestion is of nervous origin and *Origanum majorana* if gastritis or an ulcer are present.

To ease indigestion once present, the same oils can be used. Also effective at this stage are *Citrus reticulata* [MANDARIN], *Citrus limon* (per.) [LEMON] (analgesic and antacid), *Melissa officinalis*, *Mentha × piperita* and *Rosmarinus officinalis* (camphor and cineole chemotypes).

Headaches and migraines

These can occur for a number of reasons which are not always apparent, especially in the elderly. Because of this, it is important to make use of the synergy between essential oils and mix two or more together.

The oil most often used to combat headaches and migraine is *Lavandula angustifolia*. Equally effective are *Chamaemelum nobile*, *Mentha × piperita*, *Ocimum basilicum*, *Origanum majorana* and *Rosmarinus officinalis*. The choice of oil may depend on the cause, for example *Mentha × piperita* works well on a headache caused by digestive disorders.

Inhalation from a tissue (or other means—see Ch. 5) gives the speediest reaction, though massage of the neck and face, particularly the forehead (using two or three of the above oils in a carrier oil), gives the patient the additional relaxing and soothing benefits of massage. Anyone not fully qualified in massage should limit this to gentle strokes with the whole hand, as described in Chapter 6.

Pressure sores

This is an area where traditional medicine has limited success, and nurses using aromatherapy have been rewarded by the healing which has occurred with the use of essential oils.

Cicatrizant oils together with those which are strongly antiseptic can be used in a spray with water when the sores are suppurating—10 drops in 100 ml water, shaking well each time before spraying the area. If it can be touched, gently apply a little from a mix made from 5–8 drops in 50 ml oil of *Calendula officinalis* which itself has cicatrizant effects on wounds and persistent ulcers (Price 1993 p. 172). Calendula oil will also help to strengthen the skin if the mixture is massaged in gently twice a day. Compresses may be useful (see Ch. 5), but check that the dressing used is non-stick. Passant (1990) frequently used a combination of rose, geranium, lavender and marjoram (types unspecified) in inhalations to calm and comfort her patients before changing dressings (Wise 1989).

Recommended essential oils include *Boswellia carteri*, *Chamomilla matricaria*, *Lavandula angustifolia* [LAVENDER], *Lavandula × intermedia* 'Super' [LAVANDIN] and *Pelargonium graveolens*. The cicatrizant qualities of the resinoid *Styrax tonkinensis* [SIAM BENZOIN] could also play a part in healing.

Insomnia

The problem of helping an elderly patient achieve a good quality, refreshing night's sleep is a bigger problem in hospitals than when the patient is at home.

Hospital admission can disrupt sleep patterns to such a degree that a useful night's sleep can become impossible. This is especially true in the elderly, whose normal sleep pattern may already be erratic. Factors such as anxiety, lack of privacy, noise and ward activity are all contributory factors, not all of which can be totally eliminated. Often the usual nursing practices are still not sufficient to correct the problem, even when noise levels and lack of privacy are reduced to a minimum. As a result, we often find that the use of drugs is resorted to.

(Cannard 1994)

Lavender (expected to be *Lavandula angustifolia*) is the usual essential oil used to induce sleep, although Macdonald's finding (1995), that 'a few drops of the appropriate oils on the pillow helped to induce a peaceful sleep in many patients', implies the use of more than one, which is always an effective measure. Without accurately specifying lavender, the type used is unknown and the results from separate varieties of both lavenders and lavandins can give very different results. Hospital pharmacists often supply the more camphoraceous *Lavandula latifolia* rather than the French *L. angustifolia* (Buckle 1992).

Since the reduction in production of French lavender (see Ch. 1), much of the essential oil sold by that name is in fact lavandin. The variety of lavandin closest to true lavender is *Lavandula × intermedia* 'Super', though it has far fewer constituents. True lavender contains more terpenes, alcohols and esters and *L. × intermedia* 'Super' contains more camphor (around 5%). See Chapter 1 for details of the differences in properties and effects of these two plants.

Franchomme & Pénoël (1990 p. 364) indicates *Lavandula × intermedia* 'Super', *Melissa officinalis*, *Citrus bergamia* [BERGAMOT] and *Origanum majorana* for insomnia. Other effective oils are *Chamaemelum nobile*, *Citrus aurantium* var. *amara* (flos) [NEROLI BIGARADE] and *Citrus reticulata* (per.), plus *Ocimum basilicum* var. *album* for nervous insomnia (Valnet 1988 p. 97). Some sedative and calming essential oils seem to possess sleep-inducing properties, e.g. *Santalum album* [SANDALWOOD] and *Valeriana officinalis* [COMMON VALERIAN], as do some hypotensors, such as *Cananga odorata* [YLANG YLANG] and *Citrus limon*. The essential oils can be vaporized, used on a tissue, put in the bath or applied in massage.

PROJECT USING LAVENDER TO PROMOTE SLEEP

A 6-week project using vaporized essential oils to relieve insomnia was carried out at the Old Manor Hospital in Salisbury (Hardy 1991). The aim of this project was to find a natural replacement for night medication, and after consulting relatives and ward staff the project was begun. Lavender (botanical name not given) was used in a vortex unit which was activated during the last 2 weeks of the project for three periods a day: 21:00–22:30, 02:00–03:00 and 05:30–06:30.

Four male residents (referred to in this text as A, B, C and D) took part, their ages ranging from 67 to 88. Their normal medication (length of time on named medication in brackets) was as follows:

- A—Promazine 25 mg (3 years)
- B—Heminevrine 1 cap. (7 months)
- C—Temazepam 10 mg (1 year)
- D—no medication (nor previously).

The four men's sleep patterns were assessed over a 6-week period:

- Weeks 1 and 2—normal medication given
- Weeks 3 and 4—no medication was given
- Weeks 5 and 6—no medication given, but lavender oil was used.

Results

The results were split up into day and night periods, each giving the average number of hours sleep (see Table 12.1).

The total number of hours slept by the four men over the 6-week period is shown in Table 12.2:

From Tables 12.1 and 12.2 it can be seen that:

- All four men slept approximately the same number of hours with lavender oil as with medication.

Table 12.1 Average number of hours slept during night and day by 4 subjects (A, B, C and D) with medication (weeks 1 & 2), without medication (weeks 3 & 4), and without medication but with vaporized lavender oil (weeks 5 & 6)

	With medication (weeks 1 & 2)	Without medication (weeks 3 & 4)	With vaporized lavender (no medication) (weeks 5 & 6)
Night			
A	8.9	7.1	8.8
B	6.6	5.2	7.4
C	9.3	7.8	9.3
D	8.5	8.0	8.3
Day			
A	1.5	1.0	1.6
B	0.5	0.5	0.5
C	2.8	2.0	1.9
D	1.1	0.4	0.2

Table 12.2 Total number of hours slept by 4 subjects (A, B, C and D) over the 6-week period of the project

	With medication (weeks 1 & 2)	Without medication (weeks 3 & 4)	With vaporized lavender (no medication) (weeks 5 & 6)
A	125	100	123
B	94	78	103
C	132	110	130
D	117	108	116

- B slept longer with lavender and was originally the worst sleeper, with noisy, aggressive periods during the day. These moods improved considerably towards the end of the project.
- C and D no longer felt the need to sleep so much during the day, perhaps indicating that their quality of sleep during the night was improved with lavender. 4 days after the lavender was administered C reported that he had not had such a good night's sleep for years.
- The cost of essential oils was found to be 60% less than the cost of conventional drugs.

Conclusion

Lavender oil used in this manner can successfully replace medication to relieve insomnia.

ESSENTIAL OILS AS AN ALTERNATIVE TO TEMAZEPAM

The Tullamore Nursing Development Unit (NDU), The General Hospital, Tullamore, Southern Ireland has also looked at the use of aromatherapy in sleep disturbance in the elderly. In this unit, drugs are used as a last resort but, where necessary, the drug of choice for a patient with sleep disturbance is Temazepam (an intermediate acting benzodiazepine). This drug certainly has its place in the treatment of short-term sleep disturbances. However, if drugs can be avoided, especially in the elderly, then any adverse reactions, interactions and dependency can also be avoided (Storrs 1980 p. 17, Reynolds 1993 p. 590). Graham Cannard, co-ordinator in this NDU, together with his team of nurses, decided to look for an alternative to conventional medication and selected aromatherapy to augment the nursing practices already employed in an attempt to reduce the use of night sedation.

Methods

The first step was to assess the amount of night sedation being prescribed. Of the 10 patients in the NDU at that time, eight were prescribed sedation each night. These eight patients were a combination of respite and acute medical patients over the age of 70. One was a long-stay patient.

Christine Dalton, a nurse and qualified aromatherapist, was enlisted to help implement the programme. Dalton undertook the training of the NDU nurses in the correct use of one blend of essential oils to reduce levels of insomnia. Shirley Price's 'Care for Sleep' oil was used, a pre-mixed blend of oils containing European basil (low in methyl chavicol), lavender and sweet marjoram.

The other three nurses on the team (Clarke, Caffrey and Tracey) were taught the various methods of administration and the team decided that vaporization into the atmosphere and a five-minute hand-massage using the oils for those patients for whom the vaporization alone was not successful were the two methods upon which they could concentrate. Under the guidance of Dalton, guidelines for the use of aromatherapy were drawn up.

The team explained their aims and proposed methods to the Consultant Physician and received his full support. As they were concerned that the patients might be adversely affected if aromatherapy did not work for them, and the night sedation had been deleted from their prescription chart, the consultant agreed that the prescription for night sedation would be rewritten as an 'as required' medication so that if the patient were distressed by still being awake at midnight, then the medication could be administered.

Because of the potential for withdrawal symptoms, the team was advised by Dalton that for the first 2 nights the patients would be given their usual sedation (as prescribed) together with aromatherapy, in order to establish a response to the oils before withdrawing the medication. The nursing team began by surveying the medication charts of all the patients in the NDU prior to the introduction of aromatherapy (some were on regular night sedation—usually Temazepam). The sleep patterns of those patients were charted and 94 patient nights were recorded over 2 weeks—without aromatherapy.

Following the introduction of aromatherapy, sleep patterns were again recorded over 94 patient nights. Sedation was only administered when requested by the patient but treatment with essential oils was ongoing. A record was maintained for each patient, showing the name of the oil used, the amount, the method of administration and the night sedation given (if any). An evaluation of the sleep pattern was carried out and charted the following morning. The sleep pattern was assessed by the nurse, asking the patient how he/she slept and if he/she felt refreshed. The nurse's observations of the sleep patterns were also charted. These records were filled in each night for each patient and were used to obtain the data.

Results

Prior to the introduction of aromatherapy the situation was as follows:
* patients reported a good night's sleep for 69 of the 94 patient nights (73%)
* night sedation was given on 85 of the 94 patient nights (80%) to help achieve this quality of sleep.

After the introduction of aromatherapy the situation changed as described below:
* during the 2 nights where night sedation and aromatherapy were given simultaneously, all patients slept well (100%)
* following this, night sedation was only given when requested by the patients and was necessary on 34 patient nights (41%)
* the number of patients reporting a good night's sleep improved to 91 out of the 94 patient nights (97%)
* a reduction in night sedation of 49% was achieved
* some patients needed no sedation at all whilst using aromatherapy, whilst some required it periodically
* only one patient requested sedation on a regular basis.

Table 12.3 Percentage of patients sleeping well and needing medication before and with introduction of *Care for Sleep* essential oil mix

	Before essential oils	With essential oils
Slept well (%)	73	97
Needed medication (%)	80	31

This information is summarized in Table 12.3. The figures in this Table show an overall 24% improvement in sleeping and a 49% reduction in medication as a result of the use of essential oils.

Conclusion

Apart from the obvious effect on the sleep patterns of the patients, other benefits of using aromatherapy were noted. These were:
* The homely and fresh smell of the ward was very comforting; the usual 'hospital smell' that is often present had been disguised.
* Patients received more physical contact with the nurse due to receiving hand-massage with the diluted essential oils. The importance of touch is recognized as being therapeutic in itself (Price 1993b p. 196, Byass 1988). This is especially true for the elderly hospitalized patient who may receive very little physical contact that is not associated with a nursing procedure.
* It was noted that the use of the 'Care for Sleep' essential oil mix was much less expensive than the use of Temazepam.

This small-scale study has certain limitations. It did not show how much the psychological effect had on improving sleep patterns in the patients, nor did it show whether massage or vaporization was the more effective method of administration. There was also some difficulty in assessing sleep patterns: occasionally the patients and the nurses' comments were at variance.

However, the study did show that the use of this blend of oils for sleep disturbance in the elderly is of definite benefit. It is a useful adjunct to the usual nursing care given to the patient and is free of side-effects. The team are hoping to expand their knowledge of aromatherapy so that they can offer essential oils to patients with other problems, in the hope that the use of drugs may be reduced and the quality of care improved.

Respiratory problems

Elderly people suffering from catarrhal problems, such as chronic bronchitis or asthma, can benefit from a daily application of essential oils in a carrier lotion onto their chest and neck. The thin skin behind the ears also facilitates penetration by essential oils. Suitable anticatarrhal, expectorant and mucolytic oils include:

- *Boswellia carteri*—also antitussive
- *Cedrus atlantica* [CEDARWOOD]
- *Eucalyptus smithii*
- *Hyssopus officinalis* [HYSSOP]—also antitussive (but suitable only for non-epileptic patients)
- *Mentha* × *piperita*
- *Salvia officinalis* [SAGE]
- *Styrax tonkinensis* (a resinoid, so quality is of paramount importance)
- *Thymus mastichina* [SPANISH MARJORAM].

If any respiratory infection is present *Origanum majorana* and/or *Thymus vulgaris* ct. geraniol or ct. linalool [SWEET THYME] should be added to the mix, unless *E. smithii*, which has powerful disinfectant properties (Pénoël 1993 personal communication), is one of the oils used. 8 drops of essential oils in total should be added to 50 ml carrier lotion.

E. smithii is an excellent preventive measure for winter coughs and colds because it increases the resistance of the respiratory system to infection. It has a pleasant aroma, is inexpensive and can be vaporized daily in the lounge area of the ward, and/or in the ward (or bedrooms, as many of the newer hospitals name the rooms of the elderly or clients with learning difficulties).

Rheumatism and arthritis

Rheumatism is a vague term which covers various types of conditions involving pain in the muscles. The two main types are rheumatoid arthritis, which involves inflammation of the joints, and osteo-arthritis. Rheumatoid arthritis is more common in women and involves chronic inflammation of the connective tissue around the joints (normally attacking them in symmetrical pairs), which causes pain, swelling and stiffness, frequently accompanied by weight loss and fatigue. In osteo-arthritis there is a progressive wearing away of the cartilage, the connective tissue thickens and any fluid which may fill the joint causes swelling, resulting in severe pain and reduced movement. Wingate & Wingate (1988 p. 349) suggests that because there is no inflammation, the term 'osteoarthrosis' is preferred.

A change in diet has been known to bring about a noticeable improvement in people with rheumatoid arthritis and essential oils have been used successfully for many years to reduce inflammation and pain in the fibrous tissues around the joints (Price 1992), giving increased mobility. There are many different varieties of arthritis and there is no specific evidence as yet that the bone pain in osteoarthrosis can be alleviated.

Choice of oils

Although there are many essential oils indicated for muscular pain and arthritis, if it is not possible to discover the cause and deal with that first, the individual needs to be looked at for the symptoms displayed in order to make full use of the properties of the essential oils.

Pain is perhaps the most important symptom to consider and 'while conventional analgesics give some relief, they seldom give complete or sustained relief. Furthermore, where there is chronic pain, the stress associated with the anticipation of pain can increase the sensation of pain' (Macdonald 1995). It follows that stress-relieving essential oils which are also analgesic may have the strongest effect, because they deal with mind-initiated pain as well as the physical pain from the joints themselves. *Origanum majorana*, *Pelargonium graveolens* and essential oil from the branches of *Juniperus communis* have both analgesic and stress-relieving properties (juniper is also antiinflammatory, Roulier 1990 p. 268).

Many of the antiinflammatory essential oils seem to be mainly indicated for inflammation of the digestive tract, e.g. *Coriandrum sativum* [CORIANDER]. For arthritis, essential oils are required which primarily affect inflammation of the connective tissue. However, *Coriandrum sativum*, like *Melaleuca cajuputi*, does possess antiinflammatory properties effective on connective tissue, thus indirectly dulling arthritic pain (Franchomme & Pénoël 1990 p. 343).

Essential oils which are both stress-relieving and antiinflammatory include *Chamaemelum nobile* [ROMAN CHAMOMILE], *Cymbopogen citratus* and *C. flexuosus* [LEMONGRASS], *Lavandula angustifolia*, *Lavandula × intermedia* 'Super' and *Lippia citriodora* [LEMON VERBENA].

Pinus sylvestris and *Cymbopogon nardus* [CITRONELLA] are antiinflammatory (Franchomme & Pénoël pp. 389, 348). *Melaleuca viridiflora* is both antiinflammatory and analgesic; where the patient is also depressed, this is a valuable oil to use.

Other essential oils with analgesic properties are *Piper nigrum* (Roulier p. 295) and *Zingiber officinalis*. *Rosmarinus officinalis* is an effective muscle relaxant in stronger doses (Franchomme & Pénoël p. 393), and for temporary relief (but not as a regular measure) can be applied undiluted on a small area. For severe pain, *Syzygium aromaticum* (flos), *Melaleuca cajuputi* and *Myristica fragrans* may have a stronger effect.

Juniperus communis and *Rosmarinus officinalis* also help to reduce any fluid around the joints.

The most effective method of using the essential oils (diluted for regular use) is by applying them directly to the affected area or with a compress. They can be applied with or without massage, although massage can help to relax the muscles. A warm bath containing essential oils also relaxes the muscles and reduces the pain.

STUDY USING AROMATHERAPY IN RHEUMATOLOGY

A hospital study carried out in 1990/91 at the Devonshire Royal Hospital in Buxton, Derbyshire, included only patients at a noninflammatory stage of their arthritis, due to the understandable scepticism of the doctors, who were unsure of the effects of aromatherapy (Cawthorne 1991). Although it was difficult to draw conclusions from this small study, because so many different essential oils were used, it resulted in recommendations for a follow-up study to be undertaken, with patients selected at random.

In the original study, out of the 10 patients who returned the questionnaires:

- 10 enjoyed using the oils
- 7 experienced pain relief (2 were able to reduce their analgesics)
- 6 were sleeping better (1 decreasing his night sedation)
- 9 felt more relaxed.

It was interesting to note that the nurses had used all the oils in combinations of 2 or 3 oils. They were chosen in partnership with the patients. The aim was to match the patient's problem with a smell they liked. For example, if a patient was tense and depressed then both relaxing and uplifting oils were used.

(Cawthorne 1991)

Although the specific oils used on each patient were not given, the results appear to demonstrate the multitherapeutic action of essential oils and their effectiveness when selected for the individual.

SINGLE-SUBJECT PROJECT ON RELIEF OF ARTHRITIC PAIN

Macdonald (1995) carried out a single-subject project at Duncuan (Care of the Elderly Unit), Lochgilphead, Argyll, not only as a pilot study for future work but in order to see how aromatherapy could be incorporated into her working day. She states that 'large numbers of subjects are not required for single-case research, where generalisability is achieved through replication studies. ... Le Roux & Lyne (1989) have argued that single-case research designs provide firm foundation for developing sound nursing practices. ... It was decided that three patients would be a manageable number in the first instance.'

Project aim

The aim of Macdonald's project was to discover whether the use of aromatherapy enhanced conventional methods of pain relief. Informed consent was sought from the patients (three females aged between 60 and 90 selected at random), who were given written details of the intervention in addition to a verbal account. The UKCC Code of Conduct was adhered to at all times.

Method

A simple 2-phase design was used alternately. Phase A lasted 3 weeks and conventional analgesics only were given. Phase B lasted 2 weeks, and as well as conventional analgesics incorporated the topical application (without massage) twice daily of 5–10 ml of essential oils in a carrier lotion. The oils selected were eucalyptus, juniper, marjoram and rosemary (botanical names unspecified) in a 1.5% dilution. Phase A and Phase B were then repeated. The extra week in Phase A was to allow for any carry-over effect of the treatment. The Scott & Huskisson (1976) pain scale was used to measure change in the condition of the patients. Lack of time and resources prevented the measurement of pain experienced in walking, dressing or sleeping. The pain scale, which ranged from 0 (no pain) to 10 (worst possible pain) was used at each drug administration.

Results

Barthel index scores for self-care (maximum possible score 53) and mobility (maximum possible score 52) were taken on admission for assessment and again after the 10-week period (mobility score shown in brackets). The results of these are shown in Table 12.4.

For simplicity's sake, the pain scale figures are shown in as an average for each week (PSA). Table 12.5 also shows the number of times medication was administered, week by week.

Table 12.4 Barthel index scores for self-care and mobility for 3 patients (A, B and C), assessed on admission and after 10-week project

	Self-care		Mobility	
	Week 0	Week 10	Week 0	Week 10
A	24	27	10	10
B	4	7	3	10
C	53	53	28	42

Conclusions

Some interesting conclusions can be drawn from this project, and some of them are presented below.

Patient A.   In week 6, as expected, there may have been some effects of the essential oils remaining, shown by the average reduced pain scale figures compared with weeks 1–3 and 7 and 8.

Less medication was needed during weeks 4, 5, 9 and 10, when essential oils were applied daily (except for week 3, although the average number of tablets taken during weeks 2 and 3 was still less than week 1). Could it be psychological, in that she was anticipating being helped by the essential oils? Immediately the treatment stopped, the patient was in need of medication (week 6).

Weeks 9 and 10 show an accelerating reduction both in medication and pain scale readings, and it is interesting to speculate what the results would have shown had the project been extended for a further 5 weeks.

Table 12.5 Average weekly pain scale figures (PSA, where 10 = worst possible pain) and number of weekly medications (Meds) administered to patients A, B and C over course of 10-week project, without and with essential oil use

Week		A		B		C	
		Meds	PSA	Meds	PSA	Meds	PSA
1	} Medication only	14	5.28	10	5.85	21	2.14
2		12	5.71	10	5.85	21	3.71
3		8	4.71	8	5.28	21	3.71
4	} Medication plus	9	4.71	4	2.28	21	0.28
5	essential oils	6	2.57	1	0.28	21	0.00
6	} Medication only	11	3.71	5	2.71	21	1.85
7		11	5.71	5	3.00	21	1.00
8		12	5.42	7	3.57	21	2.85
9	} Medication plus	7	3.00	1	0.57	21	0.00
10	essential oils	1	1.57	0	0.00	21	0.00

Patient B. During the whole of weeks 6, 7 and 8 without essential oils, B's medication and pain scale reading were lower than during the first 3 weeks, reducing to 0 on both counts after the second intervention with essential oils. It could be that B's faith in aromatherapy after the first application period was a contributory factor (see Ch. 7).

Patient C. C's medication did not alter, although the pain scale readings were considerably reduced at each aromatherapy intervention. The reduction to 0 on the pain scale during the second intervention may suggest that C's medication could be reduced were the topical application of essential oils to be continued permanently.

Many further interesting observations were included in this project, full details of which can be found in Macdonald (1995).

Parkinson's disease

Parkinson's disease usually (but not always) affects people in later life, so this may be the place to give details of a project carried out by the authors on three groups of people with Parkinson's disease in 1992.

PARKINSON'S DISEASE PROJECT

This project was set up to determine whether or not essential oils can play a part in improving movement in a Parkinson's disease sufferer and perhaps increasing the time span before administering stronger drugs; it was intended only as a preliminary exercise for possible future research.

Objective of the trial

The objective of the trial was to discover whether daily application of essential oils without massage was as effective as full-body-massage with essential oils on a regular basis, thus making it possible for people to benefit from essential oils at a reasonable cost and without a full-body-massage (which not everyone wants because of time and cost considerations). Because the recipe of essential oils had to be identical for everyone, it was impossible to select holistically for each person.

The choice therefore was focused on lowering stress levels and loosening joints and muscles, with the hope also of relieving insomnia and perhaps constipation in those presenting such symptoms.

Method

All oils and/or lotions used, either for massage or self-application, were mixed at 1.5% concentration and supplied by the authors, to guarantee uniformity (6–8 drops of the undiluted essential oil were used in the bath where indicated). Out of the 52 people who volunteered for treatment (20 each in Groups A and B and 12 in Group C), 27 were able to complete the 9-month period. Of the rest:

- 8 found the weekly recording difficult
- 7 could not keep up the daily application (1 had chosen an oil-based mix in preference to a lotion and found it difficult to remove the vegetable oil from her clothes)
- 3 had hospital visits which interrupted the routine
- 2 changed medication, which invalidated the results
- 1 transferred to phase 2 after a 2-month period with no treatment
- 1 only applied the lotion when he remembered
- 1 stopped after 3 months because her speech problems showed no improvement, though she admitted to sleeping better and having fewer cramps during this time
- 1 had to have a mastectomy half way through the project, but commented that her balance had improved and her doctor had remarked on her increased self-confidence and positive outlook during her treatment period
- 1 died.

The trial was organized in the following way:

- Group A—10 people received a weekly massage from an aromatherapist (who gave his/her time free of charge) for 12 weeks, followed by a monthly massage for 6 months, using a specific blend of essential oils. The carer applied the same essential oil blend in a lotion base daily in between treatments.
- Group B—9 people were supplied for 9 months with pure essential oils for the bath and a lotion or oil based mix containing the same essential oils to be applied daily for 3 months and every other day for a further 6 months.

- Group C—8 people received similar treatment to Group A above except that the massage was carried out with plain vegetable oil, with no essential oils added. This was difficult because, for the project to be reliable, not even the therapists were allowed to know that there were no essential oils in the mix supplied. This was achieved by *telling* them that they were using a 0.05% concentration even though no essential oils were present.

All participants had to obtain their doctor's permission to take part and be willing to do what was asked of them, especially with regard to home use.

Oils used

The essential oils selected were:

- *Salvia sclarea* [CLARY] relaxant, nerve tonic. To aid general relaxation and relief of anxiety.
- *Origanum majorana*—analgesic, antispasmodic, digestive tonic, hypotensor, nerve tonic, relaxant. To relieve muscle pain and insomnia and improve the digestion.
- *Lavandula angustifolia*—analgesic, antispasmodic, digestive stimulant, hypotensor, sedative. To relax the muscles and relieve pain, insomnia and anxiety.

Results

A synopsis of the results of this trial is presented here. Full details can be found in Price 1993a.

The results for symptomatic relief showed very little difference between Group A and Group B, which points to the potential of baths and self-application for those who cannot afford weekly aromatherapy treatments. The results for Group C, i.e. the patients receiving massage (and home care) with a bland vegetable oil were as follows:

- 4 found the treatment relaxing and reported feeling better afterwards, although the effects were not lasting
- 2 felt brighter in themselves and in their general health
- 2 found the treatment itself relaxing but felt no other noticeable change.

The symptomatic improvements experienced by all three groups are shown in Table 12.6.

Table 12.6 Number and percentage of Parkinson's disease sufferers in Groups A and B (combined) and Group C experiencing symptomatic relief over 9-month trial period (after Price 1993). Dashes indicate that a person was not asked by the therapist if he/she suffered from that symptom

	Groups A and B (combined)		Group C	
	No.	%	No.	%
Anxiety	4	100	—	—
Constipation	5	83	1	33
Cramp	1	50	1	50
Depression	3	75	—	—
Energy lack	4	100	0	0
Insomnia	7	85	2	66
Memory loss	0	0	0	0
Muscular pain	8	100	3	60
Nightmares	2	100	—	—
Rigidity	2	50	—	—
Slurred speech	2	28	—	—
Stiffness	9	100	1	50
Swallowing difficulty	0	0	—	—
Tremors	4	33	1	16
Weak limbs	5	62	—	—

Conclusion

Group A. On the whole, an aromatherapy treatment once a month was found to be insufficient. However,

- 7 patients maintained their improvement during the last 6 months when receiving an aromatherapy treatment only once a month
- 2 were able to discontinue their medication for insomnia
- 2 did not maintain their improvement during the last 6 months, but still felt better than before treatment commenced (beneficial effects of treatment lasting 4–6 days).

It was felt that fortnightly (if not weekly) aromatherapy treatments would be preferable to monthly ones.

Group B. Essential oils without massage appear to be able to give relief in the same areas as in group A. 2 patients felt the improvement they experienced was limited.

A perceived extra benefit of Group A over Group B may be the complete relaxation derived from the massage, with improved circulation as a result (though this was not mentioned in the patient feedback).

Group C. Massage without essential oils, although beneficial on several counts, scored the lowest in lasting effects.

Dementia

Some elderly people suffer from organic deterioration of their mental faculties. They are unable to think clearly or to concentrate for any length of time, the memory may be confused and unreliable, some may hallucinate sights and sounds and others may have difficulty with their speech.

Essential oils best known for stimulating the mind and improving the memory are *Rosmarinus officinalis* and *Mentha × piperita* (van Toller & Dodd 1991). Passant (1990) used cardamom, geranium and lavender (unspecified) and Franchomme recommends *Syzygium aromaticum* (flos). For those who are depressed, essential oils which are a tonic to the nervous system may be used, such as *Boswellia carteri*, *Citrus aurantium* var. *amara* (flos) [NEROLI BIGARADE], *Ocimum basilicum* var. *album* (with a low phenolic ether content—see Ch. 8), *Origanum majorana*, *Rosa damascena* [ROSE OTTO], *Salvia sclarea*. All the oils in this section can be given by inhalation, in the bath or by scalp-, hand- or foot-massage.

Case 12.5 Aromatherapist: Marlene Cadwallader (BAppSciNursing), Australia

I provide care in Heyfield Bush Nursing Hospital, which is a 13-bed rural hospital providing care for the elderly, acute medical paediatric casualty/outpatients clinic/day surgery neonatal and palliative care. The hospital manageress, staff and doctors accept and support the provision of care using essential oils and massages and Reiki channelling, appreciating the benefits of tactile therapies. Although there is no written policy for the use of essential oils within the hospital, there is often the aroma of lavender, geranium or rosemary wafting from a vaporiser in the secretary/managers office.

a
One elderly resident always appears sleepy and lethargic. A combination of orange, lemon and lavender in a base oil has helped her immensely and other nursing staff have commented on her increased alertness and sense of humour, showing the effects of the uplifting properties.

b
An elderly male patient aged about 85 years, who had experienced several strokes, was self-caring, possessed a tremendous sense of humour and always had a smile on his face. He loved chatting, but always forgot what he was saying in the middle of a sentence, much to his annoyance. An oil blend of lemon (to uplift his spirits as he tended to fall asleep frequently), lavender and rosemary (to assist his memory) was made up in a carrier of grapeseed oil and calendula oil (to nourish his dry skin).

Foot-, hand- and back-massage were given when time permitted—mostly foot-massages, which he looked forward to with a cherubic grin. As time progressed, he developed more movement in his legs and feet, permitting increased mobility. His family were amazed at the improvement in his general health.

c
A middle-aged gentleman was admitted with an allergic reaction. Welts and rashes appeared over his body, as well as recurring swelling of his throat and lips. He was most unwell and intramuscular medication was administered on a regular basis to reduce the swelling, with cold packs, showers and calamine being applied externally to relieve the itch. I happened to be working on a night shift when we met, and he said 'this itch is driving me mad'—he was speaking literally. I made up a solution of 3 drops lavender, 2 drops tea tree and 1 drop peppermint, putting 1 drop into a small bowl of water for sponging off his body. He claimed the solution soothed his body and he certainly appeared more relaxed.

Case 12.6 Aromatherapist: Brenda Weston SPDipA, MISPA, SRN, SCM, UK

Mrs P had suffered a severe stroke the previous September, leaving her left arm completely paralyzed and with only partial recovery in her left leg. She had always been a very independent and strong-willed lady, lived alone, and at the age of 89 still ruled her children with a rod of iron. During her hospitalization, Mrs P had taken her disability very badly, resenting the loss of her independence. She became so depressed, almost suicidal, that she required the assistance of a psychiatrist.

On admission to my nursing home, Mrs P initially settled very well, enjoying the home's Christmas festivities, outings at the local church and day centres, and day out with her family. Then, during January, she became very unsettled and unhappy, realizing she was never going to go back to her own flat. She became very angry with her family for forcing her into this decision, and for selling her flat and belongings. She became determined to leave us, and actually wandered off, twice falling badly. This resulted in two periods of hospitalization for a fractured pelvis and femur.

The psychiatrist periodically reviewed Mrs P's case and changed the medication to sedate her and to relieve her depression. Mrs P became very apathetic, and due to the effects of the medication slept 20 hours out of 24, resulting in dehydration, loss of weight, anorexia and incontinence. I could not bear to watch Mrs P's condition deteriorate and decided to 'interfere'. My care plan involved daily massage of hands, legs and face with melissa (antidepressant), lavender and geranium. These were blended in a base of grapeseed oil with 25% hypericum (restorative to the nervous system). The same mixture of essential oils was used in Mrs P's bath, and periodically placed on her bed-linen prior to her returning from the bath.

Prior to starting this treatment, Mrs P's mood and behaviour was monitored for 7 days, using the Beck inventory for measuring depression, to see if there was any pattern to her distress and mood. It was noted that she appeared worse in the late mornings and in the evenings before bed. Treatments were therefore given mid-morning and at bedtime.

After 4 weeks Mrs P was more content and alert; medication had been reduced, and she was eating and drinking well, gaining weight in the process. She has even begun to take outings with her family again and is more positive about the future, planning to enjoy life as best she can.

Summary

Essential oils have wide application in the treatment of the elderly (and other) hospitalized patient, and nowhere more so than for sleep disturbance. Small-scale studies have shown the effectiveness of aromatherapy in this situation, and it is to be hoped their conclusions (and the less unequivocal results of rheumatology trials) will be corroborated by further controlled studies.

REFERENCES

Buckle J 1992 Which lavender oil? Nursing Times 88(22): August 5: 54–55

Byass R 1988 Soothing body and soul. Nursing Times 84(24): 39–41

Cannard G 1994 On the scent of a good night's sleep. Trial Project. Midland Health Board News January: 3

Cawthorne A 1991 Aromatherapy on trial. Aromanews 30: 7–8

Franchomme P, Pénoël D 1990 L'aromathérapie exactement. Jollois, Limoges

Hardy M 1991 Sweet scented dreams. International Journal of Aromatherapy 3(2): 12–13

Le Roux A A, Lyne P A 1989 Firm foundations: applying the results of research based on the clinical trial design to nursing practice. RCN Research Society Conference, Cardiff. RCN, London

Macdonald K 1993 Orange blossom cure for heart patients. Daily Mail. March 16th

Macdonald E M L 1995 Aromatherapy for the enhancement of the nursing care of elderly people suffering from arthritic pain. The Aromatherapist 2(1): 26–31

Passant H 1990 A holistic approach in the ward. Nursing Times 86(4) January 24: 26–28

Price S 1991 Aromatherapy for common ailments. Gaia, London

Price S 1992 Arthritis and rheumatism. Yoga and Health, February: 37–38

Price S 1993a Parkinson's disease project: is aromatherapy an effective treatment for Parkinson's disease? The Aromatherapist 1(1): 14–21

Price S 1993b The aromatherapy workbook. Thorsons, London

Reynolds J E F 1993 Martindale: the extra pharmacopoeia. Pharmaceutical Press, London

Roulier G 1990 Les huiles essentielles pour votre santé. Dangles, St-Jean-de-Braye

Scott J, Huskisson E C 1976 Graphic representation of pain. In: Pain, Elsevier, Holland, vol. 2, pp. 175–184

Storrs A M F 1980 Geriatric nursing. Baillière Tindall, London

Tattam A 1992 The gentle touch. Nursing Times 88(32): 16–17

Valnet J 1980 The practice of aromatherapy. Daniel, Saffron Walden

van Toller and Dodd 1991 Perfumery. Chapman & Hall, London

Wingate P, Wingate R 1988 Penguin medical encyclopedia. Penguin, London

Wise R 1989 Flower power. Nursing Times 85(22) May 31: 45–47

13

Care of the dying

Introduction

Complementary therapies have become increasingly popular since the mid 1980s, with a growing number of the general public and the nursing profession becoming aware of alternative and complementary methods of caring for people with terminal illnesses. With the help of aromatherapy hundreds of people faced with terminal illness have enjoyed a quality of life better than they might otherwise have experienced.

INTRODUCTION OF AROMATHERAPY INTO TRADITIONAL SETTINGS

Many terminally ill people are cared for in their homes through the informal carer network, and a great number are cared for in hospices. Hospices were the first healthcare establishments in Britain to welcome aromatherapy as a possible mode of relief to their patients. When the therapy was relatively unknown, aromatherapists found hospices to be the easiest point of entry for the introduction of the use of essential oils into an NHS situation. This may have been because hospices often have good resources of time and money (many being funded by charities), although most of the therapists offered their services voluntarily. It may also have been because those in charge (who had no first hand knowledge of the efficacy of massage or the use of essential oils) felt that at least it could do no harm! The help aromatherapy can offer in this field.

has been warmly received and much appreciated by both patients and staff. It has helped staff on oncology units and in hospices to provide the enhanced quality of care they seek to give their patients. In many ways it has also been the way of entry into wider acceptance in the Health Service as a whole.

(Lundie 1993)

With terminal illness, one of the primary aims is to bring about an improvement in the quality of life of the patient and essential oils have been found to be capable of this, by relieving stress, raising the spirits, strengthening and revitalizing the mind and providing comfort to the body by easing some of the distressing effects of the illness. In fact, the Director of Nursing Services at Compton Hospice states that 'we often wonder how we coped without the aid of aromatherapy' (Kensey 1986 personal communication).

In achieving this aim there is no doubt that the relief of stress is beneficial, not only for the patients themselves, but also for the relatives and loved ones who can only watch and support. The use of essential oils by an aromatologist/aromatherapist can improve the outlook and mood of the patient and relatives alike. Moreover, the nurses and carers can also benefit, for they too are under a certain amount of stress due to working continually among those who have not long to live, and having to cope with the inevitable fears, anxieties and questions of both patients and visitors.

Selecting the most effective essential oils.

An important consideration when selecting essential oils holistically is that the patient should like the aroma. Always let him/her smell a mix before using it, adjusting the aroma if necessary with an extra drop of one of the prescribed (or other) essential oils. The psychological effect of a welcomed aroma can do much to begin the healing process.

Stress

Many essential oils have the ability to relieve stress (see Ch. 10). The most popular one used by nurses in the last few years has been lavender, almost to the exclusion of others. No doubt this is on account of its pleasant aroma, long list of therapeutic

effects, known low toxicity (except *Lavandula stoechas* which is high in ketones) and reasonable cost. There have been a few studies carried out on the stress-relieving effects of lavender, but the specific variety of lavender used is not usually given—it may not even have been known (see Ch. 1 under Clones of lavender and lavandin).

Other essential oils with a wide range of therapeutic effects are being introduced more and more, sometimes in synergy with lavender, and include oils such as:

- *Chamaemelum nobile* [ROMAN CHAMOMILE]
- *Citrus limon* (per.) [LEMON]
- *Origanum majorana* [SWEET MARJORAM]
- *Pelargonium graveolens* [GERANIUM].

Stress may have different consequences for different people and when determining which essential oil(s) to use for stress, the consequential symptoms presented (e.g. insomnia, constipation) must also be borne in mind (see Ch. 10).

Stress and insomnia

- *Chamaemelum nobile* (also helpful in cases of nervous shock)
- *Cananga odorata* [YLANG YLANG]
- *Citrus reticulata* (per) [MANDARIN]
- *Lavandula angustifolia*, syn. *L. officinalis*, *L. vera* [LAVENDER]
- *Origanum majorana*.

The use of more than one of these essential oils will increase the synergy. Experience shows that the effect of two (or three) oils blended together is usually greater than that of one used alone (see Ch. 3).

Depression

The depressed state of mind of a terminally ill person may have a more detrimental effect on the body than stress, and more appropriate oils to use under these circumstances would be:

- *Ocimum basilicum* var. *album* [EUROPEAN BASIL].
- *Thymus vulgaris* [THYME], preferably one of the sweet (alcohol) chemotypes. The geraniol chemotype has a particularly gentle aroma, which may be more acceptable to the patient

than the harsher phenolic chemotypes. A sweet thyme would blend well with *Citrus bergamia* [BERGAMOT], which is also an uplifting essential oil.

- *Citrus aurantium* var. *amara* (flos) [NEROLI BIGARADE], a nerve tonic and antidepressant (Franchomme & Pénoël 1990 p. 338) is a useful essential oil to include in the mix and significantly improves the aroma, especially if one of the phenolic thymes is being used.

Depression and the immune system

It is believed that the use of certain oils may strengthen the body's resistance to secondary infection. This is an important consideration for those living with HIV-related immunodeficiency, and something for which allopathic medicine has no answer as yet (see immune system list on p. 201 and in Appendix B.9). Essential oils which may be effective for both depression and lowered immunity are:

- *Boswellia carteri* [FRANKINCENSE], an uplifting essential oil which helps to strengthen the immune system. It also relieves arthritic pain and inflammation.
- *Citrus bergamia* which will recharge the central nervous system with energy (Roulier 1990 p. 243), therefore indirectly helping to strengthen the immune system. It is also a good digestive oil.
- *Melaleuca viridiflora* [NIAOULI] which is uplifting and an immunostimulant as well as being radioprotective (Roulier 1990).

Chapter 5 gives methods of use and percentages of essential oils to be used.

These few examples should give some indication of how to select essential oils. Always make the first selection according to the emotional state of the patient concerned. From this, two or three oils may then be selected for the more specific symptoms portrayed. This synergistic selection will then have positive effects on the whole person—i.e. the choice is holistic.

Imagery and positivity

Some patients, who already know a little about complementary therapies and who have not reached the final stages of their illness (and those who can take on—with help—some responsibility for their own health) may be able to apply some of the principles of visualization and the ability of the body to heal itself through positive thoughts, helped by determination, a caring therapist and supportive relatives.

The success of a positive attitude and visualization has been observed by many nurses and aromatherapists working with different complementary therapies on patients living with cancer and HIV-related immunodeficiency. A change of attitude is naturally easier for someone in the earlier stages of a disease to accomplish, when they can learn about improved diet, positivity, reflex therapy, massage and aromatherapy before the disease has got too firm a hold (Machin 1989).

The use of touch and massage

Aromatherapy with massage is particularly suited to the terminally ill, who have a profound need for the caring and loving touch of gentle hands. Massage conveys warmth, comfort, pleasure and safety (McNamara (1993 p. 13). For these people, the use of essential oils to enhance the massage can relieve some of the anxiety in a caring way and perhaps bring about deeper, more relaxed sleep. Such treatment inspires patients (when asked to describe their reactions to their aromatherapy treatment) to utter words such as remarkable, marvellous, cheering, soothing, reassuring, comforting, etc. (Phillips 1989).

As a general rule, these reactions are heard after the use of essential oils together with massage—but comfort, touch and massage *without* essential oils would also result in the expression of similar comments. A trial carried out to assess the value of massage for patients with breast cancer showed an improvement in concentration and lessening of fatigue and stress, as well as generally feeling better, compared to a control group (Sims 1986).

Although massage is much used in aromatherapy treatments, the use of essential oils in appropriate health situations can (and should) be extended wherever possible to include other equally beneficial methods such as inhalation and compresses (see Ch. 5).

With bedridden patients a full massage is not always possible or necessary to bring about the desired improvement. The outcome of a specific-area-massage (e.g. the feet) *with* essential oils may almost be compared with that of a full-body-massage *without* them, taking much less time out of a busy nursing schedule. Any massage done should be modified to suit the needs of each individual patient, taking into account the stage of development of their illness and, in the case of people with cancer, whether or not they are receiving radiation treatment.

The essential oils and/or the massage may bring hidden emotions to the surface, even tears. Carers should be aware of and prepared for this possibility and confident that they can handle it successfully, using any counselling skills they may have or referring the patient on if they feel they cannot deal with the situation themselves.

Terminally ill patients need strong support to be able to cope with the reality (and sometimes the apparent injustice) of their illness. When it comes to understanding and soothing their fears and alleviating their mental suffering, essential oils too can play an important part. Examples of oils said to relieve fear and despair are as follows:

- *Boswellia carteri*
- *Citrus reticulata* (per.)
- *Citrus aurantium* var. *amara* (fol.)
- *Cananga odorata*.

Nurses who can carry out only a simple treatment with essential oils still have an effective tool at their disposal, which has already achieved a measure of success in the field of the terminally ill (see Ch. 13).

Cadwallader (1993 personal communication) finds working with selected essential oils in appropriate ways valuable with terminally ill patients and their families, in assisting with coping abilities and allaying the distress and anxiety associated with the dying.

CANCER

Cancer has been recorded since Egyptian times, and treatment for cancer using aromatic plants was mentioned 2000 years ago by Dioscorides in his Materia Medica. Cancer is widespread today, and although more than 200 different types have been diagnosed the reasons for its development and spread are unknown (McNamara 1993). This is in spite of great advances in the treatment of many types of cancer, and extensive research worldwide.

Fear of being diagnosed as having cancer is one of the great stresses in the lives of those who have already lost one of their family through this disease, and those with no family history of cancer can suffer shock, confusion and fear after diagnosis. Statistics show that 1 in 4 people will develop cancer at some stage, which unfortunately increases any anxiety already experienced regarding the disease.

A change in health status will result in emotional conflict which may be expressed as psychosomatic-related symptoms which may increase distress. A person's loss of control over his or her emotions may worsen feelings of hopelessness and helplessness and inhibit normal coping strategies which motivate moves towards recovery.

(Crowther 1991)

Suggestions for treatment

There are no precise guidelines concerning the employment of aromatherapy for cancer, and normally no specific oils are used by therapists, because they are generally selected by taking a holistic view of each patient. Dr. Valnet, considered to be an authority on the subject of aromatherapy, gives a selection of essential oils for the prevention and treatment of cancer. The oils he cites are as follows (Valnet 1980):

- *Syzygium aromaticum* (flos) [CLOVE BUD]
- *Cupressus sempervirens* [CYPRESS]
- *Pelargonium graveolens*
- *Hyssopus officinalis* [HYSSOP]
- *Salvia officinalis* [SAGE]
- *Artemisia dracunculus* [TARRAGON].

He also cites the essential oils of garlic and onion, but these are not generally used in aromatherapy because of the very strong odour.

Aromatherapists today may be wary of using the essential oils of *Hyssopus officinalis*, *Salvia officinalis* and *Artemisia dracunculus*. The first two contain neurotoxic constituents and are contraindicated in pregnancy; the third has a high content of methyl chavicol, although one source states that no contraindications to the essential oil are known (Franchomme & Pénoël 1990 p. 326). In the appropriately controlled dosage these oils may in future come to be accepted as useful in the treatment of cancer, when our knowledge is more advanced than it is at the moment.

Certainly, the fears (after tests on animals) that tarragon and basil might be carcinogenic (because of the similarity of the safrole molecule to that of methyl chavicol) have proved unfounded (Caldwell 1991). Well-trained aromatherapists/aromatologists need have no fears regarding the safe use of these oils (i.e. low concentration), and with due respect to any contraindications.

As well as Valnet, other writers mention essential oils they believe are effective against cancer:

- Bernadet (1983) recommends the internal use of *Cupressus sempervirens*, *Syzygium aromaticum* and *Pelargonium graveolens* for the prevention of cancer. He also states that the person with cancer can use plants to act on his general state.
- Gattefossé (1993 pp. 72, 84) cites Professor Cabbasè as suggesting that *Boswellia carteri* may be used for the prevention of smoker's cancer, and Sassard as recommending *Hyssopus officinalis* (5 drops in olive oil) three times daily for cancer of the liver.
- Bardeau (1976) mentions *Citrus limon*, *Commiphora myrrha* [MYRRH], *Lavandula officinalis* and *L. latifolia*, *Melaleuca viridiflora*, *Rosa damascena* and *R. centifolia* [ROSE OTTO], and *Styrax benzoin* [BENZOIN].
- Roulier (1990 p. 230) suggests that certain essential oils can help to improve the immune system and eliminate abnormal cells. He states that they should be determined and used by the aromatherapy practitioner following laboratory tests, and includes *Syzygium aromaticum*, *Lippia citriodora* [TRUE VERBENA], *Melaleuca viridiflora*, *Pogostemon patchouli* [PATCHOULI].

Some patients with cancer can acquire a deficiency of the immune system, especially those on chemotherapy or undergoing radiation. For these people, essential oils which are believed to strengthen the immune system, such as *Boswellia carteri* cited previously (Franchomme and Pénoël 1990 p. 328), *Melaleuca viridiflora* and *Syzygium aromaticum* (flos) (Roulier 1990 p. 230), may be useful. (See also p. 201 and Appendix B.9.)

Regarding the use of essential oils, Franchomme & Pénoël (1990 p. 88) say that it is not a question of aiming at the breakdown of a malignant tumour by recourse to them. Nevertheless, the antitumoral properties of certain sesquiterpenic lactones and certain sesquiterpenic ketones and of benzaldehyde, as well as the antiviral properties of certain ketones can be useful in expert hands to assist the prevention of certain degenerative states.

Benefits

Patients vary in their aromatherapy needs: the amount of pain suffered, the site and extent of any tumours, tenderness of specific areas, the frequency of radiotherapy if being treated, the rate of the circulation, the ability to sleep, the condition of the skin, the medication taken, whether or not they are on chemotherapy, the state of their morale, etc. Those who elect to receive aromatherapy treatment may benefit in one or more of the following ways:

- Reduction of anxiety, stress and tension (which in turn helps to reduce any blood pressure), fear (which keeps the body in a permanently tense condition), or shock.
- By gaining a feeling of wellbeing, which helps inability to cope, strengthening self-belief.
- Relief of constipation, headaches, muscular pain and insomnia, resulting in an improvement in quality of life, often followed by a reduction in medication for secondary problems such as these.
- Elevation of the pain threshold level (Barker 1993), sometimes enabling a reduction in analgesics.
- Improvement in the circulation of both blood and lymph, helping to eliminate unwanted toxins more efficiently.
- Stimulation of the immune system. 'There is ample evidence of the overall increase in

---

Case 13.1a Cancer—Aromatherapist: Jeannie Maher, Australia

This lady in her 50s had had a brain tumour removed—she still had a malignant tumour level 4 which was growing deep into the middle of the brain. She had received 6 weeks of radium treatment and was on a lot of medication. On first seeing her, she was partly paralyzed down the left side and was using a walking frame. Circulation and lymph were poor, broken sleep pattern due to arm and leg twitches, general health not good, having seizures at least once a week and increasing as time went on. She became dehydrated easily and had a very itchy scalp where her hair was growing back and the skin was very dry.

She was having physiotherapy treatments up to 3 times a week, which she found made her very tired, so they cut them back to once or twice a week. These were concentrated on exercising the partly paralyzed limbs. She was a healthy hard-working lady. The first symptoms of her disorder were loss of balance and migraines which she did not normally suffer. On visiting the doctor, he immediately did tests and referred her to a neuro-surgeon. They operated—this was not only a shock to herself but also to her family. Her daughter contacted me a few months after her mother's operation, having heard of aromatherapy in England.

Treatments were given weekly, then twice-weekly, using a base which included 5% avocado and 5% calendula to help her dry skin, with lavender essential oil (central nervous system, sedative, antiseptic, bactericidal and balancing). She was more relaxed afterwards and it helped to give her a better quality of sleep as the treatments stopped the nervous twitching of her arm and leg. On different occasions I would alternate essential oils, sometimes using mandarin for its balancing and uplifting effects, and sedative effect on the nervous system.

Her general condition was becoming worse and it was decided that aromatherapy and physiotherapy treatments should cease for a period of 1 month. At this time they also found the tumour had spread and seizures were becoming more frequent. The doctors suggested she recommence aromatherapy treatments because she had commented that they assisted in her feeling of well-being. Also, it had been found that during the course of my treatments the seizures had been of shorter duration and less violent; the treatments had also relieved some of the pain.

---

immune functioning when relaxation is achieved by soft tissue massage' (Chaitow 1987), which is believed to be enhanced by the appropriate essential oils.

Safety

There are differences in opinion on whether or not full-body-massage in the early and middle stages of cancer should be carried out. However, in all cases where full-body-massage has been used during these stages, with or without essential oils, only beneficial results have been obtained. There is abundant empirical evidence from the many aromatherapists presently working with patients living with cancer, and there is certainly no evidence after many years of aromatherapy use to substantiate the theories of opponents. Most doctors agree that although massage with essential oils cannot cure cancer, its advantages outweigh any risks (see also p. 99).

Chemotherapy

The aromatherapist's first concern is to treat the *person*, not the disease, and a person receiving radiation treatment or chemotherapy certainly needs help to cope during this stressful time. The use of essential oils with massage alongside chemotherapy treatment is an area of uncertainty. As massage helps to release and eliminate toxic waste, it could be assumed that provided the massage given is of the right type, pressure and location, it would be beneficial. For people undergoing chemotherapy, it may be preferable to administer only specific-area-massage. This releases fewer toxins at a time and at a slower rate—important, as even people *without* cancer on high medication may feel unwell for up to 48 hours after a full aromatherapy massage. A full-body-massage is therefore recommended for people on chemotherapy only if it is extremely gentle and brief.

According to a study carried out on people with Parkinson's disease (Price 1993a), patients receiving specific-area application of essential oils derived more benefit than those receiving full-body-massage *without* essential oils.

The benefits of full-body-massage to the patient receiving chemotherapy would be no greater than those gained by specific-area-massage with essential oils, therefore nothing extra would be achieved by the former (apart from the patient experiencing a caring touch for a longer period of time). When the toxic residues begin to clear after the course of chemotherapy, the area of the body massaged can be increased, slowly building up to a full-body-massage (with the consent of the patient).

When using essential oils with chemotherapy, a low concentration of essential oils in a blend is recommended: about 4 drops of essential oils in 50 ml carrier oil (or lotion) is enough. Only distilled oils should be used during this time—solvent-extracted oils (absolutes) with their impurities could produce an adverse reaction, especially on the skin. In all cases it is advisable to carry out a patch test on the client before any massage, because of possible sensitivity of the skin (Horrigan 1991). There seems to be no substantiation for the view that essential oils should not be used at all during chemotherapy treatment, nor in fact, before all the residues are cleared from the body (McNamara 1993).

Radiotherapy

Radiotherapy is another area where people are hesitant to use essential oils. For some years now essential oils have been used in France for the purpose of mitigating the side-effects of this treatment. The essential oils are used prior to treatment on the area to be irradiated, to reduce deep burning and scarring. Pénoël suggests *Melaleuca viridiflora* (Franchomme & Pénoël 1990 p. 282) and Franchomme ascribes this property to most of the Melaleuca oils, i.e. *Melaleuca alternifolia* [TEA TREE], *M. cajuputi* [CAJUPUT] *and M. viridiflora* ct. cineole (Franchomme & Pénoël 1990 pp. 368–371). As to method of use, it is recommended that the essential oil of *Melaleuca viridiflora* is applied before the radiotherapy session on the area to be irradiated to avoid or at least limit cutaneous lesions (Franchomme & Pénoël 1990 p. 263). This feature is also mentioned elsewhere:

In cases where radiotherapy is necessary, the skin can be protected by the use of niaouli on the treated areas. This essential oil minimises the severity of burning in the skin. The oil is applied neat, undiluted before the irradiation sessions, and after the session a mixture is applied. This mixture may be either a) *Melaleuca viridiflora* 50% in *Hypericum perforatum* (St. John's wort) 50% or b) *Melaleuca viridiflora* 50% in *Rosa rubiginosa* (rosehip) 50%.

(Roulier 1990 p. 230)

It may take some time before doctors accept this in Britain, but many aromatherapists (including ourselves) recommend the use of essential oils on people undergoing radiotherapy. The oils are applied routinely on a daily basis in between radiation treatments (excluding the day of the treatment), with no adverse results.

One person with cancer used *Lavandula angustifolia*, *Rosa damascena* (distilled) and *Boswellia carteri* (distilled), blended by myself (S. Price) using the dilution mentioned above in calendula carrier oil. This was not to help prevent scarring, but to lift the client out of her depression after being told she would need radiation therapy, and to help recover the positive attitude she had had towards her cancer previously. They were used at her own insistence (with the permission of her doctor) twice a day in between her radiotherapy sessions, with what she felt were positive results.

Although one case does not constitute conclusive evidence, there appears to be no evidence indicating that the use of essential oils on someone receiving radiation treatment may be harmful. As with most other essential oil treatment, there is only empirical knowledge in this area to date, and very little even of that. It is our belief that, in low concentrations, most essential oils can be used beneficially on a person receiving radiation treatment, especially on parts of the body not being irradiated, but any contraindications should be observed.

One of the side-effects of radiotherapy is that the skin may become very tender and fragile. ... This is where the application of oils rather than massage is very useful, and is used in France. The diluted essential oils (niaouli and/or tea tree) can also be sprayed onto the irradiated area. Other areas of the body may receive massage (with oil if desired).

(McNamara 1993)

Conclusions regarding use of essential oils on cancer patients can be formulated:

- in the case of weak general health, the elderly or advanced cancer, 50% normal-strength blends of oils should be used (see Ch. 2 for normal dilutions)
- massage with normal pressure (never heavy) may be used on specific restricted areas—shoulders (except on patients with breast

cancer), feet, hands, scalp, face, depending on the individual case

- only very gentle massage should be used for a full body treatment
- permission must be sought from the doctor in charge to use essential oils on a person with cancer, especially on an area receiving radiotherapy
- for a person receiving chemotherapy, specific-area or full-body massage may be given, bearing in mind the precautions indicated by the type and site of the cancer; the massage blend should be at quarter normal strength
- any suspected cancerous site should be avoided; Swiss reflex therapy (see Ch. 6) should be used instead.

Complementary approaches

One organization dedicated to helping people with cancer is Wirral Holistic Care Services, which carried out a study on cancer and complementary therapies between 1984 and 1987.

The aim was to identify the specific needs of people with cancer and to emphasize the need for patients/clients to take control of their treatment back into their own hands. The study used a basic question-and-answer format with time-evaluation tools and the self-selected patients/clients came via local cancer self-help groups or direct contact with the researchers (Crowther 1991).

The average time spent questioning patients/clients was 1 hour, depending on the identified needs of each one, which included the following, in order of importance:

- emotional support
- counselling
- education on self care
- dietary advice
- education on the disease
- education on the treatment modalities and complications and/or side-effects
- information on complementary therapy (seen as non-invasive)
- information on alternative therapy (may be invasive).

The Bristol Cancer Help Centre, set up in 1980, also gives help and encouragement to many sufferers of the disease. Despite criticism from time to time, a tremendous amount of comfort, hope and relief from pain has been given by the Centre over the years. There have been positive improvements in health in a number of patients, including some unusual remissions. As Burke & Sikora point out (1992), 'If complementary and orthodox cancer care can be provided together, it is possible that the consequent benefits would be greater than the sum of the two'.

The vast majority of patients in hospices suffer from cancer, though there is a steady increase in the number of patients with HIV-related illness being admitted. Jill Baxter was possibly the first person to work with essential oils on the terminally ill, offering her services voluntarily. R. Kensey, Director of Nursing Services at the Compton Hospice in Wolverhampton, wrote to the authors' college (where Baxter trained) about the benefits her patients received from aromatherapy:

The fact that someone cares helps patients and relatives alike to learn to accept their illness. Feelings of isolation, loneliness, depression and fear are reduced through the relaxation afforded by the gentle massage with essential oils. Pain in the bone and muscles is also relieved and we have found that movement of the limbs is easier after a treatment. Jill has certainly made a difference to our hospice.

(Kensey 1986 personal communication)

Case 13.1b Cancer—Aromatherapist Jeannie Maher, Australia

This elderly lady had lost her first husband and her son became a paraplegic at the age of 17 after being in an accident. She had remarried a few years ago. In 1977 she was diagnosed with diabetes and in December 1992 was discovered to have cancer. The scan showed a large mass in the head of the pancreas obstructing the common bile duct.

I was asked to do a treatment just before Christmas when the cancer was in the final stages. She had been given only a few weeks to live. Circulation was poor, skin dry and she was having trouble swallowing. The nail of her big toe had infection around it. For this treatment I mixed 1 drop each of frankincense and lavender in a base of almond oil and applied tea tree to the infected toe. I massaged mainly her feet, lower legs and hands, and the neck and shoulders to help with the swallowing. It was around lunchtime when I was there during the treatment—her husband and son were having a prawn sandwich. One of her greatest desires was to be able to eat a prawn sandwich—she had been eating mainly liquid foods.

Her desire was fulfilled as she got to eat and swallow her prawn sandwich following the treatment, as it relaxed the muscles with the massage. She found this very special as she had thought that would never be possible. She passed away several days later.

Case 13.2 Cancer—Aromatherapist: Helen Tuzio, UK

One of the problems we have had in offering aromatherapy here at the Neil Cliffe Cancer Care Centre is that of demand from the clients compared with the time therapists had available, so we devised a way of offering aromatherapy to many clients within these time constraints, while maintaining high standards.

Our aims for using aromatherapy are to enhance the relaxation process and promote a sense of well-being. We offer hand- or foot-massage, and feel the one-to-one contact of patient and therapist is intrinsic to the therapeutic process. Relaxation is taught in a group room, with up to eight clients and takes about 30 minutes. Aromatherapy massage is then offered on an individual basis, which takes about 15 minutes each person. There are usually three aromatherapists and an appointment system is organised so that everyone has a treatment.

Essential oils are selected and blended with a carrier oil by a qualified member of staff—nurse or occupational therapist with qualifications in aromatherapy and/or massage. Lavender is used the most because of its safe reputation, its relaxing qualities and its appeal to clients, who actually ask for it. Peppermint is used occasionally because of its antispasmodic action on the digestive system, easing nausea and vomiting. Bergamot and geranium—occasionally used for their uplifting qualities.

Case 1. Gentleman with cancer of the colon, with recurrent disease and also a colostomy. In an attempt to control symptoms of nausea, antiemetic drugs were given via syringe driver. However, the problem persisted. He agreed to attend the Centre for relaxation and aromatherapy. We decided to use *Mentha × piperita* to settle his stomach and apply this by a hand massage. The next week he reported that the feelings of nausea were eased on the evening of the treatment, and requested it again.

He attended on a weekly basis and always requested peppermint as he felt he was benefiting from it. The one-to-one attention gave him the opportunity to discuss his frustrations in no longer being able to follow his interests, and the opportunity to replace these by joining in other activities at the Centre—which he did!

Case 2. Elderly lady with diagnosis of head and neck tumour. Unfortunately, side effects of the treatment have caused a degree of deafness and she is also partially sighted. She chooses to have a hand-massage with oil of *Lavandula angustifolia*. The aim of this treatment is to stimulate her sense of smell as other senses are depleted. The one to one contact allows her to discuss her own agenda; she uses the time well knowing she has the therapist's individual attention. She says she feels more relaxed and comforted at the end of the massage. She looks happy and cheerful, as if she had had a special treatment.

Evaluation

The way in which we offer aromatherapy massage could be classed as therapeutic massage with essential oils rather than aromatherapy. This description better reflects the fact that presently we cannot undertake pre-treatment individual assessment or use specific oils to treat specific symptoms. However, the current system enables us to ensure that many people benefit from a therapeutic massage with essential oils.

Case 13.3 Cancer—Therapist: Lai Fong Cox, Hong Kong

A patient who had been admitted with a suspected bowel obstruction was vomiting heavily, producing nearly 3 l a day. He had a laparotomy and was found to have bowel cancer, which necessitated a further operation. The operation itself had no complications and the patient recovered.

By the 3rd or 4th day post-operation, the patient started having diarrhoea, producing 3 l a day. To begin with, the doctors thought that this was due to the patient fasting for some time and having intravenous fluid. The patient was therefore started on a liquid diet, gradually progressing to a soft diet. The patient tolerated the diet plan very well for 4 days, with no complaints of nausea or vomiting, but the diarrhoea did not subside, and he continued passing 3 l of faecal fluid every day. Following this, the doctors changed the diet back to intravenous infusion and the patient was given total parenteral nutrition (TPN) in order to give his bowels a rest and cease the diarrhoea. The TPN feed was carried out for another 3 days with no improvement in the patient's frequent diarrhoea and he was put back on a normal diet. By then it was more than 10 days since his operation.

I asked the primary nurse to let me try aromatherapy with him. The request was granted and I also received permission from the patient and his wife. Due to the surgical operation, I could not perform any type of body massage so I carried out Swiss reflex aromatherapy. I prepared the reflex massage cream, adding eucalyptus, lavender and chamomile. These three essential oils are able to ease diarrhoea and relax the nerves. After the first session the patient said that he had a good sleep and after 6 daily sessions said that he had not felt so well for a long time.

The amount of faecal fluid gradually reduced from day to day until the 6th day, when it was down to 900 ml. The primary nurse, patient and I were very pleased with the result. I then had a change of duty rota and a week later, when I went back to work, I was disappointed that the patient's diarrhoea had returned to 3 l a day. I started the therapy again and managed to do three daily sessions, during which time some improvement was evident to the primary nurse. Unfortunately, she could not convince the doctors of this and the patient was discharged. I could not help him further due to the distance, though I was told that he was looking for further complementary therapy to help with his cancer. About 9 months later, he was re-admitted and died soon after.

Case 13.4 Cancer—Aromatherapist:
Marlene Cadwallader (BAppSciNursing), Australia

a

A 60-year-old male had a pancreatic cancer. His pain was managed with analgesia and nausea managed by maxdon. 9 litres of fluid had been withdrawn from his abdomen (paracentesis).

I used a blend of chamomile (calming and antinausea), lavender (also calming, all-round effect) and geranium (balancing, correction of fluid retention).

I noted that the next paracentesis produced a much smaller volume of fluid—2 l or less. He looked forward to his massages over a period of a couple of months. In that time he was able to eat a light diet, relax to music and come to terms with his coming death.

Lavender was altered to neroli when signs of distress were showing. This provided a calming and peaceful effect which was useful for the family when provided with a drop on a tissue. A tissue with neroli was also placed onto shelves and drawers and one was placed inside the spygmanomake situated at the head of the bed. The family were at ease, feeling that the oils, massage and Reiki made the transition easier.

It was also noticed that the nursing staff were much happier and cheerier amongst themselves. Was it the neroli?

b

Patient B, a 61 year old male who was battling severe pain from cancer of the lung, was slowly coming to terms with the fact that his life would not be prolonged. I worked closely with him and his family in the hospital setting. His feeling of relaxation and peace was evident as he would say 'I feel really good', and he claimed he also slept well for a couple of nights after a treatment.

The essential oils I used to assist comfort were frankincense, chamomile and rose as a pure oil blend for placing on the soles of his feet and to inhale. The same mix was used in a reflex base cream mix for hand, foot and back massages.

The monoterpenes and esters in rose oil are balancing and calming, the sesquiterpenes and aldehydes in the chamomile easing anxiety, tension, anger and fear, calming the mind and providing peace. The sesquiterpenes, terpenes and alcohol in frankincense would be sedative and analgesic, creating a balance by soothing the mind, providing a feeling of calm, allaying fear and anxiety. It is possible that frankincense may have been helpful in easing his shortness of breath (Sellar 1992).

His wife carried a tissue on which was a drop of rose—she claimed it helped her accept the inevitable. To help with the bereavement I provided a mix of 1 drop melissa, 3 drops marjoram and 1 drop rose blended in 8 ml of carrier oil, which was used by the family as a self-massage around neck and shoulders.

Marjoram was chosen as it contains terpenes, alcohols, ketones and sesquiterpenes, providing an analgesic and calming effect, relieving anxiety, strengthening the mind to confront situations. It seemed to be very helpful in providing a comfort in grief.

Melissa, with its alcohols, esters, aldehydes and a high percentage of monoterpenes has a calming and 'pick-me-up' effect on the emotions. Good for shock, panic and hysteria, helping bereaved to face situations of loss and promoting positivity.

Rose oil was chosen for the reason stated above; it was generally felt that the oils were effective in providing peace and acceptance.

HIV/AIDS

Since its appearance in the 1980s the HIV virus, which causes a defect in the human immune system, has spread at an alarming rate, ruthlessly attacking even infants and the unborn (who may contract the disease in the womb or by breastfeeding). At the 9th International Conference on AIDS in Berlin in June 1993 it was revealed that 1 million babies had been infected by then. Two real needs were identified:

- to develop a vaccine that is effective and available to all
- to develop effective barrier methods under the control of women, for example a vaginal viricide (International Conference on AIDS 1993).

Conventional drugs have so far been generally unsatisfactory against viruses. Specific essential oils have already been shown in research to kill off certain viruses (see Ch. 4). None have yet been researched for their effect on the HIV virus and none are claimed by aromatherapists to treat the infection itself. Nevertheless aromatherapy care can do much to improve the quality of life, as it can for people living with cancer, and several essential oils have been found to boost the immune system (see below).

Maintaining the immune system must be of paramount importance, and therapies aimed at re-establishing the unique functional integrity of the total human being should be used. Certain essential oils … are powerful in supporting the immune system, … particularly so if used early in the treatment. This in itself could turn the tide and tip the balance between maintaining well-being or developing the opportunist infections that lead to full blown AIDS.

(Burnett 1992)

A study of the chemistry of the individual essential oils is a great help in making the choice of what to use on people with HIV, because the effects of certain chemical constituents have been researched. As with cancer patients, a holistic choice of essential oils should be made, starting in this case with those which may stimulate the immune system into action, then selecting from these the essential oils which could have a beneficial effect on other prevailing symptoms. Although several essential oils are effective on certain viruses, no research has yet been carried out regarding their effect on HIV in particular (see Ch. 4). Osato (1965) carried out research on people with cancer using the isolates of citral (by injection) and citronellal (by mouth). The results were not conclusive and the percentage of people in remission after 15 years was 5%. It may be that the whole essential oils rich in citrals (neral and geranial), such as *Cymbopogon flexuosus* [LEMONGRASS], *Lippia citriodora* and *Melissa officinalis* [TRUE MELISSA], could be added to the list of possible oils to try.

Immunostimulants

Essential oils which may benefit the immune system include:

- *Boswellia carteri* (Franchomme & Pénoël 1990 p. 328)
- *Syzygium aromaticum* (flos) (Roulier 1990 p. 230)
- *Inula graveolens* [INULA] (Roulier 1990 p. 230)
- *Melaleuca alternifolia* (Franchomme & Pénoël 1990 p. 369)
- *Melaleuca viridiflora* (Roulier 1990 p. 230)
- *Pogostemon patchouli* (Roulier 1990 p. 230)
- *Thymus vulgaris* (thymol, linalool and geraniol chemotypes). Franchomme & Pénoël (1990) give the thujanol chemotype, but this is very difficult to cultivate from cuttings (Lamy 1989).

Should any oil not on this list be thought holistically helpful for the patient, it should be added, to increase the synergistic effects.

Psychological factors

The factors of stress and depression need also to be considered in oil selection and *Thymus vulgaris* (particularly the geraniol and linalool chemotypes) is known to stimulate the immune system as well as uplift the nervous system (Franchomme & Pénoël 1990). In spite of the lack of research studies on essential oil activity against the HIV virus, there is empirical evidence from many aromatherapists and aromatologists who have had encouraging results using widely differing oils—due to the nature of holistic selection for each individual.

The psychological state of the client's carers is important too. Alan Barker (1994 personal communication) has this to say:

It is vital that we care for the carers—their 'burn out' can break a vital link in the chain of care, and to show the partners and the carers how to administer a simple massage or application of an essential oil prescription is a wonderful way of creating a bond or link with care. All too often the partners of patients feel left out and this is a great opportunity for them to be again a part of this person's life/death.

ARC symptoms

Symptoms which present themselves as a result of the progression of the virus (known as the AIDS Related Complex—ARC) are such things as infected and swollen glands, recurrent fevers, sore throat (caused by the presence of an additional virus, herpes or candida), coughing (sometimes with sputum) and severe shortness of breath (Barker 1993).

An area not often considered in connection with the HIV virus is the skin, which is very often badly affected by seborrhoeic dermatitis, atopic dermatitis, psoriasis, Kaposi's sarcoma and drug-induced eruptions (Burnett 1993). Carrier oils such as calendula, rosehip and hypericum have a beneficial effect on the skin, and should be used in conjunction with essential oils known for their affinity with the particular skin symptoms as well as stress and depression.

Once the considerations above have been noted, the treatment by aromatherapy of a patient with HIV-related symptoms can follow the normal pattern. Its effectiveness lies in the fact that the essential oils trigger natural homoeostatic principles in the body to create a healing process (see Ch. 7).

One of my HIV positive patients cried for quarter of an hour after his second aromatherapy massage and reported feeling 'as if he had let out a can of worms'. He slept better than he had since before he was first diagnosed.

(Burnett 1993)

Case 13.5 HIV/AIDS—Aromatologist: Alan Barker, UK

Mr A was diagnosed with the HIV virus (body positive) in 1988, and has for the most part been cared for in the community by a designated community-based nurse. On the occasion of any opportunistic infection that could not be dealt with within the confines of the community (through the GU out-patient department), admission to the hospital was needed.

A wide range of drug therapy has been employed depending upon the needs of Mr A, and opportunistic infections have for the most part been kept under control. This, as in many other cases, often requires long spells in hospital and, depending upon the infection/problem, may require compound drug therapy, e.g. chemotherapy or radiation therapy. Mr A had had the offer of complementary therapy in various forms (one being aromatherapy) both in the community and in a hospital situation. The aromatherapy in the home setting has been of great value, not only to Mr A but also to partners and carers.

With the amount of chemotherapy being used, Mr A was suffering from an itching dermal reaction and insomnia. Conventional options were having very little effect, apart from putting more chemicals into his body. After being asked by the consultant if I could do anything, we tried a bath oil containing 5 drops each of *Pelargonium graveolens* and *Chamomilla recutita* in 100 ml vegetable oil (90% grapeseed, 10% unrefined macerated oil of calendula—i.e. low concentration). As well as this, a cream was made up (15 drops of *Chamomilla recutita* in 30 g base cream), to apply as needed to any itching part of the body.

Because of respiratory problems Mr A (together with conventional antibiotic therapy) had a diffuser in his own room (both at home and in hospital) using *Boswellia carteri*, *Cinnamomum camphora*, *Eucalyptus smithii* and *Satureia montana*. These were varied according to his needs. Essential oils were given in a shampoo base to help his itching scalp: *Chamaemelum nobile*, *Melaleuca alternifolia*, *Rosmarinus officinalis* and *Thymus vulgaris* ct. alcohol. Generalized relaxing baths and massage (clinical areas only, i.e. foot, legs, neck and shoulder) were given, using numerous relaxing, calming and soothing essential oils.

Mr A died of pneumocystis carinii and progressive multifocal leukoencephalopathy amongst other complications, but his quality of life in the final stages was of the very highest, due in part to dedicated staff administering aromatherapy prescriptions and to a positive attitude by health care professionals to the use of this complementary medicine.

Case 13.6 HIV/AIDS—Aromatologist: Alan Barker, UK

This is a difficult case to relate but the basic problem is that A is in the last stages of full-blown AIDS. He cannot cope with baths or massage due to the onset of Kaposi's sarcoma. Added to this there is evidence of infiltration of the nervous system, due to the virus which has at this point become phagocytosed by the macrophages, allowing these cells to cross the normally impervious blood-brain barrier.

The options open to the team are very limited, but not beyond helping. There needed to be a way to get the oils into the lymphatic system in order to stimulate the growth of T-helper cells and white blood cells. We devised an effective way of applying the oils by introducing them in a lotion carrier and applying this to the main lymph nodes, i.e. armpits, thorax, groin area. The method in which the essential oils are applied may seem unorthodox, but it was necessary to adapt to the needs of the client. It is only by taking these unprecedented steps that we may be able to connect with this new challenge in health care/aromatherapy. The oils we are using are 10 drops each of *Citrus limon* (per.), *Thymus vulgaris* ct. alcohol and *Melaleuca alternifolia* in 30 ml carrier lotion. The lotion, applied in a thick smear, is easily absorbed into the skin/lymph node area without too much effort on part of the client or therapist.

At the time of writing A is stable and very well able to cope with the applications, and his T-helper cell count is rising.

Case 13.7 HIV/AIDS—Aromatherapist: Joy Burnett Borneo, UK

S is 37-years-old and was diagnosed HIV-positive in 1986. Developed pneumocystis carinii, pneumonia and various other infections early in 1991. I was contacted by the Cleveland Aids Support who had been asked by the patient's consultant if any help was available.

6.11.91 S very depressed, angry and unable to handle his own sense of helplessness. His whole body is covered with atopic dermatitis. Unable to walk because of pain in his legs and ankles—scratches constantly and legs, ankles and bottom are scratched raw. The essential oils used for his back massage were bergamot (to uplift, and to help his depression, emotional and mental weariness), German chamomile (for impatience and irritability) and sandalwood (repressed anger, emotions and fear). I mixed an oil for him to apply to himself daily (to relieve the itching and help combat the dermatitis) containing lavender, German chamomile and patchouli.

13.11.91 Skin on legs much improved (S applying it up to 6 times a day). Massaged his back, arms and hands with the same mixture as last week as he reported feeling so good after the first aromatherapy treatment. Gave him a blend of lavender, geranium and sandalwood for his bath.

27.11.91 Temperament seems to have improved (his mother's comment). Skin much better but pain and swelling in his feet considerable so concentrated on these. Used juniper (for the oedema), chamomile (antiinflammatory) and geranium (for circulation). This was gently applied to his legs and a mixture left for him to apply himself.

12.12.91 Massage as before, concentrating on his legs and feet. Generally feels much better and has managed to walk a bit this week. Skin continues to improve and is applying his original mix regularly.

27.12.91 Skin much better; ankles still red and itchy but he is no longer scratching. He is feeling generally a lot better and has been away for Christmas. His legs are less painful and he is managing to walk a little. Massage this week included frankincense—to help with the scarring.

Treatment continued successfully through the early months of 1992 and the skin problem only erupted again when he was taken into hospital in May, just before he died.

Summary

Complementary medicine has been able to offer much in the way of support to those living with diseases such as cancer and HIV-related illness. This is increasingly backed by the medical profession despite the fact that there is little in the way of published research results on the use of aromatherapy in this field. However, a few studies have been carried out which show positive results with regard to the improvement of life quality and a greater acceptance of death.

REFERENCES

Bardeau P 1976 La médecine aromatique. Robert Lafont, Paris
Barker A 1993 The clinical use of aromatherapy and the AIDS virus. Unpublished Dissertation, International Shirley Price International College of Aromatherapy, Hinckley, Leics
Bernadet M 1983 La phyto-aromathérapie pratique. Dangles, St-Jean-de-Braye
Burke C, Sikora K 1992 Cancer—the dual approach. Nursing Times 88(38): 62–66
Burnett J 1992 Using aromatherapy to enhance the immune system and alleviate symptoms for those affected by HIV and AIDS. Unpublished Dissertation, Shirley Price International College of Aromatherapy, Hinckley, Leics
Caldwell 1991 Research reports. International Journal of Aromatherapy 3(1): 6
Chaitow L 1987 Soft-tissue manipulation. Thorsons, Wellingborough
Crowther D 1991 Complementary therapy in practice. Nursing Standard 5(23): 25–27
Elliott C 1991 Cancer was a killer in the dark ages. Sunday Telegraph, December 29: 9
Franchomme P, Pénoël D 1990 L'aromathérapie exactement. Jollois, Limoges
Gattefossé R-M 1993 Aromatherapy. Daniel, Saffron Walden
Horrigan C 1991 Complementing cancer care. International Journal of Aromatherapy 3(4): 15–17

International Conference on AIDS 1993 The HIV/AIDS pandemic: global spread and global response. Berlin
Lamy R 1989 The cultivation of chemotypes of thyme and rosemary. Riverhead Publishing, Hinckley
Lundie S 1994 Introducing and applying aromatherapy within the NHS. The Aromatherapist 1(1): 283
Machin M 1989 Advanced cancer. International Journal of Aromatherapy 2(1): 19
McNamara P 1993 Massage for people with cancer: a working paper. Wandsworth Cancer Support Centre, London
Osato S 1965 Chemotherapy of human carcinoma with citronellal and citral and their action on carcinoma tissue in its histological aspects up to healing. Tohoku Journal of Experimental Medicine 96: 102–123
Phillips A 1989 Advanced cancer. International Journal of Aromatherapy 2(1): 18
Price S 1993a Parkinson's disease project: is aromatherapy an effective treatment for Parkinson's disease? The Aromatherapist 1(1): 14–21
Roulier G 1990 Les huiles essentielles pour votre santé. Dangles, St-Jean-de-Braye
Sellar W 1992 The directory of essential oils. Daniel, Saffron Walden
Sims S 1986 Slow stroke back massage for cancer patients. Nursing Times 82(13): 47–50
Valnet J 1980 The practice of aromatherapy. Daniel, Saffron Walden

Policy and practice

14

Aromatherapy in the UK

Introduction

Complementary therapies have grown in importance within the NHS during the 1980s and 1990s. Unregulated at first, there have been increasing demands that they should observe similar ethical and practical constraints to orthodox medicine. This chapter proposes a model set of policies and protocols for the professional practice of aromatherapy in UK healthcare settings.

THE GROWTH OF COMPLEMENTARY THERAPIES IN THE NHS

The ever-increasing interest by the nursing profession in complementary therapies, especially aromatherapy, has raised several issues of importance to the nursing profession. As a result, a forum within the Royal College of Nursing now introduces nurses to the various complementary therapies available, with a steering committee set up to compare results of their use by nurses in hospital situations. Where the benefits to patients can be quantified, it is hoped to use this evidence to persuade more hospital managers to fund natural therapies—including aromatherapy. The RCN has also compiled a Statement of Beliefs which reflects the principles nurses practising complementary therapies should observe.

At the same time a directive entitled the Liability of Suppliers of Service makes it clear that 'individuals should be able to justify their actions should any malpractice claim be made against them by clients' (Rankin-Box 1992). Clearly, aromatherapy as it has been implemented to date—by any nurse in any circumstance thought to be valid—cannot continue, and a number of hospital authorities have already set up (or are in the process of doing so) criteria for the practice of complementary therapies.

Aromatherapy is the most widely-used complementary therapy in the Health Service (Lundie 1994), and many nurses are now taking up training in the subject. Cawthorne (1991) states that 'aromatherapy allows nurses to practise the *art* of nursing, which over recent years, due to the increase in medical technology, has taken a secondary role to the *science* of nursing. The relaxing nature of the massage also has a calming effect on the nurse who gives it. In addition, it allows them to give true holistic care'.

Several hospitals are funding nurses of various standing on aromatherapy courses and The Ardenlea Marie Curie Centre and Help the Hospices have worked closely with The Shirley Price International College of Aromatherapy, running courses specifically for the nursing profession. In 1994 the RCN in conjunction with the Shirley Price International College of Aromatherapy produced a video which emphasizes the need for adequate training and knowledgeable use of essential oils.

Consultants and GPs today certainly have a more sympathetic and cooperative attitude towards aromatherapy than when the authors came into the profession in the early 1970s. Only since the late 1980s has there been a rapid growth in the willingness of the medical profession to listen seriously to claims of the positive and sometimes dramatic effects essential oils can have on people's overall health (see Ch. 4). One of the reasons for previous reluctance was the understandable reaction to the short length of training formerly required—only 5 or 6 days, compared with the same number of years for medical training! It was never put across clearly or knowledgeably enough in those days by enthusiastic aromatherapists that aromatherapy was not intended to supplant allopathic medicine, but to supplement it and enhance the caring work carried out by nurses—to reintroduce natural healing agents into hospitals perhaps suffering from an overdose of synthetic drugs. Another off-putting factor could have been the aromas—how

could pleasant smells affect the health in a positive way? Finally, the word 'massage' with its then sleazy connotation did not help, particularly at a time when touch was being ousted from nursing care and machines were largely replacing the healing hands of the physiotherapist. Now, however, clinical successes in hospitals where essential oils have been used and the results of projects and trials (albeit a comparatively small number) have led to a greater willingness to listen and to employ the therapy in hospitals.

At first, therapists found it easier to obtain permission to work in hospices with the terminally ill, usually on a voluntary basis (no doubt it was felt that at least no harm could be done!), but now aromatherapy is used in general hospitals too, and a number of therapists work in conjunction with their local GP on minor health problems which can be helped by essential oils. A major breakthrough for the therapy occurred in 1993, when GPs were empowered to refer patients to complementary therapists for treatment on the NHS, provided that the GP concerned remained clinically accountable for the patient.

An understanding of the attitudes of the medical and nursing profession, and of the legal and professional issues which govern their practice, are important as they all play a part in the acceptance and use of complementary therapies generally, and aromatherapy specifically. This even before consideration is given as to whether the necessary pennies are available to spend on what at first may appear to be an aromatic luxury.

(Lundie 1994)

The professionalization of aromatherapy in the UK

Aromatherapy was introduced originally through the beauty therapy world in the 1960s. Massage therapists became aware of it in the first half of the 1980s, by which time only four aromatherapy books had appeared—Robert Tisserand, *The Art of Aromatherapy* 1977; Jean Valnet, *The Practice of Aromatherapy* 1980; Shirley Price, *Practical Aromatherapy* 1983; and Raymond Lautié and André Passebecq, *The Use of Plant Essences in Healing* 1979.

In the 1980s many books on the subject appeared and nurses became conscious of the immense possibilities of this gentle therapy. Aromatherapy began creeping into the health professional's practice without due attention to the training of those using the essential oils and without Health Authority policies or hospital protocols from which to work (as is the case at present in many other countries). This was perhaps due in part to the great number of aromatherapy books written for the general public, which emphasize the ease of use and the successful effects of essential oils. However, it was probably mainly due to the strong desire of nurses to give their patients help in an area which had begun to be neglected by 20th-century medicine. Many of the original nurses who trained in aromatherapy were leaving, or were about to leave, the nursing profession because they felt their caring skills were being pushed into the background. Less and less time was available in hospital settings for the personal contact which used to be a key element of their chosen profession. There was also the hope that the use of essential oils could perhaps help to reduce the need for secondary medication given to cope with the side-effects of primary treatment.

Professional aromatherapy associations

In response to these trends, in 1985 10 aromatherapists, including the authors, met to discuss the inauguration of the first worldwide aromatherapy organization—the International Federation of Aromatherapy (IFA)—which created the first set of standards for aromatherapy in this country. A second major aromatherapy association (of which again the authors were founder members), the International Society of Professional Aromatherapists (ISPA), was launched in 1990 to give qualifying aromatherapists a choice of associations, insurance benefits and venues for meetings. These associations offer legal support and insurance, which provides cover for malpractice, public and product liability. Their aims are to develop and maintain high standards of qualification and to provide a forum for the development and exchange of knowledge and skill. Annual general meetings (in ISPA's case a weekend seminar) are held with speakers appropriate to the requirements of professional aromatherapists. There are also a number of smaller associations, such as the Aromatology Association.

The British Complementary Medicine Association

In 1990 a new consultative body for all complementary medicine was formed—the British Complementary Medicine Association (BCMA), designed to promote complementary therapies at all levels, and to represent therapies not covered by the Council for Complementary and Alternative Medicine or the Institute for Complementary Medicine. It represents around 30 therapies and, apart from aiming to integrate complementary medicine into the structure of the nation's healthcare system, it aims to encourage, through democratic process, the many individual therapy organizations to form an umbrella group for collective action.

The Aromatherapy Organisations Council

As a result of the work undertaken by the BCMA, the Aromatherapy Organisations Council (AOC) was born in 1991 and is the leading body for the aromatherapy profession in the UK. It is composed of both aromatherapy associations and training schools, but does not have individual membership. One of the main aims of the AOC is to establish common standards of training and to ensure that all organizations registered with the Council provide appropriate standards of professional practice and conduct for their members. They also aim to initiate, support or sponsor research and provide a collective voice through which to initiate and sustain political dialogue with government, civil and medical bodies, in order to enhance the best interests of professional aromatherapy.

The AOC has set a minimum standard for aromatherapy which, at the time of writing, demands an in-house training of 180 hours over a minimum period of approximately 12 months, plus a qualification in anatomy and physiology if this is not already held. (Some nurses trained under Project 2000 may need to study anatomy and physiology since there is no set syllabus and not all teaching hospitals give it the time it warrants.) Most aromatherapy schools include anatomy and physiology questions on their examination papers.

Short courses, workshops and seminars

Health professionals without complete aromatherapy or aromatology training should use essential oils only under the direction of, or after consultation with, a qualified aromatherapist or aromatologist. One- and two-day seminars in aromatherapy may be adequate for such health professionals but it should be made clear that more rigorous training is required in order to practise independently and prescribe essential oils for individual patients.

Accredited training

Aromatherapy training establishments approved or accredited by an aromatherapy organization to the minimum standards set by the AOC teach detailed chemistry and properties of essential oils, their actions on the body and mind and how to use them accurately. When a knowledgeable aromatherapist dispenses appropriate essential oils there should be little likelihood of any adverse effects. It is a question of being aware, as with any medicine, of what and how much should be administered and for how long.

In 1993 an Aromatherapy Trades Council was launched, and included among its aims and objectives:

- the establishment of guidelines for safety, labelling and packaging for the aromatherapy trade
- the promotion of responsible use of aromatherapy products.

Examples of the standards they hope to introduce include ensuring that all essential oil bottles have an integral dropper and that labelling information includes appropriate cautions and contraindications. They also aim to try and stop companies from violating the Medicines Act 1968 regarding health claims made for products. Many labels still claim that a product is 'for arthritis' or 'for breathing difficulties' etc., but this is only permitted when a therapist is making up a prescription for a client who has been seen face-to-face. It is not permitted at all on products sold off the shelf to a person unknown to the producer of that product.

Aromatherapy-in-Care

In 1988 a special group within the International Federation of Aromatherapy was established, in what must be regarded as a unique endeavour by a nonmedical profession, to introduce aromatherapy into medical establishments. Aromatherapy-in-Care (AIC) therapists introduced themselves first into hospices, as did a number of independent aromatherapists, where they all used their skills on patients with cancer. Their voluntary services were much appreciated and soon members of the AIC group (and the independent therapists) were invited into NHS hospitals, self-governing cancer care organizations, centres for people with learning difficulties and other support groups.

Members of Aromatherapy-in-Care, aromatherapy practitioners and practising health professionals qualified in aromatherapy have together been instrumental in arousing the interest and acceptance of the British medical profession, who can see for themselves the advantages of touch and essential oils. This has been supported by aromatherapists who, like the authors, have lectured in hospitals and presented papers at nursing conferences to create an awareness in this field.

RCN Special Interest Group

In 1991, a Special Interest Group was set up by the RCN to look into complementary therapies. The group has developed a Statement of Beliefs, together with guidelines for nurses looking for a complementary therapy course or practitioner. They focus on how to introduce complementary therapies into the workplace, and on the education and standardization of nurse education in this field.

One objective of the Special Interest Group is to make nurses aware of the need to check the credentials of any course in which they are interested, including the tutor/student ratio and the qualifications of the tutors. It suggests asking whether or not there is supervised practice, an anatomy and physiology examination and a practical examination in the therapy. Counselling, communication and self-development skills should be included along with support for the trainee therapist.

RCN Statement of Beliefs

The RCN Statement of Beliefs for the practice of complementary therapies (to be revised as necessary and on the advice and suggestion of members and other interested parties following discussion by the steering committee) reads as follows:

1. We believe that nurses using complementary therapies as part of their care should know and understand their responsibilities to the patient/client and the United Kingdom Central Council for Nursing, Midwifery and Health Visiting. Further we believe that the UKCC code sets the professional requirements to be met by all registered nurses using complementary therapies.
2. We believe that all patients and clients have the right to be offered and to receive complementary therapies either exclusively or as a part of orthodox nursing practice.
3. We believe that all patients have the right to expect that their religious, cultural and spiritual beliefs will be observed by nurses practising complementary therapies.
4. We believe that all complementary therapies available to patients must have the support of the collaborative care team.
5. We believe that a registered nurse who is appropriately qualified to carry out a complementary therapy must agree and work to locally agreed protocols for practice and standards of care.
6. We believe that the patient/clients, in partnership with the nurse complementary therapist, should determine the suitability of any proposed complementary therapy. Informed, documented consent should be

obtained and detailed records kept with the patient/client's care record.
7. We believe that, where possible, research based complementary therapy practices should be used. Where this is not possible then nurse complementary therapists, as accountable professionals, must be able to justify their actions.
8. We believe that nurse complementary therapists should, when appropriate, be prepared to instruct significant individuals in the patient/client's life (including the patient/ client) so that they can learn basic complementary therapy skills for self care.
9. We believe that nurse complementary therapists should seek to develop their self awareness and inter-personal skills and so enhance their role as reflective practitioners.
10. We believe that nurse complementary therapists have a responsibility to collect detailed information on all therapy sessions and to evaluate the outcomes of therapy on the patient/client.
11. We believe that the practice of complementary therapies by nurses should be the subject of at least an annual review by an appropriately constituted multidisciplinary committee. The review should take into account patient measures of satisfaction and benefit.

It is not easy to quantify complementary therapies working exclusively with energies, for example acupuncture or spiritual healing. Aromatherapy, however, is a multiple therapy embracing energies, therapeutic touch, massage and the administration of remedies—not to mention the pleasing aroma which could be partly responsible for aromatherapy possibly being the most popular complementary therapy which nurses wish to study.

The United Kingdom Central Council for nursing, midwifery and health visiting

It is advisable that nurses, as professional and accountable practitioners, should take into account the United Kingdom Central Council's (UKCC)

Code of Professional Conduct (CPC), Scope of Professional Practice (SPP) and Standards for the Administration of Medicines (SAM), since these documents govern all nursing activities.

The UKCC documents, together with appropriate and well-thought-out policies and local protocols for the use of aromatherapy (see below), are designed to lead to informed professional functioning by nurses who choose to include aromatherapy in their work.

Many issues covered in these UKCC documents are directly applicable to nurses working with essential oils, and the relevant points will be brought into focus for the purposes of this chapter. For ease of reference each document quoted will be referenced by its initials in brackets.

'The range of responsibilities which fall to individual nurses, midwives and health visitors should be related to their personal experience, education and skill' (SPP Introduction, p. 2). Experience and skill should be built upon education—a comprehensive and detailed learning base is essential.

'Just as practice must remain dynamic, sensitive, relevant and responsive to the changing needs of individual patients and clients, so too must education for practice' (SPP 3).

Many practitioners of different disciplines do not regularly update their knowledge. This is unwise since updating is of paramount importance, especially in a world where ideas and accepted behavioural patterns are changing fast. 'The practice of nursing takes place in a context of continuing change and development' (SPP Int. 1).

The CPC states that:

'As a registered nurse, midwife or health visitor you are personally accountable for your practice and, in the exercise of your professional accountability, must:

- promote and safeguard the interest and well-being of patients and clients;
- ensure that no action or omission on your part, or within your sphere of responsibility, is detrimental to the interests, condition or safety of patients and clients;

- maintain and improve your professional knowledge and competence;
- acknowledge any limitations in your knowledge and competence and decline any duties or responsibilities unless able to perform them in a safe and skilled manner.'

The registered nurse, midwife or health visitor must:

- 'take steps to remedy any relevant deficits in order effectively and appropriately to meet the needs of patients and clients' (SPP 9. 3)
- 'recognise and honour the direct or indirect personal accountability borne for all aspects of professional practice' (SPP 9. 5)
- 'avoid any inappropriate delegation to others which compromises those interests' (SPP 9. 6).

The last two points, when applied to aromatherapy, emphasize the need for suitable insurance cover specific to the use of essential oils. This can be obtained from one of the professional aromatherapy/aromatology associations on becoming a full member. ISPA and the Aromatology Association also insure student aromatherapists during their time of study.

'Patients and clients require skilled care from registered practitioners—and support staff require direction and supervision from these same practitioners' (SPP 11).

The UKCC acknowledges that nurses require support staff in their work and, although it does not have a direct role in the training of healthcare assistants, it states its position in relation to support roles:

- 'healthcare assistants to registered nurses, midwives and health visitors must work under the direction and supervision of those registered practitioners' (SPP 23.1)
- 'healthcare assistants must not be allowed to work beyond their level of competence' (SPP 23.3).

In conclusion, the Council declares that the framework and principles of Scope for Professional Practice reflect the personal responsibility and accountability of individual practitioners, entrusted by the Council to protect and improve standards of care.

With this amount of responsibility and accountability applying to the practice of aromatherapy and aromatology in hospitals, it is time for nurses suitably qualified in these professions to have the courage to say, with the following writer, 'I am an aromatherapist' first and foremost.

All too often I hear the same cry—'I am a qualified nurse using aromatherapy'. …
A nursing qualification does not make you a better aromatherapist—indeed, to some, it can be a disadvantage.
We should be proud of our profession in the use of essential oils and not need to use another profession as a crutch. Many people may say 'But a nurse will have a greater understanding of clinical matters'—this is not true at all! … If we feel inadequate with the essential oil training we have had—if it has not covered the areas needed in a clinical field—then find a course which does.
If we are insecure with our training and wish to hide behind the apron strings of another profession, this is not acceptable to either discipline; in fact, the one will strangle the other.'

(Barker 1993)

Barker goes on to say that we are competent and appropriately-trained professionals in our own right, and do aromatology/aromatherapy a great disservice by tagging it onto another discipline to give it credibility when it is already a valid system of medicine.

AROMATHERAPY, AROMATOLOGY AND INGESTION

Aromatherapy is strictly 'the use of essential oils to promote the health and vitality of the body, mind and spirit by inhalation, baths, compresses, topical application and massage'—not merely 'a massage using essential oils' (see Ch. 5) (Price 1985).

The definition of aromatology is not quite the same as that for aromatherapy; the two main differences are that (a) in aromatology, unlike in aromatherapy, full-body-massage is not an integral part of the basic training and (b) internal uses of essential oils are included in aromatology but not in aromatherapy. In France, essential oils are administered internally (pessaries, suppositories and injections as well as by mouth) by medical doctors and phytotherapists, since oral ingestion is an extremely effective method for disorders of the digestive tract, reaching the site of the problem by a direct route. Topical application (without massage), inhalation and compresses are the other methods generally used by French medical aromatologists.

The first British aromatherapists to write books on aromatherapy were Tisserand (1977) and Price (1983). Apart from Lautié & Passebecq (1984) and Valnet (1980) (both translated from French) no other books were published for a further 5 years. Tisserand was not in the beauty business and although Price was originally a beauty therapist, she found her vocation in the kind of aromatherapy advocated by Lautié & Passebecq and Valnet, and accepted ingestion, as did Tisserand, as an appropriate method of use.

The first aromatherapy organization comprised mainly beauty therapists, and the beauty therapy code of practice was taken into consideration. Since this disallows oral administration of anything, even vitamin tablets, it was written into the association's code of practice (and therefore that of every subsequent aromatherapy association) that internal use was not allowed. In one way this was providential, because there soon appeared on the market a plethora of commercial 'essential oils', most of which were (and still are) of a standardized perfume quality, not ideal for therapeutic use (see Ch. 2) and definitely not suitable for internal use. For this, only essential oils which are known not to be adulterated or 'ennobled' in any way and are from plants free from harmful herbicides and pesticides may be ingested . Wild and naturally- and organically-farmed plants are the only suitable sources—and are preferable for *all* methods of therapeutic use.

Volatile (essential) oils appear in the British Pharmacopoeia and have traditionally been used orally as expectorants, carminatives and for other digestive disorders. In this respect they are used as medicines, conform to certain standards and can be found in formulations within a recommended dose range (Farrell M 1994 personal communication)—but they are not administered by the British medical profession as medicines in their own right. However, at the time of writing there are a few hospitals in Britain which do orally administer essential oils (diluted in a suitable medium), with the consent of the consultants concerned. Some of these hospitals come under the Community Health Sheffield (NHS Trust) which employs a clinical aromatologist.

Aromatherapists give essential oils mainly by massage and inhalation. Nevertheless, inhalation is a form of ingestion in that the essential oils penetrate directly to the internal systems of the body. With massage, the essential oils pass via the skin into the blood stream and the surrounding tissues—again, a form of ingestion. Aromatherapists use gargling and suppositories as methods of penetration into the body tissues for the essential oils and this too is looked upon as a form of ingestion. Suppositories act directly on the rectum as a treatment for anal fissures and haemorrhoids or by absorption via the blood supply to the colon for systemic use. This route, giving direct access to the blood supply, avoids 'first pass' metabolism in the liver and is rapid in effect (Farrell M 1994 personal communication).

Oral ingestion should not be dismissed or feared, but to use this method (or indeed any internal method) the specialized training given on an aromatology course is required.

Standards for the administration of medicines

With respect to the above, nurse/midwife aromatherapists using essential oils, whether for baths, inhalations, topical application (including compresses), suppositories, pessaries and/or massage, should accept that they are administering medicines. Therefore, some of the Standards for the Administration of Medicines, written by the UKCC for its members, indirectly apply to them, emphasizing yet again the need for professional training or supervision:

'The administration of medicines is an important aspect of the professional practice of persons whose names are on the Council's register. It requires thought and the exercise of professional judgement' (SAM Introduction p. 2). 'The Council expects that, in this area of practice as in all others, all practitioners will have taken steps to

develop their knowledge and competence' (SAM Introduction p. 4). The document goes on to reiterate that all registered nurses, midwives and health visitors must recognize the personal professional accountability which they bear for their actions.

Medicinal preparations are prescribed by a physician, checked and dispensed by a pharmacist and administered by a nurse. An essential oil prescription is prescribed by a competent aromatherapist or aromatologist and administered by that practitioner, or by a nurse suitably trained in the method of administration, and in ideal circumstances the prescriber should not be the dispenser and the dispenser should not administer (Farrell M 1994 personal communication). The prescription of essential oil massage mixes should nevertheless satisfy the following criteria:

- 'that it is based, whenever possible, on the patient's awareness of the purpose of the treatment and consent' (SAM 6. 1)
- 'that the prescription is either clearly written or typed, and that the entry is indelible and dated' (SAM 6. 2)
- 'that the prescription provides clear and unequivocal identification of the patient for whom [it] is intended' (SAM 6. 5).

The UKCC SAM states that the nurse, midwife or health visitor must apply knowledge and skill to the situation at hand, whether administering, assisting with administration or overseeing self-administration of medicines (in this instance, essential oils). The practitioner must be confident that she or he:

- 'has an understanding of substances used for therapeutic purposes' (SAM 9.1)
- 'is able to justify any actions taken' (SAM 9.2) and
- 'is prepared to be accountable for the action taken' (SAM 9.3).

All of the above is, strictly speaking, applicable to orthodox medicinal products. However, it is the present authors' belief that it should also apply to the administration of essential oils, by whatever method.

The section in SAM dealing specifically with complementary and alternative therapies summarizes very well our selection from the documents above:

Some nurses, midwives and health visitors having first undertaken successfully a training in complementary or alternative therapy which involves the use of substances such as essential oils, apply their specialist knowledge and skill in their practice. It is essential that practice in these respects, as in all others, is based upon sound principles, available knowledge and skill. The importance of consent to the use of such treatment must be recognized. So, too, must the practitioner's personal accountability for her or his professional practice.

(SAM 39)

The hazards of unqualified practice

Many aromatherapy books give the impression that the reader can fully understand the subject after reading only one book, and the fact that local colleges offer 24-hour courses (over 12 weeks) seems to support this theory. Accredited aromatherapy schools and some NHS units using aromatherapy offer one- or two-day seminars for healthcare professionals. This is acceptable, provided adequate emphasis is placed on the necessity for such healthcare professionals to work under the supervision of a professional aromatherapist or aromatologist.

Regrettably, there are many health professionals not qualified in aromatherapy or aromatology who, because the therapy appears to be uncomplicated, have been (and in some hospitals still are) using essential oils without adequate training, insurance or supervision by an aromatherapist or aromatologist. Sue Lundie, a midwife and aromatologist, states (1993 personal communication) that this state of affairs

has resulted in some rather worrying situations and incidents arising. This has caused concern among those members of the nursing, medical, pharmaceutical and aromatherapy professions, who are well aware that essential oils are highly concentrated and potent herbal preparations which should be used with the same caution as any other medicinal or pharmaceutical product. Professionals from all areas now feel that aromatherapy (without being medicalized—which would be undesirable and regrettable) must be placed within a well structured framework.

Some instances which have arisen due to lack of qualification have led some hospitals to forbid the use of aromatherapy totally. One example occurred in a hospital before the appointment of a clinical aromatologist. A nursing assistant considered 2–3 drops of essential oil of *Mentha* × *piperita* [PEPPERMINT] to be inadequate in a bath of water, so put in more than 20, resulting in unpleasant tingling sensations in the patient's legs and burning in the genital area (Barker 1992 personal communication). The patient could not be persuaded to try essential oils again, even after explanations from the qualified aromatologist. Similar stories are common, but the authors are unaware of any lasting harm from such incidents.

It is not unreasonable to ask health professionals wishing to use essential oils on their own initiative (particularly in healthcare settings where the condition of patients may be very poor), to receive the training required to become full members of a professional association.

AREA HEALTH AUTHORITY POLICIES

In order to obtain permission from the hospital management board for the practice of aromatherapy or aromatology on the wards, a nurse should be well prepared—if necessary with research references to demonstrate the efficacy of essential oils and a draft protocol to prove that the nurse concerned is responsible, knowledgeable and keen to proceed in a correct and competent manner. He or she should be able to answer confidently any questions on why the therapy is viable and how the essential oils will affect the patient or client, e.g., what effects the constituents have on the body and what, if any, are the contraindications. A stress-relieving treatment (not necessarily full-body-massage) could be offered to a surgeon or senior consultant so that first-hand experience is available to them. A policy document can then be prepared to serve as a basis for the individual hospital protocol.

The Bath District Health Authority is believed to be the first to produce a policy statement and it has been used by many health authorities as a basis for their own, adding to it or enlarging it as they saw fit. The authors have combined all points from the Bath District Health Authority Policy, Dewsbury Health Authority Policy (based on the Bath District Policy) and the Community Health Sheffield (NHS Trust) Policy 1993 and 1994 (based exclusively on aromatherapy). Each reference to the UKCC principles will be given in full, to give as complete a picture as possible to those wishing to introduce aromatherapy into their hospitals. Where a single authority expresses a statement, the initials of the authority concerned appear in brackets.

Policy statement

Complementary therapies

These are natural and holistic therapies which may be used exclusively or in harmony with recognized nursing practice.

It is recognized that complementary therapies may enhance patient care (DHA).

Only complementary therapies approved after agreement with the Complementary Therapies Steering Committee may be used on a register held by the Steering Committee (DHA).

Some registered nurses, midwives and health visitors, having first undertaken successfully a training in complementary or alternative therapy which involved the use of substances such as essential oils, apply their specialist knowledge and skill in their practice.

It is essential that practice in these respects, as in all others, is based upon sound principles, available knowledge and skill.

The importance of consent to the use of such treatments must be recognized.

So, too, must the practitioner's personal accountability for her or his professional practice (UKCC SAM 39).

Recognized practitioners

Those who may practise are as follows:

* Accountable Practitioner:
  A registered healthcare professional holding a recognized qualification, such as:
  —Medical Practitioner (DHA)

—First Level Nurse—RGN, RMN, RSCN, RNMH, RM
—Second Level Nurse—EN(G) or EN(MH)
—Occupational Therapist (DHA)
—Physiotherapist (DHA)
who has undertaken a recognized training course leading to competence in a specific complementary therapy.
* Assistant (if appropriate):
  A healthcare worker who has attended an introductory programme in a specific therapy by a qualified practitioner employed by the health authority concerned. All participants who have completed the basic programme will be obliged to undertake training at yearly intervals to keep them up-to-date with developments and research in complementary medicine. The assistant will work *only* under the guidance of an Accountable Practitioner.

Criteria for practice

The criteria for the practice of complementary therapies are listed below.

Authorization

The accountable practitioner must have been given authorization to practise by his or her service manager (see Nurse management responsibility below).

Permission needs to be sought from the relevant Medical Practitioner before establishing a specific complementary therapy in a particular area. Should any Medical Practitioner refuse permission, his or her patients will be excluded.

Consultation

The accountable practitioner must practise the specific complementary therapy in consultation with relevant medical practitioners of the multi-disciplinary team. The practitioner should have full knowledge of the patient/client's past and present medical history.

Consent

The patient/client/relative/carer must give *informed consent* for the accountable practitioner to practise the specific complementary therapy in accordance with 'Consent for examination and treatment guidance' (HC{90}22).

Documentation

- The accountable practitioner must demonstrate and document within the patient/client care-plan or notes the relevance of the complementary therapy being used.
- The accountable practitioner should keep a record of patients/clients and the treatments given according to the training given in each specific complementary therapy (BCMA Code of Conduct).

Evaluation

- The accountable practitioner must evaluate and document the effectiveness of the specific complementary therapy being used.
- The final decision on a treatment plan when approved by all parties will be officially documented in the nursing care-plan of the named client.

Competence

The attention of accountable practitioners will be drawn to specific UKCC Professional Codes of Conduct, as well as those of the Chartered Society of Physiotherapists (DHA) and British Association of Occupational Therapists (Professional Standard 16) (DHA) where applicable:

- 'Ensure that no action or omission on your part, or within your sphere of responsibility, is detrimental to the interests, condition or safety of patients and clients' (SPP 6.2).
- 'Acknowledge any limitations in your knowledge and competence and decline any duties or responsibilities unless able to perform them in a safe and skilled manner' (SPP 6.4).

Accountability

The UKCC Exercising Accountability principles can be summarized as follows:

- The interests of the patient are paramount.
- Professional accountability must be exercised in such a manner as to ensure that the primacy of the interests of patients or clients is respected

and must not be overridden by those of the professions or their practitioners.
- The exercise of accountability requires the practitioner to seek to achieve and maintain high standards.
- Advocacy on behalf of patients or clients is an essential feature of the exercise of accountability by a professional practitioner.
- The role of other persons in the delivery of healthcare to patients or clients must be recognized and respected, provided that the first principle above is honoured.
- Public trust and confidence in the profession is dependent on its practitioners being seen to exercise their accountability responsibly.
- Each registered nurse, midwife or health visitor must be able to justify any action or decision taken in the course of her or his professional practice (UKCC 1989).
- The practitioner must accept accountability for improving and maintaining an appropriate level of knowledge and skill for the specific complementary skill practised:
  —Patients and clients require skilled care from registered practitioners, and support staff require direction and supervision from these same practitioners (SPP 11).
  —Healthcare assistants to registered nurses, midwives and health visitors must work under the direction of these registered practitioners (SPP 23.1).
  —Healthcare assistants must not be allowed to work beyond their level of competence (SPP 23.3).
- A practitioner, in the exercise of professional accountability must act always in such a manner as to promote and safeguard the interests and well-being of patients and clients (SPP 6. 1).
- The interests of the patient or client must be paramount.

Nurse management responsibility

The manager for the clinical area will be accountable for ensuring that:

- authorization has been obtained for the use of specific complementary therapies by staff

- any complementary therapy used is one approved by the health authority concerned
- the accountable practitioner has undertaken a recognized training course at an accredited training institution, to a standard entitling that practitioner to full membership of the relevant professional association
- the manager and accountable nurse make an agreement with regard to the level at which that nurse practises the specific complementary therapy (and this to form part of the individual hospital's protocol)
- permission has been sought from appropriate medical practitioners before establishing a specific complementary therapy in a particular area
- assistant practitioners have received an approved level of training by an accountable practitioner before assisting with a specific complementary therapy
- a list of assistant practitioners is maintained for reference (DHA)
- the manager and accountable practitioner review the practice of the specific complementary therapy on an annual basis (or more frequently if appropriate) to ensure (a) a quality service and (b) that administration of prescription treatments is carried out in a professional manner and to the benefit of the client.

Prescription of oils

The Medicines Act 1968 does not allow natural therapists to prescribe or supply substances freely simply because they occur naturally. In the main it is herbalists who are affected but aromatherapists and aromatologists come under the same heading, since they too prescribe herbal substances (SHA). The Act defines a herbal substance or herbal remedy (section 132.1) as 'a medicinal product consisting of a substance produced by subjecting a plant or plants to drying, crushing, or any other process, or of a mixture whose sole ingredients are one or more substances so produced, and water or some other inert substance'. This of course includes plant oils.

Conditions

The conditions of prescribing are:

- the remedy must be a herbal remedy as defined above
- the herbal remedy may be sold, supplied, manufactured or assembled without a licence in a shop or a consulting room provided that the occupier supplies to a particular person in that person's presence after being requested to use his/her own judgement as to the treatment required.

This means that a practitioner cannot supply a person, even without charge, an oil or mixture of oils without a licence—unless that person has consulted that practitioner and he or she has actually seen the person (SHA).

Labelling regulations

Since July 1977, regulations control the dispensing of products for medicinal use. The mandatory requirements for every container of medicine, lotion, ointment, tablet, etc. are as follows:

- it must have a label
- the label must contain:
  —the name of the patient for whom the medicament has been prescribed
  —the name and address of the practitioner who has supplied the product
  —directions for use and dosage, which may be omitted if the use has been explained to the patient and substituted by: 'to be used as directed'. (However, the authors feel that directions for use should always be written down.)
  —'for external use only' if it is a liquid preparation for topical use
- bottles must be fluted (ribbed) when dispensing remedies prescribed for external use only.

Summary

- A licence is necessary to supply a medicinal product unless:
  —the remedy is a herbal remedy *and*
  —the remedy is prepared for adminstration to a particular person who has consulted the

practitioner and been personally seen by them *or*

—the product is supplied in the original wrappings of the manufacturer without any claims being made by the supplier, e.g. as in a shop.

- All products supplied by the practitioner should be labelled. Labels should be typed or indelible ink used. The label must contain the following information:
  —name of the patient
  —name and address of the practitioner
  —directions for use
  —'for external use only' if it is a liquid preparation for topical use.
- Liquid preparations for topical use must be dispensed in a fluted (ribbed) bottle.

Service provision

Arrangements for the involvement of accountable practitioners in complementary therapies is subject to the needs of the service and availability of resources. Responsibility for resourcing therapies lies with individual managers (DHA).

Research

It is anticipated that clinical areas in which complementary therapies are practised will encourage a research-based approach to practice.

HOSPITAL PROTOCOLS AND GUIDELINES

A protocol, directorate or set of guidelines for the practice of aromatherapy and the specific use of essential oils within that practice is a key document required by each hospital. This document should set out which essential oils are to be used, how they are to be used, by whom and for how long.

The following, adapted from the Community Health Sheffield (NHS Trust) protocol will give the nurse aromatherapist or aromatologist wishing to prepare such a document the general guidelines to be observed. For the purposes of this document 'accountable practitioner' refers to the professional aromatherapist or aromatologist and

'healthcare assistant' refers to the person working under the supervision of the said professional aromatherapist or aromatologist.

Local protocol

1. Permission to use essential oils on a patient or client must be requested from that patient or client's GP/consultant:
   a. this must be done before commencement of the treatment
   b. this may be requested by the on-site nursing staff.

   Other members of the multidisciplinary team will be made aware that aromatherapy is being used as part of a treatment plan agreed with the patient/client and carer.
2. All patients or clients must be referred to the accountable practitioner. After receipt of the referral a letter of confirmation will be sent to the patient or client giving details of the consultation date.
3. It is essential that accountable practitioners and healthcare assistants are aware of and have studied their Health Authority policy document.
4. Persons using aromatherapy/aromatology must be one of the following:
   a. an accountable practitioner, i.e., a healthcare professional who is a full member of an aromatherapy or aromatology association, *or*
   b. a healthcare assistant, i.e.:
      (i) a healthcare professional who has attended an introductory programme on aromatherapy of at least two days if external to the hospital plus extra tuition by the accountable practitioner *or*
      (ii) a healthcare professional who has attended an introductory programme on aromatherapy of at least two days run by an accountable practitioner.

   A healthcare assistant may give massage to the parts of the body listed in 7.d below, except for the back, face and full-body-massage, which may only be given if the said assistant already holds a qualification in full-body-massage.

5. The patient/client approach must satisfy or include all of the following points:
   a. Aromatherapy treatments will only be offered after full consultation with and acceptance by the patient/client, together with the healthcare assistant if required.
   b. An assessment, including the plan of treatment, will be offered and fully explained to the patient/client; this may include any one or more of the methods of approach mentioned in 8 below. The final decision on a treatment plan when approved by all parties will be officially documented in the nursing care plan of the named patient/client.
   c. Before using any essential oils on a client or patient, they should be tested on that patient/client in the dilution—and carrier—which will be used for the treatment. To do this, place a small amount of the mix on one of the following places: inner elbow, inside wrist, in the groin, behind the knee or just behind the ear. It should be left for 12–24 hours, covered with a light porous dressing if necessary. If there is no irritation or reddening of the skin, treatment may proceed.
   d. At all times the dignity of the patient or client shall be respected. When giving massage, any part of the body not being massaged shall be covered in accordance with the ethics and code of professional conduct set out in the professional practice document of the ISPA Code of Practice, and that of the European Aromatology Association.
   e. The location of treatment will vary according to each patient/client's needs. If a full-body-massage is entailed this should normally be given in the patient/client's private room (using curtains in a ward situation). The possible exception to this may be a hand massage, but the wishes of the patient/client should be respected with regard to privacy if required.

6. The treatment should be allocated for each named client for a period of no more than three weeks, when the prescription/treatment should be re-assessed.

7. Types of treatments will be selected from the following list according to the individual patient or client's needs, using essential oils appropriate to that patient or client:
   a. inhalation (dry or with steam), with or without an electric room diffuser. Electric diffusers must meet the requirements of the Health and Safety at Work Act. No night light vaporizers or ceramic rings are to be used because of fire risk
   b. baths—foot-, hand-, sitz- or full-body-. Oil prescriptions should be added after the bath has been run
   c. topical application, without massage
   d. massage—full-body, arm, hand, leg, foot, back, face, neck, shoulders, scalp. Relevant contraindications to full-body-massage will be taken into account
   e. compresses
   f. ingestion
      (i) anal suppositories
      (ii) vaginal pessaries
      (iii) orally for digestive disorders: only with the consultant's permission and only if insured for the internal use of essential oils with the Aromatology Association or the RCN.

8. Essential oil prescriptions must satisfy the following requirements:
   a. Only genuine therapeutic quality essential oils are to be used; i.e. not essential oils of perfume quality, but only those which can be traced to source and which originated from plants grown by natural farming methods or from biologically-grown or wild plants—this is the responsibility of the accountable practitioner.
   b. Only unrefined or cold pressed and unrefined carrier oils are to be used, from plants grown using natural farming methods.
   c. The accountable practitioner will use the number of drops and amount of carrier oil laid down by the accredited aromatherapy or aromatology course followed.
   d. The prescription bottle must be made up only by the accountable practitioner for a named patient/client's use only—it is not to be used on any other patient or client.

e. A prescription card must be allocated to each patient or client, recording the following:
   (i) name of patient or client
   (ii) address or ward number/name
   (iii) date of birth
   (iv) name of GP/consultant
   (v) details of prescription, including carriers where used
   (vi) details of administration of prescription
   (vii) frequency of administration of prescription.

   The prescription/administration card must be signed on application of the prescription, by the authorized accountable practitioner or healthcare assistant.

f. The bottle label must contain:
   (i) the name of the patient or client
   (ii) the date of expiry (i.e., 3 weeks)
   (iii) the directions for administration.

g. The prescription will not be added to, substituted or changed in any way without consultation with the accountable practitioner.

h. Any change of prescription must be noted on the prescription card by the accountable practitioner; and the old treatment-bottle is to be returned to the accountable practitioner.

i. Re-assessment of all aromatherapy prescriptions must take place within the 3-week period of the prescription date on the label.

j. All treatment bottles are to be returned to the accountable practitioner (regardless of a review) after the expiry date.

9. Recording of clinical data
   Patient or client response (positive and/or negative) to the prescription is to be clearly and informatively recorded on the named patient or client's nursing care plan.

10. The safety aspects of using essential oils must be observed (see also COSHH regulations):
   a. Storage of all essential oil prescriptions must take place in
      (i) the locked external medicine/dangerous drug cupboard *or*
      (ii) the locked external preparations cupboard *or*
      (iii) a locked cupboard in the occupational therapy department.

   All essential oil prescriptions must be treated with the same respect as any other prescribed medicine.

   b. The toxicity of, and reactions to, essential oils must be borne in mind at all times by accountable practitioners and healthcare assistants who must be aware of the following possible hazards and the consequences of their abuse:
      (i) neurotoxicity
      (ii) dermal toxicity
      (iii) dermal sensitivity
      (iv) possible respiratory sensitivity
      (v) phototoxicity.
   [Authors' note: see Ch. 3 and Appendix B.]

   c. In incidents with essential oils requiring first aid, the following points must be observed:
      (i) should a patient or client accidentally swallow any pure essential oil, contact the emergency services (999) then contact the accountable practitioner at once
      (ii) should a patient or client get any pure essential oil into the eye, wash the eye immediately with vegetable oil only—not saline solution—then contact the accountable practitioner at once
      (iii) should any adverse reaction be presented, stop using the prescription and contact the accountable aromatherapist or aromatologist.

   d. Prohibited or restricted essential oils. It is important that accountable practitioners and healthcare assistants are aware of essential oils which:
      (i) must not be used at all
      (ii) must be used with caution. If it is found possible to purchase these over the counter, this should be reported to the Aromatherapy Trades Council.
   [Authors' note: see Appendix B.4 and B.5.]

11. General points to bear in mind include the following:

   a. Essential oils must not be used undiluted over a large area of skin.

   b. Essential oils must never be used undiluted on or near the eyes.

   c. It must be understood that excess use, i.e. too high a concentration, may lead to headaches or nausea, or can lead to the opposite effect to that intended (e.g., a high concentration of *Lavandula angustifolia* can produce insomnia instead of sleep).

   d. It is suggested that a limited range of essential oils be selected carefully and specifically to cover the requirements of the health conditions and side-effects from orthodox drugs found in a healthcare situation. Further essential oils can always be added if or when found to be necessary. The following have proved to be the most useful and cover all health topics mentioned in this book:

- *Boswellia Carteri* [FRANKINCENSE]
- *Cananga odorata* [YLANG YLANG]
- *Chamaemelum nobile* (= *Anthemis nobilis*) [ROMAN CHAMOMILE]
- *Chamomilla recutita* (= *Matricaria chamomilla*) [GERMAN CHAMOMILE]
- *Citrus bergamia* [BERGAMOT]
- *Citrus limon* [LEMON]
- *Citrus reticulata* [MANDARIN, TANGERINE]
- *Citrus aurantium* var. *amara* (flos, fol. and per.) [NEROLI BIGARADE, PETITGRAIN BIGARADE, ORANGE BIGARADE]
- *Cupressus sempervirens* [CYPRESS]
- *Eucalyptus globulus* (if unrectified) [TASMANIAN BLUE GUM]
- *Eucalyptus Smithii* [GULLY ASH]
- *Foeniculum vulgare* [FENNEL]
- *Hyssopus officinalis* [HYSSOP]
- *Juniperus communis* (fruct. and ram.) [JUNIPER BERRY and TWIG]
- *Lavandula angustifolia* [LAVENDER]
- *Lavandula intermedia* × 'Super' [LAVANDIN]

- *Melaleuca alternifolia* [TEA TREE]
- *Melaleuca viridiflora* [NIAOULI] (if genuine)
- *Mentha* × *piperita* [PEPPERMINT]
- *Ocimum basilicum* var. *album* [EUROPEAN BASIL]
- *Origanum majorana* [SWEET MARJORAM]
- *Pelargonium graveolens* [GERANIUM]
- *Piper nigrum* [BLACK PEPPER]
- *Rosmarinus officinalis* ct. cineole, ct. camphor [ROSEMARY]
- *Salvia sclarea* [CLARY]
- *Santalum album* [SANDALWOOD]
- *Syzygium aromaticum* (flos) (formerly *Eugenia caryophyllata*) [CLOVE BUD]
- *Thymus vulgaris* ct. alcohol [SWEET THYME]
- *Zingiber officinale* [GINGER].

Guidelines

Together with a protocol, each hospital usually has guidelines on the specific uses of essential oils within their field of care. An example of such guidelines can be found on page 140, and typical inclusions in a general set of guidelines would be:

- local contraindications
- conditions which can be treated
- essential oils which can be used for these conditions, including sample prescriptions
- methods by which, in that particular hospital, the selected essential oils can be administered for the specified conditions
- method of recording treatments and prescriptions of essential oils.

Summary

This chapter has shown the great steps that have already been taken towards self-regulation of aromatherapy in the UK, alongside the practice guidelines created by several health authorities. It is to be hoped that more health provision agencies will welcome these positive moves, and the suggested policies and protocols will be adapted and applied where appropriate.

REFERENCES

Barker A 1993 ISPA AGM and Conference October 30–31 Aromatherapy in a hospital setting

Cawthorne A 1991 Aromatherapy on trial. Aromanews 30: 7–8

Lautié R, Passbecq A 1979 Aromatherapy: the use of plant essences in healing. Thorsons, Wellingborough

Lundie S 1994 Introducing and applying aromatherapy within the NHS. The Aromatherapist 2: 30–35

Price S 1983 Practical aromatherapy. Thorsons, Wellingborough

Price S 1985 Aromatherapy training notes. Shirley Price International College of Aromatherapy, Hinckley

Rankin-Box D 1992 Appropriate therapies for nurses to practise. Nursing Standard 6(50) Complementary Therapies Special Supplement: 51–52

Tisserand R 1977 The art of aromatherapy. Daniel, Saffron Walden

United Kingdom Central Council June 1992 Code of professional conduct. UKCC, 23 Portland Place, London

United Kingdom Central Council June 1992 The scope of professional practice. UKCC, 23 Portland Place, London

United Kingdom Central Council October 1992 Standards for the administration of medicines. UKCC, 23 Portland Place, London

Valnet J 1980 The practice of aromatherapy. Daniel, Saffron Walden

15

Aromatherapy worldwide

Introduction

The practice of aromatherapy varies widely across the globe. In some countries, such as France, phytotherapy (which includes aromatology) is an established branch of medicine, and essential oils may be prescribed only by qualified doctors. In other countries, such as South Africa, aromatherapy is in its infancy, and is practised in hospitals on a voluntary basis only by aromatherapists and interested nurses.

This chapter examines aromatherapy use within the health-care systems of seven countries, representing a range of different stages of development, implementation and style of practice.

FRANCE

In France aromatherapy is a branch of medicine, generally included with medical herbalism (phytotherapy) and used by medical doctors already involved in alternative or complementary medicine. Thousands of doctors, hundreds of pharmacies and some analytical and bacteriological laboratories are involved in aromatherapy/aromatology and phytotherapy. The profession of aromatherapist does not really exist in France and the use of essential oils in body massage, as it is practised in the UK style, has only recently started to become known.

The development of natural therapies

In order to understand its medical development, it is necessary to view the position of aromatherapy in the larger context of the range of the different natural therapies in France.

The first form of natural therapy to be practised in France was homoeopathy, and all French homoeopaths are medical doctors. Natural therapies are taught as a medical speciality, over 3 years, at Bobigny Medical University near Paris. Doctors who follow this teaching are called *naturothérapeutes*, in order to distinguish them from *naturopathes*, i.e. naturopaths who are not medical doctors. Such naturopaths, like osteopaths, are not legally allowed to practise—though many do. Several other university medical departments organize postgraduate teaching in different alternative fields, including phyto-aromatherapy.

The Institut Méditerranéen de Documentation, d'Enseignement et de Recherche sur les Plantes Médicinales (IMDERPLAM) runs regular study courses on the medicinal properties of plants, including the medicinal properties of essential oils; one of the courses covers this theory together with massage and holistic oil selection (taught by the authors). The publication in 1993 and 1994 of two of Shirley Price's books in French has aroused great interest in the UK style of aromatherapy in France. This, together with the aromatherapy taught at IMDERPLAM and the UK-style aromatherapy courses which aromatologist Dr D Pénoël hopes to initiate in 1995, suggests that aromatherapy as practised in the UK has begun its growth in France. Already the general public can buy essential oils in health food stores there, and from many markets in the south of the country.

At the time of writing, those doctors already practising a form of natural therapy are the ones using essential oils and, in most cases, they use medical aromatherapy along with phytotherapy. This means that the final prescription will generally include different plant extracts (e.g. tinctures or a concentrated form in gelules) and essential oils to be taken internally (orally and/or as suppositories) or to be applied externally. The external application usually involves much higher concentrations than are used in the UK, ranging from the neat essential oils to a 5–10% dilution for good penetration of the skin, for example on the thoracic area (see Dr Pénoël's Case Study in Ch. 4).

Patients take their prescription to the local pharmacist, and phytoaromatic preparations are made up either there or by one of the larger pharmacies which supply the smaller pharmacies. There are several hundred pharmacies which stock a range of essential oils of therapeutic quality.

Homoeopathy is still largely refunded by the national health system and although phyto-aromatic preparations were refunded until 1990, the law was then altered to change this situation. The price paid by the patients to the pharmacist for phytoaromatic preparations can no longer be claimed back from the insurance system, thus the individual now has to bear the total cost.

Main medical applications of essential oils

Should anyone who is aware of aromatherapy in the UK be asked its main purpose, the answer would probably include the relief of stress and nervous tension. In France the question would bring answers relating to the principal use of essential oils there, i.e. for infectious conditions mainly pertaining to the respiratory system. Other infections often treated with essential oil prescriptions are those of the skin, digestive system, urinary tract and genital area, and common viral diseases.

A significant step in the fine tuning of the struggle against infection was the introduction of the aromatogram. This involves the testing of individual essential oils or blends against specific strains of bacteria or fungi taken from the patient (see Ch. 4). Several bacteriological laboratories perform aromatograms and prescriptions are made in accordance with the results of the tests, ensuring that the oils used by the pharmacist are the same as those tested by the laboratory.

The amount of data accumulated from aromatograms over the years sheds new light on the way microbes are considered and individual susceptibility, not only in directly related infectious disease, but also in a subtle and hidden manner in different pathologies, like inflammatory and even autoimmune diseases, as well as psychological problems.

Another interesting approach in France involves the analysis of different blood proteins and the comparison of two tests, one taken before and the other after a period of treatment with essential oils (in this instance it is better to use one essential oil rather than a blend). Here again, a wealth of biochemical data has been accumulated by different laboratories, which confirm the powerful action of essential oils. By treating the underlying chronic and hidden infection, if present, results can be obtained in many different pathological areas.

Aromatherapy is implemented in all medical fields, including allergies, inflammatory and immune dysfunctions, rheumatology, dermatology, gynaecology and hormonal imbalances, cardiovascular disease, digestive system problems, nervous, psychological and sexual dysfunctions. In each case, the level of action of essential oils will vary both according to the specific diagnosis and to the way the patient is prepared to become involved in the healing process itself.

Another important use of aromatherapy in France, and one where no placebo or psychological effect can be said to intervene, is in emergency situations involving burns, wounds, external trauma, etc. The successful use of essential oils in such acute cases provides strong confirmation of their efficacy.

The doctor's frame of reference

In daily medical aromatherapy practice, it is important to distinguish between the different ways of prescribing essential oils that vary according to the frame of reference chosen by the practitioner—allopathic, naturopathic etc. Essential oils can be considered as blends of natural molecules and prescribed by a doctor in the same way as any other pharmaceutical drug. In a very first approach, any allopathic physician can be taught to use a specific essential oil for a specific condition. An acute disease, tonsillitis for example, can be successfully treated by an essential oil like *Melaleuca alternifolia* [TEA TREE]. But when dealing with chronic cases or repetitive acute ones, keeping to this allopathic frame of reference, even though using essential oils, will soon reach a limit of effectiveness.

Long experience by Pénoël and Verdet, both doctors and phytotherapists, shows clearly that essential oils give the best therapeutic results when used in the frame of reference of natural medicine (see Ch. 4). Pénoël has always taught that aromatherapy is the spearhead of natural medicine, and that refusing to take a holistic approach eventually leads to disappointment, as does the use of poor quality essential oils.

For instance, seeking to improve an allergic condition without paying attention to nutrition represents a loss of time for the therapist and a waste of money for the patient. Similarly, endeavouring to help scar tissue formation on a leg ulcer oozing pus, without understanding that this ulcer might represent an effort by the organism to expel toxins, would be tantamount to 'setting the fox to mind the geese'.

In France only doctors trained as *naturothérapeutes* take the time to analyze all the elements of the lifestyle of their patients so that they can give advice on how to correct those that seem to play a role in the occurrence or the continuation of the disease. Their use of esssetial oils is part of this overall holistic approach, with great attention paid to the patient's state of mind.

The way ahead

To establish in France the profession of aromatherapist as it exists in the UK is at least as large and important a task as that of opening the British medical profession to clinical aromatherapy/aromatology. In France, however, there are certain obstacles to be overcome. The word massage is reserved for those who have a diploma of physiotherapy (called *masseurs/ kinésithérapeutes*). Graduates of IMDERPLAM and SPICA who already hold this qualification may practise aromatherapy legally but those without it cannot advertise their skills and can only use it legally on family and friends.

What is needed is a change in the educational and legal systems to enable people who are neither medical personnel nor beauty therapists to receive full training in aromatherapy and to practise the profession. The successful UK model could serve as a prototype for creating aromatherapy training schools in France and establishing this valuable profession there. It is to be hoped that, as a result, aromatherapy will become available in French hospitals in the same way as it is in the UK.

A close collaboration between UK and French aromatherapy professionals will not only be of benefit to those two countries, but to other countries wishing to establish aromatherapy as part of their healthcare system.

REPUBLIC OF IRELAND

Complementary therapies are used in Irish hospices, AIDS clinics and some hospitals. A tremendous amount of interest in aromatherapy is shown by nurses, as in the UK, and it is appreciated that teaching/learning guidelines and a Code of Practice are needed, with direction from the Irish Nursing Board.

At the time of writing, the situation is comparable to the UK in that each hospital needs to discuss the introduction of aromatherapy with its Board of Management and Department of Nursing. Many doctors are slightly sceptical, although several take a pragmatic approach. It is easier for them to see the benefits of massage, and this points to the fact that much education, with back-up from research, is called for in the field of essential oils.

Aromatherapy is used in a limited way by palliative nurses and pre-student nurses both in vaporizers and hand massage. A trial study was carried out by Tullamore General Hospital in 1994 regarding the use of essential oils in assisting sleep for the elderly (see Ch. 12).

The Irish Province of the Hospitaller Order of St John of God (a worldwide religious organization within the Catholic Church dedicated to service in the community) is an Order which recognizes the value of complementary medicine. The Order provides psychiatric health services, services for the elderly and those with learning difficulties, and it supports, as far as is practicable, staff who wish to train in aromatherapy, massage and reflexology. These therapies are used in the Order's work and they are recognized as bringing positive benefits to patients and clients.

The use of aromatherapy is growing rapidly in Ireland and will no doubt soon reach the same level as in the UK.

AUSTRALIA

Although aromatherapy is not widely used in Australian hospitals and nursing homes, there are a few nurses who are interested in aromatherapy and have attended workshops or completed a diploma who carry out treatments in healthcare settings. Because hospital budgets have been cut drastically in recent times, essential oils are mostly provided by the nurse-aromatherapist giving the treatment.

Despite the cuts, much work has been started—and is on the increase—by the Australian branches of the two professional associations, the International Federation of Aromatherapy (IFA) and the International Society of Professional Aromatherapists (ISPA). The IFA formed an Aromatherapy Incare group on the lines of its mother association in the UK, and the ISPA has formed its own group, Aroma-Care, just ahead of its mother association in the UK.

Aromatherapy Incare

Although at an early stage, aromatherapy has been enthusiastically received in nursing homes for the elderly and in at least one obstetrics and gynaecology hospital (in Melbourne), where it gained access via the Aromatherapy Incare programme. The Incarers give their time voluntarily and spend approximately 2 hours a week giving treatments to patients.

There is an Incare package, which gives therapists wishing to take part guidelines on what to do, a letter of introduction and copies of various articles to show how Incare is used to good effect in hospitals and nursing homes.

In very few cases would it be appropriate to give full-body-massage—hand and arm treatments, a foot massage or scalp and neck would be the wisest way to begin. Remember, we must be seen as Carers, who are treating stress and promoting emotional well-being. Discretion must be used in regard to the remedial properties of essential oils.

(Barrett 1993)

Staff in a number of nursing homes in Australia have shown interest in learning how aromatherapy can be incorporated into nursing care and to this end have attended workshops and seminars. Some nursing homes have purchased essential oils as recommended by the aromatherapists, but in many the therapists provide their own. At least one nursing Sister is known to have organized ongoing funding for this type of care in her nursing home.

Aroma-Care

Aroma-Care began its work in March 1994, mainly as a result of the invaluable help given by Marlene Cadwallader (B.App.Sci. Nursing, trained in aromatherapy at the Australian School of Awareness—ASA), who approached the Directors of Nursing in many hospitals. Gail Graham, the Director of Nursing at the Knox Private Hospital in Victoria met with the Director of Studies of the ASA, together with interested therapists from this School. These therapists were asked to enter the hospital system as voluntary workers in the psychiatric ward and also in the Knox Private Hospital's 11 affiliated establishments.

Cadwallader herself uses essential oils and massage at the Hayfield Bush Nursing Hospital. Although no formal policy exists as yet, the management, staff and doctors accept and support her provision of care through aromatherapy and 'there is often the aroma of lavender, geranium or rosemary wafting from a vaporizer in the secretary or manager's office' (Cadwallader 1994 personal communication).

In Tasmania another ASA therapist, Mary Evans, has been offered a paid position at the Queen Victoria Hospital, Launceston, in the birthing centre, under a programme created by the midwives themselves. In Queensland Sisters-in-charge (Bost and Davies) have been given permission to use essential oils on their wards at the Southport Hospital.

Many other organizations, such as Health Link, run by the Monash University, are promoting aromatherapy very strongly with the medical profession. The School of Health Sciences at Monash University is holding workshops run by Cadwallader, who has also researched the field of aromatherapy and its application in aged care at home and in institutions (Cadwallader 1993). The aim of her workshops is to:

- introduce and increase the carers' understanding of complementary therapies and their uses when caring for the elderly at home, in special accommodation hostels and nursing homes
- discuss how aromatherapy, massage, reflexology, reiki and visualization can assist the person who is confused, anxious, restless, low in spirits, constipated or nauseous
- discuss appropriate courses that carers may undertake, to develop further skills and knowledge in aromatherapy and related complementary therapies.

Methods of approach

Vaporization is particularly popular in nursing homes, where the antiseptic properties of the essential oils are valuable. They are also used in this way for their calming and uplifting properties. Massage of the hands, feet, shoulders and face are more popular than full-body massage; abdominal massage has been used successfully to relieve constipation. Essential oils such as lavender are added to baths and sponge bowls and are used in compresses for relieving headaches.

The way ahead

It appears that aromatherapy has reached the stage where growth in the 1990s will accelerate as it did in the UK in the 1980s, and it will be used more and more in healthcare settings. To date, it is believed that no trials have been carried out or papers presented on aromatherapy in Australia, but a seminar on complementary therapies was held in Melbourne in 1993 'for all nurses who want to know more about the role of this increasingly important area of aromatherapy, music, relaxation and massage in the aged care setting'. Policies and protocols are to be written, and will no doubt follow the same lines as those in the UK, not only to safeguard the interests of the patients, but to ensure professionalism and confirm high standards by aromatherapists in their approach to aromatherapy in hospitals and nursing homes.

UNITED STATES OF AMERICA

Aromatherapy is believed to have made its first US appearance in the state of California, where many workshops and seminars were held from the mid-1980s. California housed most, if not all, of the companies selling essential oils, mainly by mail order. During the 1980s interest in aromatherapy grew nationally—the authors, for example, introduced aromatherapy to a number of states including Pennsylvania, Colorado, Montana and Delaware. A national association was set up in California in the late 1980s, which showed great promise, holding a world conference in 1990 in Los Angeles. Unfortunately, administration difficulties later led to its demise and it was replaced by the National Association for Holistic Aromatherapy (NAHA), founded in 1990 in Boulder, Colorado. In 1993, the Aromatherapy Association of North America (AANA) was launched, holding a world conference on aromatherapy in New York in 1994.

Into healthcare settings

As there is no National Health Service in the United States, healthcare is paid for by private health insurance. Insurance companies do not cover the use of complementary therapies and so as a rule, hospitals do not provide them. However, there is an increasing awareness amongst those working in the health field of the value, both therapeutic and financial, of complementary forms of medicine.

One such form of medicine which is gaining ground is massage. This is due in part to dramatic research findings, such as those from the University of Miami School of Medicine's Touch Research Institute. Research begun there in the early 1980s looked at the effects of massage on premature babies. The results from over 10 years' study show that premature babies who are

massaged have a 47% greater weight gain and 6-day shorter stay in hospital than babies who are not. This represents a cost saving of $3000 per baby (Cohen 1994).

The National Association of Nurse Massage Therapists, founded in 1987 by a small Atlanta group of nurse massage therapists, was officially recognised by the National Federation for Specialty Nursing Organisations in 1992. As has been shown by Passant (1990) in Britain, it is a comparatively easy step for massage therapists to enhance the techniques they have already mastered by the introduction of essential oils. It is probable therefore that these nurses will be the ones who, having studied essential oil use, will go on to introduce aromatherapy into the mainstream in the United States.

Essential oil use

The use of essential oils in healthcare settings is already beginning, albeit in isolated instances. Many US-based aromatherapists estimate the development of aromatherapy in their country to be approximately 5 years behind the UK in its level of integration into the clinical healthcare setting. A professional aromatherapy practice standard, for example, is only just being developed (by Laraine Kyle, an aromatherapist nurse educator for behavioural health at Boulder Community Hospital, Colorado).

Nevertheless, aromatherapy is beginning to make an impact in healthcare. In Boulder, Colorado, a nurse massage therapist is using lavender on her Alzheimer unit and lavender has also been shown to be effective as an intervention for sundowning effect (a form of dementia in which the symptoms are worse at night) and patients are now rarely given hypnotics to regulate sleep patterns. Another, working on an acute care psychiatric unit has developed a stress management module using essential oils. The same nurse prepared a blend for the staff psychiatrist to assist him with mental alertness during the day.

Kaiser, a prominent educator, acknowledged authority on the changing healthcare system and publisher of the *Healing Health Care Network*

Newsletter, states that leading healthcare institutions are now using the power of aromatherapy to promote patient healing (Kaiser 1993). The vision the Healing Health Care Network has of the future of aromatherapy is illustrated in the following extract from their Newsletter:

Picture a nurse preparing to pass daily medications. Next to each dispensing cup she places a cartridge filled with natural essential oils. She heads down to Mr Scott's room, hands him his oral medicine and places the cartridge into an atomizer which disperses a therapeutic lavender aroma into the air to help Mr Scott's migraine. Next door, three year old Stephanie's atomizer will be filled with peppermint oil to help her asthma and Mrs Roth will receive the scent of orange blossom to help alleviate stress and anxiety the night before her open heart surgery.

(Horzely 1993)

Synthetic aromas

The use of synthetic aromas in place of genuine essential oils is growing in the United States, and is a cause for concern in some circles. In 1991 for instance, a so-called 'aromatherapy' trial was conducted at the Sloane Kettering Cancer Center using a synthetic heliotrope. The aim of the trial was to establish whether the heliotrope's fragrance could reduce anxiety levels in patients before and whilst they were undergoing a—very stressful—Magnetic Resonance Imaging scan. Spielberger test results of pulse and blood pressure readings and the patients' own reports indicated that this was indeed the case (Taylor 1993).

Another use of synthetic aromas is in environmental fragrancing, which is becoming popular in hospitals and other public buildings. But experts disagree about the effects of synthetic aromas. Many chemists believe that a synthetic copy of an essential oil will have identical effects to those of the genuine essential oil. All professional aromatherapists disagree vehemently, arguing that synthetic aromas can produce increased side-effects such as headaches, breathing problems and nausea. No research has been carried out which could resolve this difference of opinion. Until it has been, it is important to be able to distinguish between synthetic aromas and the genuine essential oils used in aromatherapy. This might best be achieved by reserving the terms fragrancing and fragrance for synthetic aromas.

SOUTH AFRICA

Aromatherapy in South Africa is being practised within hospital and hospice situations on a voluntary basis. Most of this is organized through the Association of Aromatherapists Southern Africa (AOASA) Aroma Care Plan, although there are other areas where nurses and aromatherapists have been using essential oils, e.g. in hospice care and midwifery, independently of the association.

The Aroma Care Plan provides a weekly service of aromatherapy at the haematology unit, Groote Schuur Hospital, Cape Town. This is a large government-funded teaching hospital and the haematology unit provides care for patients receiving chemotherapy and radiotherapy, mainly for the treatment of leukaemia for up to 6 weeks. The patients here also undergo bone marrow transplants.

Although no formal studies at the hospital have been carried out, a survey among staff and patients of the unit in 1993 showed the weekly aromatherapy treatments were considered to be positively beneficial to patients, helping to reduce stress levels and muscular tension as well as providing relaxation and a feeling of well-being. Sessions mainly consist of foot and hand or back and shoulder massage.

At the Nursing College attached to Groote Schuur Hospital there is increasing interest in aromatherapy among the nurses, shown by requests for lectures to post-basic students.

At St Luke's Hospice, Cape Town, where Aroma Care therapists first began working at the beginning of 1993, the demand for their services has grown considerably. Here, all aromatherapists in the Aroma Care Plan are required to do the hospice counselling course before having contact with the patients. The aromatherapists make weekly visits to St Luke's, working on the wards and in the day-care centre, where a number of patients come specifically for aromatherapy. Many of them come for massage of oedematous limbs, some for the easing of specific aches and pains associated with bone metastasis. Shoulder massage is of great relief for those suffering from lung cancer and the associated dyspnoea and many come just for the benefits of the touch therapy itself.

The essential oils which appear to be used most often on the wards are:

- benzoin
- lavender
- frankincense
- rose otto.

Aroma Care Plan therapists in Cape Town are now moving into the field of AIDS care and workshops are being held for the participating therapists to share information and provide a support system. Karen Ten Velden, Aroma Care Plan Coordinator, hopes shortly to begin the groundwork for a research study within the field of rheumatology.

GERMANY

The word aromatherapy became known in Germany in the mid-1980s, but therapy with essential oils is still very young. Essential oils can, however, be bought in all pharmacies and in many shops, tea shops and markets. Many of these are of very poor quality and are only used in aromalamps. An association, *Forum Essenzia*, has been set up for aromatherapists and gives therapeutic workshops on aromatherapy in which the necessity of using quality essential oils for therapeutic purposes is emphasized. Many of these workshops are directed at nurses, *Heilpraktiker* (those qualified in natural medicine) and physiotherapists.

However, aromatherapy can only be practised legally by doctors and *Heilpraktiker*. Other health professionals, such as nurses and occupational therapists, working in hospitals are allowed to use essential oils to alleviate minor conditions, e.g. dry skin or headache, but must have permission from the doctor in charge of the patient if they wish to use essential oils for more serious medical conditions. Doctors tend to leave the choice of oils

to the nurse concerned, as they themselves are unlikely to know very much about them—although there are some doctors who use essential oils in their own practices. The nurse must keep an updated written progress report of which essential oil is used, how often and how many drops. Any changes in treatment must also be recorded and all improvements shown.

Conditions treated in hospitals include anxiety, difficult breathing, pneumonia, scars and wounds, digestive problems, sleeping problems, varicose ulcers, terminal illness and birth. Nurses also work in the fields of endocrinology, psychocancer-therapy, and with patients in psychosomatic wards. The essential oils most often used are:

- *Chamaemelum nobile* [ROMAN CHAMOMILE] for allergies and indigestion
- *Citrus limon* (expressed) [LEMON] for fever, influenza and bronchitis
- *Foeniculum vulgare* [FENNEL] for flatulence
- *Lavandula angustifolia* [LAVENDER] for sleeplessness, headache and herpes simplex
- *Melaleuca alternifolia* [TEA TREE] for herpes simplex and herpes zoster, ulcera cruris, decubitus and candida
- *Melaleuca leucadendron* [NIAOULI] for neuralgia and respiratory tract diseases
- *Pelargonium graveolens* [GERANIUM] for depression
- *Rosa damascena* (distilled) [ROSE OTTO] for women's complaints and skin diseases
- *Rosmarinus officinalis* [ROSEMARY] for headaches
- *Thymus vulgaris* ct. alcohol [SWEET THYME] for laryngitis.

Methods used

Massage is only one of the methods used in aromatherapy nursing care, and the technique is not that of classical massage but gentle stroking or embrocation. This means that nurses trained in aromatology can apply the essential oils to the body without having a recognized qualification in massage.

Other methods include inhalation, sponge baths (in cases of fever), compresses and foot massage—and foot baths for pain control.

Training and standards

Using complementary medicine in conjunction with conventional medicine, nurses hope to provide their patients with additional optimum care. However, there is no set training for nurses using essential oils and most nurses acquire their knowledge from weekend workshops and by reading aromatherapy books. There is, though, a school for midwives in Bavaria which includes instruction on aromatherapy in its curriculum.

Some nurses in Munich meet regularly to work out a Code of Practice for the use of essential oils, combined with the ADL code (Activities of Daily Living). Nursing care plans help nurses to see the patient as a holistic being and the ADL code is the basis for everyday living. There is no general policy on the use of essential oils in a hospital setting, but there is a move to adapt the UK policy and protocol standards for use in Germany.

SWITZERLAND

Except in certain cantons (e.g. Appenzell) the term therapist is reserved in Switzerland for those in a profession approved by the Federal Government, such as physiotherapy and psycho-therapy. The term aromatherapist can therefore only be used by a therapist with medical qualifi-cations. People trained in essential oil use who have no medical qualifications are called aroma-tologists. In 1993 an association called VEROMA was set up for both aromatherapists and aromatologists, to provide support and regulate standards across Switzerland, Germany and Austria.

There is scant awareness in Switzerland, either amongst the public or the medical profes-sion, of the therapeutic uses of essential oils. Consequently, it is difficult to introduce aroma-therapy into hospitals, which are very conser-vative institutions. Not even traditional therapies such as homoeopathy are available to patients in general hospitals. Only some private doctors practise it.

There is however an increasing interest, in particular amongst many nurses, in the possible benefits of complementary forms of therapy. Those interested in essential oil use would like to see a nationally recognized training in aroma-tology and more research to provide a sound basis for discussion with classical medicine. The Nursing Research Institute established in Switzerland in 1992 researches exclusively areas of orthodox medicine.

Because there is no aromatherapy training either included in basic nursing training (con-trolled by the Swiss Red Cross) or recognized nationally in the Swiss public health service, there is no official place yet for the use of essential oils in hospitals and nursing homes.

Some basic nursing courses include a general overview of complementary therapies (including aromatherapy) and some postgraduate training, such as that given in Hofa 1 schools, includes essential oil use. Where this is the case, the following points are covered:

- history of essential oils and aromatherapy—limits and potential
- properties and action of essential oils
- production and quality of essential oils
- mode of action, effects and dangers of essential oils
- nursing competency and cooperation with the doctor
- basic rules for essential oil use
- application potential in nursing practice.

The SBK, the professional nursing association, also organizes training in the use of essential oils, both at home and in hospitals (see National procedural principles below). The introduction of essential oils into nursing as promoted by the SBK has two main objectives:

1. that essential oils be used in a caring manner to support and promote the well-being of the patient
2. that the use of essential oils by nurses be understood to be complementary to orthodox medicine.

These objectives provide a clear framework within which some hospitals do allow nurses to use essential oils, though others still do not.

Training outside SBK

Essential oils are used in some hospitals where there is no clear framework. In such instances it is most commonly nurses who introduce them, after reading about aromatherapy and using it at home. As therapeutic massage may not legally be practised by nurses, the method of use they generally choose is airborne inhalation. Most hospitals forbid the burning of candles, so aroma-lamps cannot be used. Instead absorbent stones saturated with essential oils are put on patients' night tables to help with conditions such as tension, anxiety, sleeplessness, fear, stress, apathy and depression.

Hospice use

The following is an account of Ueli Morgenthaler's work as a nurse and aromatologist at a hospice for AIDS patients in Zurich, where, at the time of writing, the SBK aromatherapy module is not known. When starting the job in 1992, Morgenthaler put a small selection of useful oils in the physiotherapy room next to the massage table. He mentioned his wish to start some aromatherapeutic activities in the hospice, and the doctor-in-charge was very encouraging. Whenever there was a problem ordinary medication could not solve satisfactorily, he would ask Morgenthaler to suggest a choice of essential oils, the methods of use and either to carry out the massage treatments or to supervise the correct adminstration of the mix as inhalations, compresses or skin care and aromalamps (candles are not prohibited in this hospice). Permission was given to use the oils in any external form but there was no policy as such.

Problems tackled in this way included:

• itching and very dry skin
• coughs and shortness of breath
• muscular pain
• fever
• eczema
• rampant thrush
• mood changes, depression, debility, fatigue and anxiety
• diarrhoea and vomiting.

As the nurses in the hospice became more interested in the essential oils (paid for by a special donation fund), they began to use them in aromalamps for their fragrancing action and for the effect they have on the mind.

At the beginning of 1994 the doctor-in-charge at the hospice mentioned the need to channel the healing arts knowledge of some individuals working at the hospice, so that it could be more professionally available to the patients. As a result, a number of these individuals founded an alternative therapies project group, aimed at selecting what could be passed on to other nurses in the form of continuing education. The continuing education package formulated consists of the following: each specialist (in aromatherapy, herb teas, compresses, homoeopathy, massage and touch, reflexology) prepares a tutorial session presenting his/her particular field in a simplified manner, giving examples of procedures that other nurses can independently implement with patients in their everyday work. Each field aims to create a nursing standard with guidelines to which the nurses can refer.

Morgenthaler is creating such a standard for aromatherapy practice. It aims to contain the following:

• descriptions of about 12 essential oils, including the necessary precautions, especially in potentially skin irritating oils, as well as the normal precautions of aromatherapy
• instructions for mixing a massage oil, adding essential oils to a bath correctly and administering a compress and an inhalation
• a list of the most common problems and symptoms together with suggested essential oils and method of use
• a special section dedicated to the mind and mental problems, blending and aromalamps
• descriptions of how to store essential oils correctly, and where they can be ordered.

Hospital use

The use of aromatherapy varies between institutions, depending to a large extent on the level of acceptance of the medical staff. Described here is one instance of its use in a hospital.

Bethenia Hospital is a private institution in Zurich, where 80% of the patients come for surgery and 15–20% come for medical treatment, including chemotherapy.

In this hospital, aromatherapy is present in a very limited form. It started with a difficult, elderly insomniac who seemed immune to the strongest of hypnotics/sedatives. Some nurses interested in aromatherapy read that lavender could be used to calm and induce sleep, so they bought a bottle, and placed two saturated stones near to the head of the nervous patient—who promptly fell asleep till dawn. This episode marked the start of essential oils in that ward, and later in others. The oils have since been used on patients receiving surgery, those with cancer and elderly people with bad odours.

No protocol has arisen yet out of this particular work, no nurse on the ward is trained in aromatherapy and no questions have been asked about interactions between the essential oils and conventional medicine. However, guidelines do exist for the use of essential oils in the hospital as a whole, written by two of the nurses who provide advice and reference books to other nurses, and it is hoped that continuing education courses in aromatherapy will soon be introduced. The guidelines include the following:

1. The patient must be informed about the procedures of aromatherapy.
2. The effects and results must be documented. The goal is to have a positive influence on the body, spirit and mind through essential oils.
3. The methods of use are claystone, fragrant bath and massage oils:
   - Claystone. Place the claystone on a plate onto the night table of the patient, putting 3–4 drops of the chosen essential oil on it once or twice daily (mixtures of two or more essential oils are possible). The correct effect of the essential oil depends on the time of administration and the oil selected—an oil could be sleep-inducing in the evening and activating in the morning. After use the stone should be baked, cleaned and reused.
   - Fragrant bath. Add up to 15 drops of essential oils to a full bath tub [Authors' note: 15 is too great a quantity; 4–5 drops is more than adequate].
   - Massage oils. Add up to 20 drops to one bottle of almond oil and massage the appropriate part of the body with this oil. [Authors' note: size of bottle and quantity of carrier oil not mentioned.]
4. Oils are to be ordered from the central pharmacy (number of stones and drops to be specified).
5. Essential oils to be used on the ward [most botanical names not given] are:
   - blood orange—calming, relaxing, uplifting
   - fennel—aids digestion, for flatulence, helps with nausea and vomiting
   - Siberian fir—liquifies lung secretions, expectorant, cleanses the air
   - geranium—balancing, fortifying, calming
   - lavender—cleansing, brings peace, dissolves nervous tensions, helps with insomnia, antidepressive
   - lime—refreshing, stimulates imagination and creativity
   - juniper berry—cleansing, sudorific, good for lack of energy
   - lemongrass—helps to promote psychological strength, acts as stimulant and tonic on the whole organism
   - *Litsea cubeba*—strengthens capacity for inspiration, promotes happiness
   - myrtle—very cleansing, especially for infections and the urinary tract and respiratory system
   - peppermint—for cases of lack of energy, tiredness, dizziness, cooling, antispasmodic, antiinflammatory, febrifuge
   - rosemary—backs up concentration and memory, circulatory, disinfecting, kills parasites
   - thyme—nervine, good with physical and mental weakness.
6. The teamwork mixture consists of 4 drops lemongrass, 4 drops myrtle and 4 drops lime, and is used to promote team work and concentration.

National procedural principles

The Swiss professional nursing association (SBK) has established principles of procedure and basic rules for the handling of essential oils for institutions in which aromatology—sanctioned by doctors—is allowed. A number of the areas covered by these rules are outlined here, beginning with the principles for procedure, which are as follows:

- Nurses must possess minimal technical knowledge (e.g. Hofa 1) and be able to justify nursing procedures using essential oils. Their knowledge must include the risks and limitations as well as the potential.
- There must be clarification with the nursing directors/matron and doctors. It must be clear in which areas of this special field of medicine essential oils are used in nursing.
- The patient or relatives are to decide whether or not therapy with essential oils is tried (the nurses will provide them with the relevant information).

The principal essential oils to be used are (no botanical names given):

- bergamont
- cedar
- eucalyptus
- lavender
- lemon
- melissa 30% [Authors' note: 30% dilution]
- orange
- peppermint
- rosemary
- tea tree.

Additional oils the association suggests considering are:

- clary
- frankincense
- immortelle
- petitgrain
- rose
- sandalwood.

Nursing is to be carried out using the following methods:

- inhalation (oil vaporizer, handkerchief, steam)
- lavage/douches

- baths
- compresses
- dressings
- application
- massage
- swabs.

The fields of application in nursing are:

- disinfection of rooms
- personal hygiene, hair care
- fever
- colds
- disturbed sleep, relaxation
- pain (headache, backache, stomachache)
- mycosis
- insect bites
- healing of wounds, care of scars, burns, sunburn
- fear, anxiety, confusion
- comfort for the dying.

Important base rules include the following:

- No synthetic oils are to be used. Simulated oils may smell similar, but never have the same effect as pure oils and may cause side-effects such as headaches and nausea.
- An oil rejected by the patient but still used by the nurse may have no therapeutic effect; the mental processes are involved in the mode of action to a greater extent than with traditional medicine.
- Essential oils are concentrates and although they are natural substances, they are by no means innocuous. Risks include sensitivity, irritation and possible toxic effects.
- Essential oils should never be brought into contact with the eyes.
- No oral application is permitted since this form of administration is in the exclusive domain of medically-trained aromatologists.
- Essential oils should always be diluted before use—less is more. Exceptions are swabs in mycosis.

Recommended doses are:

- vaporizer: 1–5 drops in water
- massage/application: 1–3 drops emulsified [quantity of carrier not specified]
- dressings/compresses: 1–3 drops in water or oil [quantity of carrier not specified]

- inhalation: 1–2 drops in water
- full bath/douches: maximum 10 drops (adults) or maximum 5 drops (children) always emulsified [the authors feel both these doses are too high, especially for hospital patients].

The emulsifiers to be used are:

- neutral liquid soap
- honey
- vinegar
- neutral body milk
- almond oil
- jojoba oil
- almond oil cream.

Other important base rules are listed below.

- A sensitivity test should be carried out before each application of a new oil, a small amount being applied direct to the skin inside the elbow. If the area turns red or itches, care should be taken.
- An essential oil should not be used continuously for more than 3 weeks, since the effect diminishes. An equivalent oil with the same effect can always be used after this time. [The authors have never found this to be the case. Any essential oil should be *ingested* for no longer than 3 weeks, not because the effect may diminish, but because of toxic build-up in the liver.]
- Care should be taken if the patient is taking a homoeopathic remedy, because of possible interferential action.

The way ahead

Essential oils are used in some hospitals and hospices, but aromatherapy as it is practised in the UK will probably not be able to enter the Swiss healthcare system before more established and widespread therapies like homoeopathy and acupuncture. Those therapies in turn can only fully enter the hospital setting when those responsible for healthcare change their attitude towards alternative and complementary therapies and show an active interest in them.

Summary

It is clear that interest in the use of aromatherapy in a health-care setting is growing rapidly worldwide. There is scope in all countries for the introduction of both the French model—i.e. aromatherapy as a branch of medicine—and of the English model—i.e. aromatherapy as the therapeutic use of essential oils by trained non-medical and interested medical personnel. In order that both these models develop according to the best possible practice it is vital that aromatherapists in different countries communicate with each other, sharing their experience and expertise to the benefit of all.

Acknowledgements

The people who helped the authors compile this chapter have been acknowledged at the beginning of this book.

REFERENCES

Barrett S 1993 Aromatherapy Incare. Simply Essential 10(October): 16
Cohen J 1994 The healing touch. Longevity January: 26
Horzely J M 1993 The art of aromatherapy: an olfactory map toward healing and wellbeing. Healing Healthcare 4(1): 3–5
Kaiser L 1993 Follow your nose. Healing Healthcare 4(1): 2

Passant H 1990 A holistic approach in the ward. Nursing Times 86(4): 26–28
Price S 1993 Aromathérapie guide pratique. Amrita, Plazac-Rouffignac
Price S 1994 L'aromathérapie au quotidien. Amrita, Plazac-Rouffignac
Taylor L 1993 Aromas and anxiety at Memorial Sloan-Kettering. Healing Healthcare 4(1): 1

Appendices, Glossary and Useful addresses

OILS CONTAINED IN APPENDIX A

Botanical name [COMMON NAME]

Achillea millefolium [YARROW]
Boswellia carteri res. dist. [FRANKINCENSE, OLIBANUM]
Cananga odorata flos [YLANG YLANG]
Carum carvi fruct. [CARAWAY]
Cedrus atlantica lig. [ATLAS CEDARWOOD]
Chamaemelum nobile (= *Anthemis nobilis*) flos
  [ROMAN CHAMOMILE]
Chamomilla recutita (= *Matricaria chamomilla*,
  M. recutita) flos [GERMAN CHAMOMILE]
Citrus aurantium var. *amara* flos [NEROLI BIGARADE]
Citrus aurantium var. *amara* fol. [PETITGRAIN BIGARADE]
Citrus aurantium var. *amara* per. [ORANGE BIGARADE]
Citrus bergamia per. [BERGAMOT]
Citrus limon per. [LEMON]
Citrus reticulata per. [MANDARIN]
Coriandrum sativum fruct. [CORIANDER]
Cupressus sempervirens fol., strob. [CYPRESS]
Eucalyptus globulus fol. [TASMANIAN BLUE GUM]
Eucalyptus smithii fol. [GULLY ASH]
Foeniculum vulgare var. *dulce* fruct. [SWEET FENNEL]
Hyssopus officinalis flos, fol. [HYSSOP]
Juniperus communis fruct. [JUNIPER BERRY]
Juniperus communis ram. [JUNIPER TWIG]
Lavandula angustifolia (= *L. officinalis*, *L. vera*) flos
  [LAVENDER]
Lavandula × *intermedia* 'Super' (= *L. burnatii*) flos
  [LAVANDIN]
Melaleuca alternifolia fol. [TEA TREE]
Melaleuca leucadendron (= *M. cajuputi*) fol. [CAJUPUT]
Melaleuca viridiflora (= *M. quinquenervia*) fol. [NIAOULI]
Melissa officinalis fol. [MELISSA]
Mentha × *piperita* fol. [PEPPERMINT]
Myristica fragrans sem. [NUTMEG]
Nardostachys jatamansi (= *N. grandiflora*) rad.
  [SPIKENARD]
Nepeta cataria var. *citriodora* flos, fol. [CATNEP OIL]
Ocimum basilicum fol. [EUROPEAN BASIL]
Origanum majorana flos, fol. [SWEET MARJORAM]
Ormenis mixta flos [MOROCCAN CHAMOMILE]
Pelargonium graveolens fol. [GERANIUM]
Pimpinella anisum fruct. [ANISEED]
Pinus sylvestris fol. [PINE]
Piper nigrum fruct. [BLACK PEPPER]
Pogostemon patchouli fol. [PATCHOULI]
Ravensara aromatica fol. [AROMATIC RAVENSARA]
Rosa damascena, *R. centifolia* flos (dist.) [ROSE OTTO]
Rosmarinus officinalis ct. cineole, ct. camphor fol.
  [ROSEMARY]
Rosmarinus officinalis ct. verbenone fol. [ROSEMARY]
Salvia officinalis fol. [SAGE, DALMATIAN SAGE]
Salvia sclarea flos, fol. [CLARY]
Santalum album lig. [SANDALWOOD]
Satureia hortensis fol. [SUMMER or GARDEN SAVORY]
Satureia montana fol. [WINTER or MOUNTAIN SAVORY]
Syzygium aromaticum (formerly *Eugenia caryophyllata*)
  flos [CLOVE BUD]
Thymus mastichina flos, fol. [SPANISH MARJORAM]
Thymus vulgaris herb. [THYME]
Thymus vulgaris (alcohol chemotypes) [SWEET THYME]
Thymus vulgaris (phenol chemotypes) [RED THYME]
Vetiveria zizanioides rad. [VETIVER]
Zingiber officinale rhiz. [GINGER]

Appendix A

ESSENTIAL OILS FOR GENERAL USE IN HEALTHCARE SETTINGS

This Appendix is not intended to be a comprehensive list of essential oils and their properties. It is designed with healthcare situations in mind, and includes enough information to cover most eventualities where treatment with essential oils is appropriate. Several essential oils mentioned in the text of this book which do not appear here are shown in the chart in Appendix B.9.

It is not possible in a general list such as this to give precise figures for the presence of a component in a given essential oil, particularly when the essential oils used in aromatherapy are not standardized but are taken directly from the still and used without any further treatment. The factors which affect the variability of components have been discussed in Section 1, Essential oil science. Authors also give widely varying information—and sometimes fail to identify accurately the plant being discussed. It cannot be ruled out that some sources may be referring to standardized or adulterated oils.

An asterisk (*) is used to indicate where the authors have found essential oils to be particularly effective.

ACHILLEA MILLEFOLIUM herb. [YARROW] ASTERACEAE

Representative constituents

Hydrocarbons
monoterpenes α-pinene 1.5–3.5%, β-pinene 6–12.3%, camphene <2.5%, sabinene 7.5–41.5%, myrcene 0.6–2%, α-terpinene 0.5–1.1%, limonene 0.4–1%, γ-terpinene 1.3–3.6%, terpinolene 0.2–0.6%, *p*-cymene 0.1–1.2%
sesquiterpenes chamazulene 5–33.2%, dihydroazulenes, caryophyllene 2.7–4.9%, germacrene D 9.3–13.6%

Alcohols
monoterpenols terpinen-4-ol 2.1–5.6%, borneol 0.2–9.5%
sesquiterpenols cadinols 0.4–1.1%

Oxides
1,8-cineole 1.9–11%, caryophyllene oxide 0.4–1.7%

Ketones
monoterpenones isoartemisia ketone 9%, camphor <2.9%, thujone

Esters
bornyl acetate <2.2%

Lactones
achilline

Phenols
eugenol

Properties and indications

analgesic	neuralgia, sprained ankle, sprains
anticatarrhal*	colds, catarrh
antiinflammatory*	prostatitis, neuritis, rheumatism
antiseptic	urinary infections
choleretic*	hepatobiliary deficiency, poor digestion
cicatrizant*	
decongestant	dysmenorrhoea
digestive stimulant	
diuretic	
emmenagogue*	oligomenorrhoea, amenorrhoea
expectorant	
febrifuge	fevers
hypotensor	hypertension
litholytic	kidney stones
vulnerary	varicose ulcers

Observations

- not normally used for babies, children and pregnant women
- neurotoxic and abortive (Franchomme & Pénoël 1990)
- yarrow contains little or no thujone (Leung 1980)
- some individuals show positive patch test reactions to yarrow
- cross-sensitivity between other Asteraceae members and yarrow has been demonstrated (Duke 1985)
- yarrow oil is obtained from the *Achillea millefolium* complex, a group of hardly separable species or subspecies of Compositae found throughout the temperate and boreal zones of the northern and southern hemispheres; the taxonomic problem is extensive and confusing (Lawrence 1984) and what is known as yarrow oil may come from one of several species
- at least 14 different chemical races have been identified in Europe (Mills 1984)
- yarrow has been universally used for the treatment of rheumatism, colds, catarrh, fevers, hypertension and amenorrhoea (Wren 1988)
- yarrow is diaphoretic, a peripheral vasodilator (Mills 1984)
- persons known to be allergic to ragweeds should be cautious about drinking chamomile or yarrow teas (Tyler 1982)
- isoartemisia ketone 9% is listed by Franchomme & Pénöel (1990) for this oil, but not by Lawrence; according to Guenther (1948–1952) it is found in *Artemisia annua*

BOSWELLIA CARTERI res. dist.
[FRANKINCENSE, OLIBANUM] BURSERACEAE

Representative constituents

Hydrocarbons
monoterpenes (40%) α-pinene 21%, α-thujene 24%, limonene 8%, *p*-cymene 6%, sabinene 6%, camphene, myrcene, α-terpinene, β-pinene, caryophyllene, γ-terpinene, terpinolene
sesquiterpenes α-gurjunene, α-guaiene, α- and β-phellandrene, copaene

Alcohols
borneol, terpinen-4-ol, trans-pinocarveol, farnesol

Ketones
verbenone

Esters
octyl acetate

Properties and indications

analgesic	rheumatism, sports
anticatarrhal*	asthma, bronchitis*
antidepressive*	nervous depression*
antiinfectious	respiratory tract
antiinflammatory	rheumatism
antioxidant	combats ageing process
cicatrizant	scars, ulcers, wounds
energizing	
immunostimulant*	immunodeficiency*

Observations

- no contraindications yet known for this gentle, effective, distilled oil
- olibanum absolute produces no skin irritation or sensitization reactions at 8% dilution when tested on humans, no phototoxic effects when undiluted (Opdyke 1978 p. 835)
- the leaf oil of *Boswellia serrata* has antifungal effects (Garg 1974)

CANANGA ODORATA flos [YLANG YLANG] ANNONACEAE

Representative constituents

(Percentage composition figures are given as a rough guide—ylang ylang is an oil of variable makeup.)

Hydrocarbons
monoterpenes α-pinene, β-pinene
sesquiterpenes α-farnesene and γ-cadinene 6.5–17.4%, β-caryophyllene 15–22%, germacrene D 15–25%, δ-cadinene 2–4.7%, α-humulene 0.9–2.5%

Alcohols
monoterpenols linalool 11.6–30%, geraniol, nerol
sesquiterpenols farnesol
aromatic benzyl alcohol

Phenols
eugenol, isoeugenol

Esters (15%)
geranyl acetate 5–10%, benzyl acetate 3–8%,
benzyl benzoate 5–12%, methyl benzoate 1–5.5%,
methyl salicylate 1–10%, methyl anthranilate,
cresyl acetate, farnesyl acetate 1–7%,
benzyl salicylate

Phenyl methyl ethers
paracresyl methyl ether 15%, safrole, isosafrole,
methyl eugenol

Properties and indications

antidiabetic	diabetes
antiseptic	intestinal infections
antispasmodic*	
balancing*	
calming	tachycardia*, hyperpnoea
hypotensor*	hypertension
tonic	scalp, hair growth
reproductive tonic	frigidity, impotence
sedative	

Observations

- no contraindications known to normal aromatherapy use
- ylang ylang oil has been recognized as an allergen and removed from certain cosmetics (Mitchell & Rook 1979)
- no sensitization reactions at 10% dilution (Draize 1959); no irritation when tested at 10% dilution on humans (Opdyke 1974 p. 1015)
- no phototoxic effects reported (Opdyke 1974 p. 1015)
- can produce dermatitis in sensitized individuals (Duke 1985)
- the oil has been suggested as a possible substitute for quinine in malaria (Burkhill 1966)
- an essential oil is also prepared from the leaves

CARUM CARVI fruct. [CARAWAY] UMBELLIFERAE (APIACEAE)

Representative constituents

Hydrocarbons
monoterpenes (38–45%)   limonene 10–45%, carvene 30%,
caryophyllene 0.1%, terpinolene 0.2%, myrcene, *p*-cymene

Monoterpenols (2–6%)
cis-carveol 5.5%, cis-perillyl alcohol 0.1%, dihydrocarveol,
cuminyl alcohol

Monoterpenones (50–60%)
carvone 45–80%, dihydrocarvones 0.7%

Aldehydes
cuminaldehyde 0.1%

Coumarins
herniarin trace

Properties and indications

antibacterial	see Table 4.4
antihistaminic	hay fever
antispasmodic*	gastric spasm*, large intestine spasm, intestinal problems
aperitive	loss of appetite
carminative*	flatulence*, aerophagy*
cholagogic, choleretic	insufficient bile, indigestion
diuretic	
emmenagogic	
larvicidal	
mucolytic*	bronchitis*
stimulant	scalp problems
calming	anger

Observations

- although caraway oil contains a substantial proportion of carvone, tests have proved that the whole oil is safe in normal use: however it is best not used on infants under 3 or expectant mothers
- in excessive dose it is neurotoxic and abortive
- no irritation or sensitization when tested at 4% dilution on humans (Opdyke 1973 p. 1051)
- has a low level of phototoxicity (Opdyke 1973 p. 1051)
- carvone and limonene have recently been shown to have an experimental cancer chemopreventative effect (Zheng et al 1992)
- the seeds are chewed to relieve toothache and for carminative effect (Foster 1984)
- it is a well-known digestive stimulant and this property is made use of in drinks such as Benedictine, Grand Chartreuse and Izarra
- caraway seeds have been found in 3000-year-old Egyptian tombs

CEDRUS ATLANTICA lig. [ATLAS CEDARWOOD] PINACEAE

Representative constituents

Hydrocarbons
sesquiterpenes (50%)   cedrene

Alcohols
sesquiterpenols (30%)   atlantol, α-caryophyllene alcohol,
epi-β-cubenol

Ketones
sesquiterpenones (20%)   α-atlantone, γ-atlantone

Other
α-ionone, epoxy–β–himachalene and its epimer deodarone

Properties and indications

antibacterial	see Table 4.4
antiseptic	skin problems, scalp (with cade oil), urinary tract, eczema, pruritis (with bergamot oil)
arterial regenerator*	arteriosclerosis*

cicatrizant	skin problems, wounds
lipolytic*	cellulite*
lymph tonic*	cellulite*, lymph circulation problems
mucolytic	bronchitis*
stimulant	scalp problems

Observations

- it is important to specify this oil accurately: the term cedarwood oil has little meaning, because many oils are sold under this name, many of them from the Cupressaceae family
- considered in France to be neurotoxic and abortive, and not normally used there for pregnant women and infants
- Duraffourd (1982) recommends leaving internal use of this oil to a doctor
- the Moroccan oil *Cedrus atlantica*
  —showed no irritation or sensitization at 8% dilution when tested on humans (Opdyke 1976 p. 709)
  —has no phototoxic effects reported, although the use of toilet preparations containing unspecified cedarwood oils followed by exposure to various wavelengths sometimes causes dermatitis (Winter 1984)

CHAMAEMELUM NOBILE
(= ANTHEMIS NOBILIS) flos
[ROMAN CHAMOMILE] ASTERACEAE

Representative constituents

Hydrocarbons
monoterpenes α-terpene 0–10%, α-pinene 0–10%, β-pinene 0–10%, sabinene 0–10%, camphene, myrcene, γ-terpinene, *p*-cymene
sesquiterpenes sabinene 0–10%, caryophyllene 0–10%, chamazulene, copaene, β-copaene, δ-cadinene

Alcohols
monoterpenols trans-pinocarveol 5%
sesquiterpenols (5–6%) farnesol, nerolidol

Aldehydes
myrtenal 0–10%

Ketones
monoterpenones pinocarvone 13%

Esters (75–80%)
2-methylbutyl 2-methyl propionate 0.5–25%,
2-methylpropyl butyrate 0.5–10%,
2-methylbutyl 2-methylbutyrate 0.5–25%,
2-methylpropyl 3-methylbutyrate 0–10%,
propyl angelate 0.5–10%, 2-methylpropyl angelate 0.5–25%,
butyl angelate 0.5–10%, 3-methylpentyl angelate 0–10%
(Nano et al 1974).
Also given: isobutyl angelate 36–40%,
isobutyl isobutyrate 4%, 2-methylbutyl methyl-2-butyrate 3%,
isoamyl methyl-2-butyrate 3%, propyl angelate 1%,
hexyl acetate 0.5–10%

Oxides
1,8-cineole 0–25%

Coumarins
scopoletin-7-β-glucoside

Properties and indications

antianaemic	anaemia
antiinflammatory*	eczema, gout, inflamed skin, rheumatic pain, urticaria, skin irritation after shaving, cracked nipples, inflamed gums, neuritis
antineuralgic	
antiparasitic*	
antispasmodic*	migraines, headaches, (relaxes neuromuscular tension), infantile diarrhoea
calming	insomnia*, irritability, migraine, nervous depression*, nervous shock*
carminative	gas, intestinal colic
digestive	indigestion, loss of appetite
emmenagogic	nervous menstrual problems
menstrual	menopause, amenorrhoea, dysmenorrhoea
ophthalmic	conjunctivitis, sore tired eyes
stimulant	
sudorific	
vulnerary	boils, burns, wounds

Observations

- no contraindications known
- no irritation or sensitization at 4% dilution when tested on humans (Opdyke 1974 p. 853)
- no phototoxic effects reported (Opdyke 1974 p. 853)
- chamomile tea may cause anaphylaxis, contact dermatitis or other hypersensitivity reactions in allergic individuals; persons known to be allergic to ragweeds should be cautious about drinking chamomile or yarrow teas (Tyler 1982)
- the oil mixed with flour is a folk remedy for indurations of the liver, stomach and spleen (Duke 1985)

CHAMOMILLA RECUTITA (= MATRICARIA
CHAMOMILLA, M. RECUTITA) flos
[GERMAN CHAMOMILE] ASTERACEAE

Representative constituents

Hydrocarbons
monoterpenes α-terpinene trace, limonene, *p*-cymene, ocimene 1.7%
sesquiterpenes chamazulene 1–35%, bisabolenes, trans-β-farnesene 2–13%, trans-α-farnesene 27%, δ-cadinene 5.2%, α-copaene 0.2%, caryophyllene 0.5%, γ-muurolene 1.3%, α-muurolene 3.4%

Alcohols
sesquiterpenols α-bisabolol 2–67%, spathulenol, farnesol

Oxides
α-bisabol oxide A 0–55%, α-bisabolol oxide B 4.3–19%, epoxybisabolol, bisabolone oxide A 0–64%, 1,8-cineole

Coumarins
herniarin (7-methoxycoumarin), umbelliferone (7-hydroxycoumarin)

Ethers
en-yn-dicycloether 0.7%

Properties and indications

antiallergic	
antiinflammatory*	eczema, gastritis, skin problems, rheumatism
antispasmodic	gastric spasm
cicatrizant	infected wounds, ulcers
decongestant	dysmenorrhoea
digestive tonic	duodenal ulcers, gastric ulcers, indigestion, morning sickness, nausea
hormonal	amenorrhoea, PMS

Observations

- no known contraindications
- there are several chemotypes of this plant, hence the wide limits for the constituents quoted
- no irritation or sensitization at 4% dilution when tested on humans (Opdyke 1974 p. 851)
- no phototoxic effects reported (Opdyke 1974 p. 851)
- bisabolol-type chamomile extracts have low sensitizing activity but there are reports of allergenic properties perhaps due to a linear sesquiterpene lactone (anthecotulide) (Hausen et al 1984)
- the azulenes and bisabolol are antiinflammatory and antispasmodic, reducing histamine-induced reactions such as anaphylaxis and hay fever, allergic asthma and eczema (Mills 1991)
- (-)-α-Bisabolol possesses low acute toxicity after oral administration in mice, rats, dogs and rhesus monkeys (Habersang 1979)
- the sesquiterpenol (-)-α-bisabolol has been found to possess ulcer protective (Szelenyi et al 1979), spasmolytic (Achterrath-Tuckermann et al 1980), antiphlogistic (Jakovlev et al 1983) and antiinflammmatory (Tubaro et al 1984) properties
- Foster (1991, 1993a) says that it is now generally believed that the chief pharmacological benefits are primarily due to α-bisabolol
- bisabolol has been shown to reduce the amount of proteolytic enzyme pepsin secreted by the stomach without any change occurring in the amount of stomach acid (Szelenyi et al 1979); it has also shown antiinflammatory action on granulomas, and shortens the healing time of cutaneous burns (Isaac 1979)
- chamazulene is anodyne, antispasmodic, antiinflammatory and antiallergenic (Foster 1993b); azulenes reduce histamine induced tissue reactions, calm the nervous system both peripherally as in visceral tension

and centrally as in anxiety, nervous tension and headaches; their activity also extends to reducing the anaphylaxis due to the allergic response and so are indicated for hay fever, allergic asthma and eczema (Mills 1991)
- included in the pharmacopoeia of 26 countries (Saloman 1992)
- it has been shown that the use of the herbicide Propyzamide caused an increase in essential oil content; it has also been stated that the use of herbicides over extended periods could readily affect the plant's metabolism and it is recommended that all medicinal and essential oil plants be screened against a number of herbicides to see if there is any long term effect on seondary product metabolism; it is noteworthy that the effects under discussion were found in plants in which residual amounts of the herbicide were absent (Reichling et al 1978, Vömel et al 1977)

CITRUS AURANTIUM VAR. *AMARA* flos [NEROLI BIGARADE] RUTACEAE

Representative constituents

Hydrocarbons
monoterpenes (35%) α-pinene, β-pinene 13%, limonene 12–18%

Alcohols
monoterpenols (40%) linalool 30–35%, α-terpineol 2–5%, geraniol 2–3%, nerol 1–3%
sesquiterpenols (6%) trans-nerolidol, 3–6%, farnesol
aromatic phenyl ethyl alcohol, benzyl alcohol

Esters (7–21%)
linalyl acetate 4–7%, neryl acetate 3%, geranyl acetate 1%, methyl anthranilate B

Aldehydes (2.5%)

Ketones
jasmone

Other
cis-heptadec-8-ene, 2.5-dimethyl-2-vinyl-hex-4-enal (Corbier & Teisseire 1974)

Properties and indications

antibacterial	see Table 4.4
antidepressive*	nervous depression, neurasthenia, lightly tranquillizing
antiinfectious	colitis
antiparasitic*	
antitumoral	
digestive	liver and pancreas (diabetes)
hypotensor	hypotension
neurotonic*	fatigue, aids sleep, sympathetic nervous system imbalance, spasms, cardiovascular erethism, sustains uterus tone
phlebotonic	haemorrhoids, varicose veins
unspecified	bronchitis
unspecified	tuberculosis

Observations

- no known contraindications
- no irritation or sensitization at 4% dilution when tested on humans (Opdyke 1976 p. 813); devoid of irritating properties (Peterson & Hall 1946)
- it is essential to use the genuine version of this much adulterated and simulated oil. NEROLI PORTUGAL, the oil distilled from the flowers of the sweet orange tree, is of a lesser quality
- the vapour of neroli showed strong in vitro antibacterial activity against one of five bacteria (Maruzella & Sicurella 1960)
- a 1:50 dilution of neroli oil exhibited antifungal activity against all of a group of eight phytopathogenic fungi (Rao & Joseph 1971)
- no phototoxic effects reported (Opdyke 1976 p. 813)

CITRUS AURANTIUM VAR. *AMARA* fol.
[PETITGRAIN BIGARADE] RUTACEAE

Representative constituents

Hydrocarbons
monoterpenes (10%)   myrcene 1–6%,
cis- and trans-β-cymenes 3–5%, *p*-cymene 1–3%,
β-pinene 0.7–1.7%, sabinene <0.4%,
α-phellandrene trace–0.2%, limonene 0.7–1.1%,
cis-ocimene trace–1.1%, γ-terpinene 0.5–1.1%,
trans-ocimene trace–3.3%, terpinolene trace–0.1%,
α-pinene trace, α-terpinene trace

Alcohols
monoterpenols (30–40%)   linalool 20–27.9%,
α-terpineol 4.6–7.6%, nerol 1–2%, geraniol 2–4%,
terpinen-4-ol 0.5–0.8%, citronellol trace–0.2%

Esters (50–70%)
linalyl acetate 44–55%, neryl acetate 0.55–2.6%,
geranyl acetate 2–3%, α-terpinyl acetate 0.2–2.2%

Aldehydes
decanal trace, neral trace, geranial trace

Phenols
thymol trace

Coumarins
citropten, bergapten

Properties and indications

antiinfectious	boils, infected acne*, respiratory infections
antiinflammatory	acne
antibacterial	see Table 4.4
antispasmodic*	
balancing*	calming, energizing to sympathetic nervous system

Observations

- no known contraindications

- no irritation at 5% dilution when tested on humans (Fujii et al 1972)
- no irritation at 8% dilution when tested on humans (Ford et al 1992a)
- no phototoxic effects when tested on mice (Forbes et al 1977)
- the common name petitgrain is used as a general term for oils distilled from the leaves of citrus trees, and so should be qualified to indicate from which tree the oil was obtained—orange (bitter or sweet), lemon, mandarin, etc.

CITRUS AURANTIUM VAR. *AMARA* per.
[ORANGE BIGARADE] RUTACEAE

Representative constituents

Hydrocarbons
monoterpenes (90–98%)   limonene 98%, myrcene 1–2%,
terpinolene, α-pinene 0.1–1%, camphene
sesquiterpenes   caryophyllene, copaenes, farnesene,
α-humulene

Alcohols (0.3–0.5%)
citronellol, α-terpineol, nerol, linalool, nerol

Aldehydes (0.9–3%)
geranial, neral, undecanal, sinensal

Esters (2%)
linalyl acetate 1%; geranyl acetate, neryl acetate,
citronellyl acetate

Coumarins (<1%)
osthol (7-methoxy-8-isopentenoxycoumarin), auraptenol
(7-methoxy-8-(2-hydroxy-3-methyl-3-butenyl) coumarin),
bergapten (5 methoxypsoralen), 7-geranoxycoumarin,
7-hydroxycoumarin, 5-isopentenoxypsoralen

Properties and indications

antiinflammatory	
anticoagulant	poor circulation
calming*	gastric spasm, nervousness, sympathetic nervous system, vertigo, palpitations
cholagogic	
digestive	constipation*, liver stimulant, indigestion*
sedative*	anxiety
tonic*	excellent tonic for the gums, mouth ulcers

Observations

- no irritation or sensitization at 10% dilution when tested on humans (Opdyke 1974 p. 735); cutaneous irritation has been reported (Schwarz et al 1947)
- a case of dermatitis has been reported in a girl employed to peel bitter orange (Murray 1921)
- phototoxic effects have been reported (Opdyke 1974 p. 735)
- it is lightly hypnotic (P. Collin, personal communication)
- the majority of the compounds in this oil are present at less than 1%

CITRUS BERGAMIA per. [BERGAMOT] RUTACEAE

Representative constituents

Hydrocarbons
monoterpenes   α-pinene 0.5–1%, camphene trace–0.03%, limonene 26.7–42.5%, β-pinene 2.9–5.1%, sabinene 0.6–0.7%, myrcene 0.4–1.4%, δ-3-carene 0–2%, *p*-cymene 0.1–3.6%, γ-terpinene 1.2–4.8%
sesquiterpenes   β-bisabolene 0.02–0.9%

Alcohols
monoterpenols (45–65%)   linalool 11–22%, nerol, geraniol 0–5.6%, α-terpineol
aromatic alcohols   dihydrocumin alcohol

Esters
linalyl acetate 30–60%, geranyl acetate 0.6–1.3%, neryl acetate 0.5–0.9%

Aldehydes
geranial 0.1–0.5%, neral 0.04–0.4%

Coumarins, furocoumarins
bergamottin,
bergapten 5% (5-methoxyfurano-2, 3, 6, 7-coumarin)

Properties and indications

antiinfectious	wounds
antiseptic*	intestinal, gas, colic, gargles for mouth and throat
antispasmodic*	colic, indigestion
antiviral	Herpes simplex I
antibacterial	see Table 4.4
calming*	insomnia
cicatrizant	
sedative	agitation
stomachic*	loss of appetite
tonic	digestive system, central nervous system
photosensitizer	vitiligo
unspecified	psoriasis

Observations

- not normally used prior to exposure to UV because it is phototoxic to human skin on account of the bergamottin and bergapten compounds which accelerate suntanning (Musajo et al 1953, 1954, Pathak & Fitzpatrick 1959)
- for the same reason some perfumes (e.g. eau de Cologne) should be used with care
- a rectified oil did not exhibit any phototoxic effects; berloque dermatitis is due to bergapten (5-methoxypsoralen) and this must be reduced to 0.001% to obviate bergapten dermatitis (Marzulli & Mailbach 1970)
- no sensitization at 30% dilution when tested on humans (Opdyke 1973 p. 1031)
- undiluted oil is slightly irritating to skin

CITRUS LIMON per. [LEMON] RUTACEAE

Representative constituents

Hydrocarbons
monoterpenes (90–95%)   limonene 55–80%, α-pinene 1.9–2.4%, β-pinene 10–17%, γ-terpinene 3–10%, sabinene 2%, α-thujene 0.01–0.4%, myrcene, α-phellandrene, α-terpinene 0.2–0.4%, *p*-cymene 1%
sesquiterpenes   β-bisabolene 0.5–4%, α-bergamotene 0.4%, β-caryophyllene 0.2%

Alcohols
aliphatic alcohols   hexanol, n-heptanol, octanol, nonanol, decanol
monoterpenols   linalool 0.1%, terpinen-4-ol 0.05%, α-terpineol 0.1–0.2%

Aldehydes
geranial 0.9–1.6%, neral 0.5–1%, citronellal 0.1%, nonanal, octanal, decanal 0.05%

Esters
neryl acetate 0.5%, geranyl acetate 0.5%, α-terpinyl acetate 0–0.7%

Coumarins, furocoumarins
bergamottin 0.2%, citropten, bergaptol trace, phellopterin, bergapten 0.6%, oxypeucedanin, imperaterin, isoimperaterin

Properties and indications

antianaemic	anaemia
antibacterial*	see Table 4.4
anticoagulant	hypertension, phlebitis, poor circulation, thrombosis, varicose veins
antiinfectious	respiratory system
antiinflammatory	boils, gout, insect bites, rheumatism
antifungal	thrush
antimelanistic	brown skin spots
antisclerotic	combats ageing process
antiseptic* (air)	crêches, burns units, hospital wards
antispasmodic	diarrhoea
antiviral	colds, herpes, veruccas, warts
astringent	diarrhoea, nosebleeds, seborrhoea (scalp and face), skin, broken capillaries
calming	headache, insomnia, nightmares
carminative	flatulence
digestive	nausea, painful digestion, aerophagy, loss of appetite
diuretic	obesity, oedema
immunostimulant	white cell deficiency
litholytic*	gallstones, urinary stones
pancreatic stimulant*	diabetes
phlebotonic	
stomachic	gastritis, stomach ulcers

Observations

- no irritation or sensitization at 10% dilution when tested on humans (Opdyke 1974 p. 725)
- no phototoxic effects reported for distilled lemon oil (Opdyke 1974 p. 727)
- the expressed oil is phototoxic (Opdyke 1974 p. 725), therefore exposure to sunlight is to be avoided for 1 hour after skin application
- in the case of expressed oils it is very important to ensure that the fruits have not been sprayed with chemicals
- nonvolatile constituents make up about 2% of expressed lemon oil

CITRUS RETICULATA per. [MANDARIN] RUTACEAE

Representative constituents

Hydrocarbons
monoterpenes limonene 65–77%, α-pinene 1.5–3%, β-pinene 1.3–2.5%, myrcene 1.6–2.2%, γ-terpinene 13.7–20.9%, terpinolene 0.6–1%, *p*-cymene 1.2–3.6%, α-phellandrene 0.05–0.1%

Alcohols
aliphatic alcohols nonanol, octanol 1%
monoterpenols citronellol, linalool 1–5%, α-terpineol 0.1–0.25%

Aldehydes (1%)
decanal 0.05–0.17%, α-sinensal 0.15–0.3%, perillaldehyde <0.1%, octanal 0.1%

Phenols
thymol <0.1%

Esters
methyl N-methyl anthranilate 0.1–0.7%, benzyl acetate

Properties and indications

antiepileptic
antifungal
antispasmodic   hiccoughs, stomach cramp, spasm
calming*   insomnia, nervous tension, cardiovascular erethism, excitability
cholagogic
eupeptic   indigestion, constipation
hepatic
stomachic   stomach pains

Observations

- because this oil may be phototoxic, exposure to sunlight should be avoided for 1 hour after skin application
- no irritation or sensitization at 8% dilution when tested on humans (Ford et al 1992b)
- no coumarins were detected in this oil by Shu et al (1974) but Franchomme & Pénoël (1990) identify a presence

CORIANDRUM SATIVUM fruct. [CORIANDER] UMBELLIFERAE

Representative constituents

Hydrocarbons
monoterpenes (10–20%) γ-terpinene 1–8%, *p*-cymene trace–3.5%, limonene 0.5–4%, α-pinene 0.2–8.5%, camphene trace–1.4%, myrcene 0.2–2%

Alcohols
monoterpenols (60–80%) linalool 60–87%, geraniol 1.2–3.3%, terpinen-4-ol trace–3%, α-terpineol <0.5%

Ketones (7–9%)
camphor 0.9–4%

Esters
geranyl acetate 0.1–4.7%, linalyl acetate 0–2.7 %

Coumarins, furocoumarins
umbelliferone trace, bergapten trace

Properties and indications

antibacterial*   see Table 4.4
analgesic   osteoarthritis, rheumatic pain
antiinfectious*   cystitis, influenza, gastroenteritis
antispasmodic   digestive, uterine
carminative*   flatulence, aerophagy
euphoric*   sadness
larvicidal
neurotonic*   anorexia, debility, general fatigue, mental fatigue
stomachic   indigestion, sluggish digestion

Observations

- no irritation or sensitization at 6% dilution when tested on humans (Opdyke 1973 p. 1031)
- weakly cytotoxic
- the linalool content depends upon the ripeness of the fruits and the geographical source, as do the proportions of the constituents
- coriandrol is a synonym for δ-linalool (Foster 1993b)
- the leaf oil has the fragrance of decylaldehyde and other fatty aldehydes (Prakash 1990)
- experimentally coriander is antiinflammatory and hypoglycaemic (Foster 1993b)

CUPRESSUS SEMPERVIRENS fol., strob. [CYPRESS] CUPRESSACEAE

Representative constituents

Hydrocarbons
monoterpenes α-pinene 35–55%, β-pinene 3%, δ-camphene 0.5%, δ-3-carene 15–25%, limonene 2.5–5%, terpinolene 2.4–6%, *p*-cymene 0.2–1.5%, sabinene 0.1–3%, γ-terpinene 0.3%
sesquiterpenes α-cedrene 0.4%, δ-cadinene 1.5–3%, ocimenes 0.4%, β-cedrene 0.3%

Alcohols
monoterpenols   terpinen-4-ol, α-terpineol 1–2%,
borneol 1–8.7%, linalool 0.8%, sabinol
sesquiterpenols   cedrol 5.3–21%
diterpenols (trace)   manool, abienols, pimarinols, totarol

Oxides
1,8-cineole 0.3%, manoyl oxide 0.5%

Esters
α-terpenyl acetate 4–5%, terpinen-4-yl acetate 1–2%

Other
sandaracopimara-8(14), 15-diene 1.3%

Properties and indications

antibacterial	see Table 4.4
antiinfectious	bronchitis, influenza
antispasmodic	cramp
antisudorific	excessive perspiration
antitussive	whooping cough, bronchitis
astringent	broken capillaries
calming	regulates sympathetic nervous system, irritability
deodorant	sweaty feet
diuretic	oedema, rheumatic swelling
neurotonic*	debility
phlebotonic*	varicose veins, haemorrhoids, poor venous circulation, protects capillary circulation

Observations

- no contraindications known
- has a very remarkable astringent action, much superior to that of witch-hazel (Duraffourd 1982)
- oil of cypress is a homologue of the ovarian hormone (Valnet 1980)
- no irritation or sensitization at 5% dilution when tested on humans (Opdyke 1978 p. 699)
- no phototoxic effects reported (Opdyke 1978 p. 699)

EUCALYPTUS GLOBULUS fol.
[TASMANIAN BLUE GUM] MYRTACEAE

Representative constituents

Hydrocarbons
monoterpenes   α-pinene 3–27%, p-cymene 1.2–3.5%,
limonene 1.8–9%, camphene 0.2–0.4%
sesquiterpenes   aromadendrene 0.1–6%, α-phellandrene 0.2%

Alcohols
monoterpenols   α-fenchyl alcohol 1–2%, α-terpineol 0.1–0.6%,
myrtenol 1.3%
sesquiterpenols   globulol 0–6%, ledol 1–2%,
trans-pinocarveol 0.8–4.5%, viridiflorol, epi-globulol

Ketones
monoterpenones   pinocarvone 1–2%, carvone 0.1%,
fenchone 0.4%

Oxides
1,8-cineole 60–85%, α-pinene epoxide 0.2%

Aldehydes
myrtenal, geranial, valeric aldehyde, butyric aldehyde,
caproic aldehyde

Esters
α-terpenyl acetate 0.1–2%

Properties and indications

antibacterial	see Table 4.4
anticatarrhal	coughs, sinusitis
antifungal	candida
antiinfectious	acute bronchitis, coughs, influenza, pneumonia, respiratory tract infections, sinusitis, laryngitis
antiinflammatory	pleurisy, bronchitis, sinusitis, laryngitis, cystitis
antiseptic*	cystitis, urinary tract infection
antiviral	colds, influenza
balsamic	combats fever and acts like a balm
decongestant	asthma, headaches, migraine
expectorant*	bronchitis, cough
insect repellent	gnats, mosquitoes
mucolytic	cough, sinusitis
rubefacient	subcutaneous infection, arthritis

Observations

- contraindicated for very young children and babies because of the high cineole content
- as with many essential oils in excessive dose, eucalyptus oil has caused fatalities from intestinal irritation (Morton 1981); death is reported from ingestion of 4–24 ml of essential oil, but recoveries are also reported for the same amount (Duke 1985)
- eliminated from the body via the respiratory tract
- it may be necessary to rid certain eucalyptus oils of some short chain aldehydes (e.g. valerian aldehyde, butyraldehyde, capronaldehyde) which are irritant and tussigenic (Belaiche 1979, Wagner et al 1984)
- no irritation or sensitization at 10% dilution when tested on humans (Opdyke 1975 p. 107)
- hypersensitivity has been reported (Goodman & Gilman 1942, Löwenfeld 1932, Schwartz & Peck 1946, Schwartz et al 1947)
- no phototoxic effects reported (Opdyke 1975 p. 107)
- there is a difference between the oils from the young leaves and the old

---

EUCALYPTUS SMITHII fol. [GULLY GUM]
MYRTACEAE

Representative constituents

Hydrocarbons
monoterpenes (20%)   limonene 9–10%, α-pinene 7%,
p-cymene

Alcohols
monoterpenols terpineol, terpineol-4, geraniol, linalool
sesquiterpenols eudesmol

Oxides
1,8-cineole 70–80%

Esters
small quantities

Aldehyde
isovaleraldehyde

Properties and indications

analgesic	painful joints and muscles
anticatarrhal	bronchitis, coughs
antiinfectious	respiratory system
antiviral	colds, influenza
balancing	calming (evening use), stimulant (morning use)
decongestant	asthma, headaches
digestive stimulant	sluggish digestion
expectorant	bronchitis, coughs
prophylactic	colds, influenza

Observations
- no contraindications known
- the oil has great synergistic and quenching properties (Pénoël 1993)
- an effective chest rub; may be used undiluted

FOENICULUM VULGARE VAR. *DULCE* fruct. [SWEET FENNEL] UMBELLIFERAE (APIACEAE)

Representative constituents

Hydrocarbons
monoterpenes α-pinene 1.4–10%, limonene 1.4–17%, α-phellandrene 0.2–4%, α-thujene 0.2%, camphene 0.2%, β-pinene 0.3–1%, sabinene 2%, myrcene 0.5–3%, α-terpinene 0.5–1%, β-phellandrene 0.4–2.6%, γ-terpinene 10.5%, cis-ocimene 12%, terpinolene trace–3.3%, p-cymene 0.4–4.7%

Alcohols
monoterpenols fenchol 3–4%

Ketones
fenchone trace–22%

Phenolic ethers
methyl chavicol 2–12%, cis-anethole trace–1.7%, trans-anethole 50–90%

Aldehydes
anisaldehyde trace–0.5%

Oxides
1,8-cineole 1–6%

Coumarins, furocoumarins
bergaptene, umbelliferone

Properties and indications

analgesic	backache, gout, painful menstruation
antibacterial	see Table 4.4
antiinflammatory	cystitis, gout
antiseptic	urinary tract infections
antispasmodic	gastric enteritis
cardiotonic	heart palpitations
carminative*	flatulence
cholagogue	
circulatory stimulant	
decongestant	breast engorgement, bruises
digestive	indigestion, loss of appetite
diuretic	cellulite, oedema
emmenagogic	lack of, irregular or scanty menstruation*
hormonal	
lactogenic*	lack of milk in breastfeeding mothers*
laxative	constipation
litholytic	urinary stones
oestrogenlike*	ovary problems, PMS, menopause
respiratory tonic	rapid breathing

Observations
- must be well diluted for young children and is best avoided in pregnancy until last 2 months
- if the oil is given in excessively high dose it may cause disturbance of the nervous system, but is safe when used in the amounts normally employed in aromatherapy
- no irritation or sensitization at 4% dilution when tested on humans (Opdyke 1974 p. 879)
- no phototoxic effects reported (Opdyke 1974 p. 879)
- large doses of oil reduced the body weight of mice
- has an epileptic action at high dose (Roulier 1990)
- special consideration must be given to the amount used when treating young children (note: it is an ingredient of Gripe Water)
- has caused pulmonary edema, respiratory problems, and seizures in quantities of 1–5 ml; for this reason, self medication with fennel should be restricted to moderate use of the fruits (seeds), and the volatile oil should not be used (Tyler 1982)
- anethole is reported to have allergenic and toxic properties; its structural similarity to catecholemines (adrenaline, noradrenaline, dopamine) may help to explain its ephedrine-like bronchodilator action and amphetamine-like facilitation of weight loss; similarity of anethole to the psychoactive compounds mescaline, asarone and myristicin has been noted (Mills 1991)
- therapeutic doses of the distilled oil of fennel occasionally induced epileptiform madness and hallucinations; dill, anise and parsley (plants) all have similar oils, and it has been demonstrated that in vivo amination of these ring-substituted oils can result in a series of three hallucinogenic amphetamines (Emboden 1972)

HYSSOPUS OFFICINALIS flos, fol.
[HYSSOP] LABIATAE

Representative constituents

Hydrocarbons
monoterpenes (25–30%)   β-pinene 8.8–22.9%,
phellandrene, limonene 0.7–1%, α-pinene 0.7–1.4%,
camphene 0.1–0.4%, α-phellandrene 0.03–0.3%,
sabinene 1.5–2%, myrcene 0.7–2%,
cis–ocimene 0.1–3.6%, trans–ocimene 0.3–0.5%,
p–cymene 0.1–0.9%
sesquiterpenes (12%)   β-caryophyllene 0.4–3.2%,
germacrene D 0.4–2.8%, allo-aromadendrene 0.5–0.8%,
δ-cadinene 0.1%, calamenene trace, α-humulene

Alcohols
monoterpenols (5–10%)   nerolidol 0.1–1%,
spathulenol 0.7–2.2%, borneol, geraniol, terpinen-4-ol 0.1%,
α-terpineol 1–1.8%, myrtenol 0.4–2.2%, linalool
sesquiterpenols   elemol 0.4–1.7%
other   1-octen-3-ol 0.1%

Esters
bornyl acetate, methyl myrtenate 2%

Ketones
monoterpenones (45–58%)   α-thujone trace-0.08%,
β-thujone 0.1–0.3%, camphor, pinocamphone 12–58%,
iso-pinocamphone 25–32.6%,
2-hydroxy-isopinocamphone 0.3–0.7%

Phenols
carvacrol trace

Phenolic ethers (4%)
myrtenyl methyl ether 0.8–3.9%, methyl chavicol 0.1–1.3%,
methyl eugenol 0.1–0.5%

Oxides
1,8-cineole 0.6%, caryophyllene oxide 0.2%

Properties and indications

antibacterial	see Table 4.4
anticatarrhal	bronchitis, coughs
antiinfectious	colds, coughs, influenza
antiinflammatory	bronchitis, rhinopharyngitis, sinusitis, emphysema, cystitis, rheumatism
antitussive	coughs, influenza
astringent	
cicatrizant	wounds, bruises*, scars, eczema
decongestant	
digestive	loss of appetite, dyspepsia, sluggish digestion
diuretic	
emmenagogue	scanty periods, irregular periods
expectorant	
hypertensor	hypotension
lipolytic	
litholytic	urinary stones
mucolytic*	bronchitis, coughs, sinusitis, pneumonia, asthma*, hay fever, dyspnoea
sudorific	
tonic	asthenia
vermifuge	intestinal parasites
unspecified	multiple sclerosis
unspecified	leucorrhoea

Observations
- this oil can be neurotoxic and abortive in overdose
- not normally used on babies, children, pregnant women and the elderly
- no irritation or sensitization at 4% dilution on humans (Opdyke 1978 p. 783)
- no photoxic effects reported (Opdyke 1978 p. 783)
- makes a synergistic mix together with *Eucalyptus globulus*, *Ravensara aromatica* and *Melaleuca viridiflora* for respiratory problems (Roulier 1990)
- maximum dose is 4 drops per day for a 70 kg adult
- may cause epileptic attack in those so predisposed (Valnet 1980)
- high dose of the essential oil can cause muscular spasm (Bunny 1984)
- eliminated via the lungs
- the essence neutralizes the tuberculosis bacillus at 0.2 parts per 1000 (Valnet 1980)
- extracts of hyssop have had antiviral effects against herpes virus (unspecified) (Foster 1993b)
- also mentioned for leprosy and scrofula (Gattefossé 1937)
- plant extracts and the essential oil, used in minute amounts as commercial flavourings in foods, are generally recognized as safe
- the essential oil is used to flavour Benedictine and Grand Chartreuse

JUNIPERUS COMMUNIS fruct.
[JUNIPERBERRY] CUPRESSACEAE

Representative constituents

Hydrocarbons
monoterpenes (60–80%)   α-pinene 26.5–70%,
β-pinene 1.7–13.6%, limonene 2.5–40%, camphene 0.3–0.8%,
α-thujene 1.2–3%, sabinene 0.3–8.8%, myrcene 2.6–9.5%,
γ-terpinene 0.3–4%, α-terpinene 0.1–2.2%, *p*-cymene 1.3–2.4%,
δ-3-carene 0.03%, terpinolene 0.3–1.8%, α-phellandrene 0.3%,
β-phellandrene 0.7%, 2-*p*-tolylpropene 0.3%, α-cubebene 0.4%,
α-*p*-dimethylstyrene 0.2%
sesquiterpenes   β-caryophyllene trace–2%, α-copaene 0.1–0.4%,
δ-cadinene 0.2–2.9%, α-humulene 1.9%, germacrene D 2.7%

Alcohols
monoterpenols   terpinen-4-ol 2.1–9.5%, α-terpineol 0.5%,
borneol 0.08%, geraniol 0.1%
sesquiterpenols   elemol, α-eudesmol, α-cadinol 0.7%

Oxides
caryophyllene oxide 0.1%

Esters
bornyl acetate, terpinyl acetate

Coumarins
umbelliferone

Properties and indications

analgesic	articular pain
antidiabetic	diabetes, pancreatic stimulant
antiseptic	cystitis
depurative	skin affections, articular pain
digestive tonic*	cirrhosis, loss of appetite
diuretic*	cellulite, oedema
litholytic	bladder and kidney stones
soporific	insomnia

Observations

- not to be used where there is inflammation of the kidneys. 4-terpineol and terpinen-4-ol are diuretic principles, and excessive doses may produce kidney irritation
- the diuretic action is due to a direct irritation of the urinary tubule wall by terpineol (Mills 1991)
- this oil has a general augmenting action on mucous secretions; elimination by all natural paths; aids active elimination of unwanted material which then cannot be deposited in the joints
- juniper and extracts should not be used by expectant mothers
- symptoms of external poisoning caused by the essential oil on the skin include burning, redness, inflammation with blisters and swelling (Duke 1985, List & Horhammer 1969–1979)
- undiluted oil when patch tested on 20 subjects showed two irritant reactions (Opdyke 1976 p. 333)
- no irritation or sensitization at 8% dilution when tested on humans (Opdyke 1976 p. 333)
- no phototoxic effects reported (Opdyke 1976 p. 333)
- makes a synergistic mix with rosemary
- juniper berry oil imparts to the urine a smell of violets (Mabey 1988)

JUNIPERUS COMMUNIS ram. [JUNIPER TWIG] CUPRESSACEAE

Representative constituents

Hydrocarbons
monoterpenes α-pinene 35%, β-pinene, limonene 3–40%, camphene 0.3%, thujene 3%, sabinene 5%, myrcene 9%, γ-terpinene 4%
sesquiterpenes β-caryophyllene 2%

Monoterpenols
terpinen-1-ol-4

Properties and indications

analgesic	
anticatarrhal*	bronchitis, rhinitis
antiinflammatory	
antiseborrhoeic	greasy scalp

antiseptic*	acne, cystitis, weeping eczema
depurative	kidneys, digestive system, urinary stones
diuretic*	gout, rheumatism* (uric acid excretion)
expectorant	
neurotonic	debility, fatigue
unspecified	arteriosclerosis

Observations

- no known contraindications
- see also notes on *Juniperus communis* fruct. [JUNIPER BERRY]

LAVANDULA ANGUSTIFOLIA (= *L. OFFICINALIS, L. VERA*) flos [LAVENDER] LABIATAE

Representative constituents

Hydrocarbons
monoterpenes (4–5%) α-pinenes 0.02–1.1%, cis-ocimene 1.3–10.9%, trans-ocimene 0.8–5.8%, limonene 0.2–7%, β-pinene 0.1–0.2%, camphene 0.1–0.3%, δ-3-carene 0.5%, allo-ocimene <1%
sesquiterpenes β-caryophyllene 2.6–7.6%, β-farnesene 1%

Alcohols
monoterpenols linalool 26–49%, terpinen-4-ol 0.03–6.4%, α-terpineol 0.1–1.4%, borneol 0.8–1.4%, geraniol 1%, lavandulol 0.5–1.5%
aliphatic cis-3-hexen-1-ol trace

Esters (40–55%)
linalyl acetate 36–53%, lavandulyl acetate 0.2–5.9%, terpenyl acetate 0.5%, geranyl acetate 0.5%, 2,6-dimethyl-3, 7-octadiene-2-ol-6-yl acetate

Oxides (2%)
1,8-cineole 0.5–2.5%, linalool oxide, caryophyllene oxide

Ketones (4%)
camphor <1%, octanone-3 0.5–3%, *p*-methyl-acetophenone

Aldehydes (2%)
myrtenal 0.1%, cuminal 0.4%, benzaldehyde 0.2%, neral and geranial 0.4%, trans-22-hexanal 0.4%

Lactones, coumarins (0.3%)
herniarin trace, butanolides trace, coumarin 0.04%, umbelliferone, santonin

Properties and indications

analgesic*	arthritis, muscular aches and pains, rheumatism
antibacterial	see Table 4.4
antifungal	candida, tinea pedis (including infection of the nails)
antiinflammatory	eczema (dry), insect bites, phlebitis, sinusitis, otitis, cystitis, bruises, sprains, acne, herpes, pruritis

| antiseptic | acne, bronchial secretions, cystitis, otitis, infectious skin complaints, influenza, sinusitis, tuberculosis, pityriasis |

antiseptic — acne, bronchial secretions, cystitis, otitis, infectious skin complaints, influenza, sinusitis, tuberculosis, pityriasis

antispasmodic — cramp, spasmodic coughing

calming, sedative — headaches*, migraines, insomnia, sleep problems, anxiety, nervous system regulator, (opposite effect at high dose)

cardiotonic — tachycardia

cicatrizant* — burns, scabs, scars, varicose ulcers, wounds

emmenagogic — scanty periods

hypotensive* — hypertension

tonic — debility, melancholy

unspecified — leucorrhoea

Observations

- no known contraindications
- a remarkable balancing effect on the CNS (Duraffourd 1982)
- no irritation or sensitization at 16% dilution when tested on humans (Opdyke 1976 p. 451)
- the oil can cause dermatitis (Duke 1985)
- no phototoxic effects reported (Opdyke 1976 p. 451)
- fine lavender oils have ketones belonging to the amyl group, while in the hybrids and lavender species other than *Lavandula angustifolia* the ketones take on the form of camphor (Foster 1993b)
- there are more than 30 different types of lavender oils traded on commercial markets; buying a high quality one is an art known only to a few experienced specialists (Foster 1993b)
- Prager & Miskiewicz (1979) came to the conclusion that two oils imported as lavender oils were in fact blends of lavender oils and lavandin oils, while one further sample was found to be a blend of spike lavender oil and lavender oil
- Bulgarian lavender oils have 35.2–37.6% linalyl acetate (Ognyanov 1984)

LAVANDULA × INTERMEDIA 'SUPER' flos [LAVANDIN] LABIATAE

Representative constituents

Hydrocarbons
monoterpenes α-pinene 0.05–0.5%, β-pinene 0.05–0.4%, myrcene 0.4–2.5%, limonene 0.2–1.6%, camphene 0.2%, sabinene 0.06%, δ-3-carene 0.02%, cis-ocimene 1.3%, γ-terpinene 0.02%, *p*-cymene 0.7%, terpinolene 0.1%
sesquiterpenes caryophyllene 0.6–1.7%

Alcohols
monoterpenols linalool 23–48%, lavandulol 0.2–1%, α-terpineol 0.5–6.3%, nerol 0.05–0.6%, geraniol 0.2–1.3%, 1-octen-3-ol 0.2%, terpinen-4-ol 0.4%, borneol 2.27%

Esters (25%)
linalyl acetate 32–52%, neryl acetate 0.1–0.5%, geranyl acetate 0.4–2%, hexyl isobutyrate 0.1%, 1-octen-3-yl acetate 0.5%, hexyl butyrate 0.6%, lavandulyl acetate 1.5%

Oxides
1,8-cineole 1.8–10.8%, trans-linalool oxide 0.2%, cis-linalool oxide 0.08%

Ketones
camphor 5–14.8%

Coumarins
coumarin, dihydrocoumarin, 7-methoxycoumarin and others

Properties and indications

anticatarrhal — bronchitis, pharyngitis

antifungal — athlete's foot, candida

antimigraine — chronic migraine

antiviral* — enteritis

expectorant — bronchitis, coughs

neurotonic — nervous debility, listlessness

sedative — postcardiac surgery (Buckle 1993)

Observations

- no known contraindications
- no irritation or sensitization at 5% dilution when tested on humans (Opdyke 1976 p. 447)
- no phototoxic effects reported (Opdyke 1976 p. 447)
- see notes on *Lavandula angustifolia*: *Lavandula × intermedia* 'Super' is a lavandin clone which is close to *Lavandula angustifolia* in its constituents, and therefore in its properties and effects

MELALEUCA ALTERNIFOLIA fol. [TEA TREE] MYRTACEAE

Representative constituents

Hydrocarbons
monoterpenes (25–40%) α-pinene 0.8–3.6%, β-pinene 0.1–1.6%, α-terpinene 4.6–12.8%, γ-terpinene 9.5–28.3%, *p*-cymene 0.4–12.4%, limonene 0.4–2.77%, terpinolene 1.6–5.4%, α-thujene 0.1–2.1%, sabinene 0–3.2%, myrcene 0.1–1.8%, α-phellandrene 0.1–1.9%, β-phellandrene 0.4–1.6%, terpinolene 3%
sesquiterpenes β-caryophyllene 1%, aromadendrene 0.1–6.6%, viridiflorene 0.3–6.1%, δ-cadinene 0.1–7.5%, allo-aromadendrene 0.3%, α-muurolene 0.1%, bicyclogermacrene 0.1%, α-gurjunene 0.2%, calamenene 0.1%

Alcohols
monoterpenols terpinen-4-ol 28.6–57.9%, α-terpineol 1.5–7.6%
sesquiterpenols globulol 0.1–3.0%, viridiflorol 0.1–1.4%, cubenol 0.1%

Oxides
1,8-cineole 0.5–17.7%, 1,4-cineole trace

Properties and indications

analgesic	
antibacterial	see Table 4.4
antifungal	candida*
antiinfectious*	abscesses, skin infections, intestinal infections, bronchitis, genital infections
antiinflammatory	abscesses (including dental), pyorrhoea, vaginitis, sinusitis, otitis
antiparasitic	lamblias, ascaris, ankylostoma
antiviral	viral enteritis
immunostimulant	low IgA and IgM
neurotonic	debility, depression, PMS, anxiety
phlebotonic	haemorrhoids, varicose veins, aneurism
radioprotective	radiotherapy burns (preventative)

Observations

- no known contraindications
- no irritation or sensitization at 1% dilution when tested on humans (Ford et al 1988)
- no phototoxic effects reported (Ford et al 1988)
- said to prevent post-operative shock due to anaesthetic (Franchomme & Pénoël 1990)
- tea tree oil has a low cineole content and is nonirritant to the skin or the mucous surfaces
- in a single blind randomized study on 124 patients with mild to moderate acne, tea tree oil was compared with benzoyl peroxide: both treatments produced a significant improvement, while fewer patients using the tea tree oil reported unwanted effects (Bassett et al 1990)

MELALEUCA LEUCADENDRON (= *M. CAJUPUTI*) fol. [CAJUPUT] MYRTACEAE

Representative constituents

Hydrocarbons
monoterpenes α-pinene 4%, β-pinene 35%, limonene 7%
sesquiterpenes β-caryophyllene 5.9%

Alcohols
monoterpenols (−)-α-terpineol 6.4%
sesquiterpenols (+)-viridiflorol, nerilodol

Oxides
1,8-cineole 50–75%

Aldehydes
valeric, butyric, benzoic aldehydes

Esters
terpineol acetate

Properties and indications

analgesic	earache, gout, painful periods, rheumatism, toothache, earache, painful joints, neuralgia, arthritis, gout

Properties and indications

antibacterial	see Table 4.4
antiinfectious	bronchitis, colds, coughs, enteritis
antiseptic	intestines, urinary tract, cystitis, respiratory tract, cholera, pityriasis, psoriasis
antispasmodic	gastroenteritis, colic
decongestant	haemorrhoids, varicose veins
expectorant	bronchitis, coughs, lungs
hormonal	
insect repellent	mosquitoes, lice, fleas
phlebotonic	varicose veins, haemorrhoids
radioprotective	radiotherapy burns (preventative)
sudorific	helps influenza

Observations

- no known contraindications, but care is advisable with pregnancy
- no irritation or sensitization at 4% dilution when tested on humans (Opdyke 1976 p. 701)
- no phototoxic effects reported (Opdyke 1976 p. 701)

MELALEUCA VIRIDIFLORA (= *M. QUINQUENERVIA*) fol. [NIAOULI] MYRTACEAE

Representative ingredients

Hydrocarbons
monoterpenes α-pinene 7.5%, β-pinene 3%, l-limonene 4–8%
sesquiterpenes β-caryophyllene 2%, aromadendrene, allo-aromadendrene, viridiflorene, α-humulene, δ-cadinene

Alcohols
monoterpenols linalool, α-terpineol 9–14%, terpinen-1-ol-4 2%
sesquiterpenols viridiflorol 6–15%, globulol, nerolidol 1–7%

Aldehydes
isovaleraldehyde, benzaldehyde <1%

Oxides
1,8-cineole 38–65%, epoxycaryophyllene

Other
sulphur constituents

Properties and indications

analgesic	labour
antibacterial	see Table 4.4
anticatarrhal	chronic catarrh
antiinfectious	respiratory infections, skin fungal infections, insect bites, boils
antiinflammatory	sinusitis*, rhinopharyngitis, bronchitis*, blepharitis, vulvovaginitis, urethritis, prostatitis, inflammation of coronary arteries
antiparasitic	
antipruritic	insect bites
antirheumatic	rheumatoid arthritis
antiseptic	infected wounds, respiratory

antitumoral	breast cancer (nonhormonal), rectal cancer, fibroma (some)*
antiviral*	viral hepatitis*, viral enteritis, genital herpes*
digestive	aerophagy, gastritis, gastric and duodenal ulcers, diarrhoea
expectorant*	bronchitis*, coughs, colds
febrifuge	fevers
hepatic stimulant	
hormonal	amenorrhoea, oligomenorrhoea, irregular menses
hypotensor	atherosclerosis, hypertension
immunostimulant	activates defences and augments leucocytes and antibodies in infected areas
litholytic	gall stones
phlebotonic	varicose veins*, haemorrhoids*
radioprotective	preventative for radiotherapy burns
skin tonic	psoriasis, boils, wrinkles, fungal infections
tonic	post viral nervous depression
unspecified	leucorrhoea

Observations

- no known contraindications but care is advised for pregnant women and children
- used in New Caledonia to purify air (Duraffourd 1982)
- procuring the genuine natural oil is not easy
- the French pharmacopoeia lists natural niaouli and purified niaouli; only the latter can be used in anticatarrhal preparations or for applications for use on burns or on wounds (Belaiche 1979)

MELISSA OFFICINALIS fol. [MELISSA] LABIATAE

Representative constituents

Hydrocarbons
monoterpenes trans-ocimene 0.2%, β-bourbonene 0.3%, limonene 0.2%
sesquiterpenes β-caryophyllene 8–10%, α-copaene 4–5%, β-elemene <1%, α-humulene <1%, δ-cadinene 1%, γ-cadinene 1%

Alcohols
monoterpenols linalool 0.4–1.3%, nerol <1%, geraniol <1%, citronellol <1%, isopulegol <1%
sesquiterpenols α-cadinol 0.3%, elemol <1%, (Z)-3-hexanol 0.1%, 1-octen-3-ol 1.3%

Ketones
6-methyl-5-hepten-2-one 4.5%, hexahydrofarnesyl-acetone 0.2%

Esters
geranyl acetate <0.5%, neryl acetate, citronellyl acetate

Oxides
1,8-cineole, caryophyllene oxide 2.5–3.6%

Aldehydes
neral 22–24%, geranial 32–37%, citronellal 0.7–2.2%

Coumarins
aesculetine

Other
3-octanone 0.6%, methyl heptanone 0.6%

Properties and indications

antiinflammatory	
antispasmodic	stomach cramp
calming	hysteria, palpitations, headaches, vertigo*, erethism
choleretic	regularizes secretions (bile, stomach)
digestive	indigestion*, nausea, morning sickness*, sluggish liver
hypotensor*	hypertension
sedative	insomnia, calming to CNS
vasodilator (capillaries)	palpitations, angina

Observations

- no known contraindications, but care may be necessary in sunlight
- often adulterated or reconstructed: caution is advised when procuring it, because the properties given above relate only to the true oil; melissa is frequently adulterated by mixing with lemongrass or citronella to increase its bulk, but is more usually totally simulated; these reconstructed oils have a similar 'lemony' aroma and contain some of the compounds found in natural melissa oil, e.g. citral, citronellal
- citronellal is the terpene to which sedative action is primarily attributed (Foster 1993b)
- skin allergies and respiratory problems are often made worse if not treated with a suitably low concentration of melissa oil (usually less than 1%)
- a powerful choleretic which triples the volume of bile in 30 min (Duraffourd 1982)
- the hydrosol is useful for regulating fever in children (Roulier 1990)
- studies have indicated that a cream with lemon balm (available in Germany) reduces the healing time of Herpes simplex I lesions and lengthens the time before recurrence (Tyler 1992)
- two chemotypes of melissa are known to exist, citral (as above) and citronellal (Lawrence 1989b)

MENTHA × PIPERITA fol. [PEPPERMINT] LABIATAE

Representative constituents

Hydrocarbons
monoterpenes (3–18%) α-pinene 0.2–2%, β-pinene 0.3–4%, limonene 0.6–6%, menthene, phellandrene, sabinene <1%, myrcene <1%, cis-ocimene trace–1.5%, p-cymene trace–0.5%, terpinolene trace–0.2%, α-terpinene <1%, γ-terpinene <1%

sesquiterpenes β-caryophyllene <1%,
trans-β farnesene trace–0.5%, α-muurolene trace–0.5%,
germacrene D 2.1–4.3%, γ-cadinene trace–0.7%,
β-bourbonene <1%

Alcohols
monoterpenols (50%) menthol 28–46%, isomenthol,
neo-menthol 2–7.7%, piperitol, piperitenol, isopiperitenol,
α-terpineol 0.1–1.9%, linalool <1%, terpinen-4-ol 0–2.4%
sesquiterpenols viridiflorol 0.5–1.3%, 10-α-cadinol trace–0.3%

Other
3-octanol <1%

Ketones
menthone 16–36%, iso-menthone 4–10.4%,
neomenthone 2–3%, piperitone 0.5–1.2%,
isopiperitone, pulegone <1%

Oxides
1,8-cineole 3–7.4%, menthofuran <3%,
piperitenone trace–0.7%, trans-piperitonoxide 0.5–3.1%,
caryophyllene oxide trace–0.5%

Esters
menthyl acetate 1.6–10%, neomenthyl acetate,
isomenthyl acetate, menthyl butyrate, menthyl isovalerate

Coumarins
aesculetine

Other
menthofuran 0.1–5.7%, trans-sabinene hydrate 0.2–1.4%,
cis-sabinene hydrate trace–0.8%

Properties and indications

analgesic	migraine, neuralgia, sciatica
antibacterial	see Table 4.4
antifungal	ringworm, skin infections
antiinfectious	
antiinflammatory	bronchitis, colitis, cystitis, eczema*, enteritis, gastritis, hepatitis, laryngitis, sinusitis, urticaria*
antilactogenic	prevents milk forming
antipyretic	fever
antispasmodic	colic, gastric spasm
antiviral	herpes, viral hepatitis
carminative	flatulence
decongestant	cirrhosis
digestive stimulant	indigestion, nausea, painful digestion, digestive problems
expectorant	bronchial asthma, bronchitis
hepatic stimulant	cirrhosis, jaundice
hormonal	irregular periods (ovarian stimulant)
hypertensor	hypotension
insect repellent	gnats, mosquitoes
mucolytic	bronchial asthma, bronchitis
neurotonic	apathy, nervous vomiting, travel sickness, palpitations, vertigo, (excites the motor nerves but damps the excitation of sensor nerves)
reproductive stimulant	impotence
soothing	skin irritation, rashes, redness
uterotonic	facilitates delivery

Observations

- contraindicated for babies and young children, where it can produce reflex apnoea or laryngospasm; an ointment containing menthol applied to the nostrils of infants for the treatment of cold symptoms has been reported to cause instantaneous collapse (Tester-Dalderup 1980)
- may cause allergic reactions such as contact dermatitis, flushing and headache in some individuals
- skin irritations may be made worse unless used in suitably low concentration
- should not be used externally in high concentration (i.e. low dilution) as in certain adults it may result in sleep disturbance
- peppermint oil is reported to be effective as an analgesic when used in conjunction with *Ravensara aromatica* (Roulier 1990)
- helps local circulation in the head
- there is a consensus of opinion that peppermint should not be used concurrently with homoeopathic treatment, although reasons vary
- menthol is cooling and anaesthetic when applied to the skin, increasing blood flow to the area to which it is applied (Mabey 1988)
- whole peppermint has more antispasmodic effect than menthol alone (Trease & Evans 1989)
- oil of peppermint is experimentally antispasmodic (Leung 1980); studies have shown peppermint oil to inhibit gastrointestinal smooth muscle spasms and reduce colonic motility (Duthie 1981, Sigmund & McNally 1969, Taylor et al 1983)
- *Mentha × piperita* is a hybrid of *Mentha spicata* [SPEARMINT] and *Mentha aquatica* [WATERMINT]

MYRISTICA FRAGRANS sem. [NUTMEG]
MYRISTICACEAE

Representative constituents

Hydrocarbons
monoterpenes (70–75%) α-pinene 14–25%,
β-pinene 10–15%, myrcene 2%, sabinene 14–35%,
α-terpinene 2–4%, γ-terpinene 1.9–7.7%,
limonene 3.7–4%, β-phellandrene, camphene <1%,
α-phellandrene 0.7–1%, *p*-cymene 1.1–3.1%,
terpinolene 0.9–1.7%
sesquiterpenes β-caryophyllene 0–1%

Alcohols
monoterpenols terpinen-4-ol 4–8.2%, α-terpineol 0.4–1.2%

Phenolic ethers
safrole 0.7–1.7%, myristicin 2.9–10.4%, elemicin 0.4–2.1%,
eugenol 0.2%, methyl eugenol 0.6%

Oxides
1,8-cineole 2–3%

Other
trans-sabinene hydrate <1%, cis-sabinene hydrate <1%

Properties and indications

analgesic	aches and pains, rheumatism, sprains, toothache, neuralgia
antibacterial	see Table 4.4
antiseptic	chronic diarrhoea
carminative	flatulence
circulatory stimulant	
digestive stimulant	loss of appetite, sluggish digestion, difficulty with starches and heavy meals, speeds up intestinal transit
emmenagogic	scanty periods
neurotonic	debility
reproductive tonic	impotence, frigidity
uterotonic	facilitates delivery

Observations

- requires great care in use on account of the myristicin content (a hallucinogen); ingestion of an overdose may produce epileptiform convulsions, coma and death (Åkesson & Wålinder 1965, Dale 1909)
- doses exceeding 5 ml take effect within 2–5 hours, producing time-space distortions and sometimes visual hallucinations accompanied by dizziness, headache, illness and rapid heartbeat (Duke 1985)
- it has been hypothesized that myristicin and elemicin can readily be modified in the body to amphetamines (Duke 1985)
- no irritation or sensitization at 2% dilution when tested on humans (Opdyke 1976 p. 631)
- Valnet (1980) lists the monoterpenols linalool, geraniol and borneol as constituents of this oil

NARDOSTACHYS JATAMANSI (= *N. GRANDIFLORA*) rad. [SPIKENARD] VALERIANACEAE

Representative constituents

Hydrocarbons
monoterpenes α-pinene 0.1%, β-pinene 0.1%, limonene 0.1%
sesquiterpenes aristolene 5%, dihydroazulenes, α-gurjunene 0.6%, β-gurjunene 29%, α-patchoulene 29%, β-patchouline 0.7%, seychellene 1.7%, β-maaliene

Alcohols
sesquiterpenols calarenol, nardol, valerianol, patchouli alcohol 6%, maaliol

Aldehydes
sesquiterpenals valerianal

Ketones
sesquiterpenones valeranone, β-ionone 1.4%, 3,4-dihydro-β-ionone trace, 1-hydroxyaristolenone 6%, aristolenone 0.7%

Oxides
1,8-cineole 0.2%

Coumarins
coumarin

Properties and indications

antispasmodic	convulsions, intestinal colic
calming	tachycardia, epilepsy, hysteria
cardiotonic	arrhythmia
phlebotonic	varicose veins, haemorrhoids
stimulant	anaemia, ovarian insufficiency
unspecified	psoriasis*

Observations

- no known contraindications
- it is sometimes used in place of valerian
- a history of religious use; used in meditation

NEPETA CATARIA VAR. *CITRIODORA* flos, fol. [CATNEP OIL] LABIATAE

Representative constituents

Hydrocarbons
monoterpenes myrcene trace–1.5%, limonene trace–0.4%, ocimenes trace–0.7%
sesquiterpenes β-caryophyllene 1.1–6.8%, α-humulene trace–4.3%

Alcohols
monoterpenols geraniol 13.7%, citronellol 48.3%

Esters
acetates, valerates, butyrates

Aldehydes
neral 4.9%, geranial 5.6%

Lactones
nepetalactone 9.4%, epinepetalactone 1.6%, dihydronepetalactone 1.2%

Properties and indications

antiinfectious	urinary infections
antiinflammatory*	irritable bowel syndrome, rheumatism*, arthritis
antiviral*	herpes
calming*	anxiety
litholytic	gall stones
sedative*	nervous depression

Observations

- no known contraindications
- the nepetalactone chemotype is described as diaphoretic and expectorant (Secondini 1990)
- the chemical structure of nepetalactone is similar to the valepotriates, the sedative principle in valerian

OCIMUM BASILICUM fol. [EUROPEAN BASIL] LABIATAE

Representative constituents

Hydrocarbons
monoterpenes (2%) α-pinene, β-pinene, camphene, limonene, cis-ocimene, *p*-cymene, γ-terpinene
sesquiterpenes isocaryophyllene, β-caryophyllene 2–3%, β-elemene

Alcohols
monoterpenols linalool 40–55%, α-fenchyl alcohol 3–12%, terpinen-4-ol 1.6%, α-terpineol 2%, citronellol 1.5%, geraniol 1.2%

Other
cis-3-hexanol

Esters
linalyl acetate, α-fenchyl acetate <1%, methyl cinnamate 0.1–7%, α-terpinyl acetate trace

Phenols
eugenol 1–19%, iso-eugenol 2%

Phenolic ethers
methyl chavicol 3–31%, methyl eugenol 1–9%

Oxides
1,8-cineole 2–8%

Ketones
camphor 0.1%

Properties and indications

analgesic	gout, migraine, rheumatoid arthritis
anthelmintic	threadworms
antibacterial	coliform cystitis; see Table 4.4
antiinflammatory*	gout, wasp stings
antiseptic	intestinal infections, gastritis
antispasmodic	gastric spasm, muscle cramp
antiviral	viral hepatitis
cardiotonic	arrhythmia, arteriosclerosis, tachycardia
carminative, eupeptic	flatulence, sluggish digestion
digestive tonic	stimulates digestive secretions, ulcers
fungistatic	
hypertensor	hypotension
insecticidal	
liver stimulant	hepatobiliary deficiency
nervous system regulator	anxiety*, epilepsy, nervous insomnia, nervousness, travel sickness, vertigo
neurotonic	debility, mental strain, convalescence, depression
reproductive decongestant	uterine and prostatic congestion
unspecified	dry eczema

Observations

- no known contraindications
- no irritation or sensitization at 4% dilution when tested on humans (Opdyke 1973 p. 867)
- no phototoxic effects reported (Opdyke 1973 p. 867)
- this oil may be used with safety when the methyl chavicol content is low
- the fact that it is a uterine decongestant does not mean that it is emmenagogic
- there is a natural variation in the chemical constituents of this essential oil both between plants and according to where the plant is grown

ORIGANUM MAJORANA flos, fol. [SWEET MARJORAM] LABIATAE

Representative constituents

Hydrocarbons
monoterpenes (40%) sabinene 2–10%, myrcene 1–9%, *p*-cymene 1–6%, terpinolene 1–7%, α-pinene 1–5%, β-pinene 0.2–2.5%, ocimene 6.4%, cadinene 4.2%, 3-carene 6.2%, α-terpinene 6–8%, γ-terpinene 14–20%, α-phellandrene, β-phellandrene 0.9%, myrcene, limonene 0.6%
sesquiterpenes β-caryophyllene 2–4.6%, α-humulene 0.1%

Alcohols
monoterpenols (50%) terpinen-1-ol-4 14–20%, cis-thujanol-4 4–13%, trans-thujanol-4 1–5%, linalool 2–9.5%, α-terpineol 7–27%, cis-*p*-menth-2-en-1-ol 2%, trans-*p*-menth-2-en-ol 2%, cis-piperitol 0.5%

Esters
terpenyl acetate 0–3%, geranyl acetate 1–7.8%, linlyl acetate 0.1%

Aldehydes
citral 5.4%

Other
trans-sabinene hydrate 1%, cis-sabinene hydrate 4%

Properties and indications

analgesic*	arthritis*, migraine, muscular pain*, rheumatism*, toothache
antibacterial	see Table 4.4
antiinfectious	whooping cough, bronchitis, headaches, respiratory infections, rhinitis, sinusitis
antispasmodic	colic, muscles, respiratory spasm, nervous spasm
calming	ether addiction, psychoses, agitation, anxiety, epilepsy, insomnia, migraine, sexual obsessions, vertigo
digestive stimulant	flatulence, gastro-duodenal ulcers, indigestion
diuretic	
expectorant	catarrh, coughs, bronchitis
hormonal	hyperthyroidism

hypotensor	hypertension, tachycardia, palpitations, fainting
neurotonic	debility*, mental instability, nervous spasm (by balancing the parasympathetic nervous system), anguish, agitation, nervous depression
respiratory tonic	nervous breathing
stomachic	diarrhoea, enteritis
vasodilator	

Observations

- no known contraindication at normal dose
- marjoram oil stimulates the vagus (parasympathetic) nerve and does not act on the sympathetic nerve, therefore its action is tranquillizing and lightly narcotic, a nervous sedative (Duraffourd 1982)
- no irritation or sensitization at 6% dilution when tested on humans (Opdyke 1976 p. 469)
- used in vermouth
- the naming and correct identification of this group of herbs presents difficulties even to the expert: there are some 30 species of marjoram with the family name origanum

ORMENIS MIXTA flos [MOROCCAN CHAMOMILE] ASTERACEAE

Representative constituents

Hydrocarbons
monoterpenes   α-pinene 15%, camphene 0.4%, limonene 8%, γ-terpinene 0.1%, terpinolene 0.25%
sesquiterpenes   germacrene 5%, β-caryophyllene 1.5%, bisabolene 2.5%, δ-elemene 0.7%

Alcohols
α-terpineol, santolina 32%, yomogi 2.4%, artemisia 2.3%, linalool 0.3%, borneol 1%, ormenol, trans-pinocarveol 3%

Ketones
camphor, pinocarvone 0.5%

Oxides
1,8-cineole

Esters
bornyl acetate 2.2%, bornyl butanoate 1.3%

Properties and indications

antibacterial*	see Table 4.4
antiinfectious	acne, cysts
antiinflammatory	dermatitis, eczema, rheumatism, colitis, cystitis
antiirritant	pruritis
hepatobiliary tonic	gall bladder and pancreas, sluggish liver
neurotonic*	nervous depression*
sexual tonic	

Observations

- no known contraindications

PELARGONIUM GRAVEOLENS fol. [GERANIUM] GERANIACEAE

Representative constituents

Hydrocarbons
monoterpenes (1–2%)   α-phellandrene trace, β-phellandrene, α-pinene 1%, β-pinene 0.2%, myrcene 0.2%, limonene 0.2%, cis-ocimene 0.2%
sesquiterpenes (1–2%)   guaia-6,9-diene 3.9–5.3%, guaiazulene, α-copaene, δ-cadinene, γ-cadinene, α-bourbonene, β-bourbonene, caryophyllene 0.7%

Alcohols
monoterpenols (55–65%)   citronellol 21–45%, geraniol 17–25%, linalool 1–13%, nerol 1.2%, α-terpineol 0.7%
sesquiterpinols   10-epi-γ-eudesmol 1%
aromatic   phenyl ethyl alcohol <1%

Esters (15%)
citronellyl formates 8–18%, geranyl formates 1–6%, citronellyl proprionates 1–3%, geranyl proprionates 0–1%, geranyl tiglates 1–2%, geranyl acetate 0.4%, citronellyl butyrate 1.3%, geranyl butyrate 1.3%, phenyl ethyl isobutyrate, phenyl ethyl tiglate

Aldehydes (Bourbon variety) (0–10%)
neral, geranial 0–9%, citronellal 0–1%

Ketones (1–8%)
menthone 0.6–3%, isomenthone 4–8.4%, piperitone, methylheptanone, furopelargone 0.4%

Oxides (only in Chinese variety) (2–3%)
cis-rose oxide 2–25%, trans-rose oxide 1%, cis-linalool oxide 0.6%, trans-linalool oxide 0.2%

Properties and indications

analgesic	facial neuralgia, osteoarthritis, rheumatism
antibacterial*	see Table 4.4
antidiabetic	sluggish pancreas, diabetes
antifungal*	athlete's foot and other skin and nail fungi, candida
antiinfectious	infectious colitis, acne, cuts, wounds, impetigo, infectious skin diseases
antiinflammatory	arthritis, colitis, pruritis, rheumatism, tonsillitis
antiseptic	
antispasmodic	colic, cramp, gastroenteritis, painful menstruation
astringent	diarrhoea, haemorrhoids, varicose veins
cicatrizant	burns, cuts, ulcers, uterine haemorrhage, stretch marks, wounds
decongestant	breast congestion, lymph congestion
digestive stimulant	jaundice, sluggish liver

haemostatic	burns, cuts, ulcers, uterine haemorrhage, wounds
insect repellent	gnats, mosquitoes
phlebotonic* (lymph*)	haemorrhoids, varicose ulcers, varicose veins
relaxant*	agitation, anxiety, debility, nervous fatigue

Observations

- no known contraindications
- to be used with care on the skin of hypersensitive individuals (Winter 1984)
- no irritation or sensitization at 10% dilution when tested on humans (Opdyke 1974 p. 883)
- no phototoxic effects reported (Opdyke 1974 p. 883)
- contact with the leaves of the plant has been reported to cause vesicular dermatitis

PIMPINELLA ANISUM fruct. [ANISEED] UMBELLIFERAE (APIACEAE)

Representative constituents

Hydrocarbons
sesquiterpenes γ-himachalene trace, β-caryophyllene

Alcohols (0.5–4%)
anisol 0.5–4%, linalool <1.5%, α-terpineol <1.5%

Phenols (0.5%)
isochavibetol 0.5%

Phenolic ethers (90–95%)
cis-anethole 0–1%, trans-anethole 90–93%, methyl chavicol 0–2%, myristicin trace

Aldehydes
aniseed aldehyde 1–2%

Ketones
p-methoxyphenylacetone

Coumarins, furocoumarins
umbelliferone, scopoletine

Properties and indications

analgesic	arthritis, backache, nauseous migraine, period pains, rheumatism, sciatica, vertigo
antispasmodic	bronchial spasm, colic, enteritis, flatulence, indigestion, infantile colic, vomiting (of nervous origin), painful periods
aperitive	stimulates digestive juices
cardiotonic	cardiovascular erethism, palpitations, tired heart
carminative*	flatulence, indigestion
diuretic	oliguria
emmenagogic	amenorrhoea, oligomenorrhoea*
expectorant	catarrh
lactogenic	lack of milk

narcotic (gentle)	
oestrogenlike*	menopause, PMS
psychoactive*	
respiratory tonic	asthma, bronchitis, congestion in lungs, nervous breathing
sexual tonic	frigidity, impotence
uterotonic	facilitates delivery

Observations

- not normally used on babies, young children and pregnant women
- like fennel oil, anise oil contains compounds that can be aminated in vivo resulting in a series of three dangerous hallucinogenic amphetamines (Emboden 1972)
- the major component of aniseed oil, anethole, can cause dermatitis (erythema, scaling and vesiculation) in some individuals
- anethole has two isomers, the cis isomer being 15 to 38 times more toxic than the trans isomer (Leung 1980)
- several cases of sensitization have been reported (Loveman 1938, Schwarz 1934, Tulipan 1938), and attributed to the presence of anethole (Schwarz et al 1947)
- no irritation or sensitization at 4% dilution when tested on humans (Opdyke 1973 p. 865); not a primary irritant to normal skin (Harry 1948)

PINUS SYLVESTRIS fol. [PINE] ABIETACEAE (PINACEAE)

Representative constituents

Hydrocarbons
monoterpenes (60–70%) α-pinene 22–43%, β-pinene 3–33%, limonene 0.7–4.1%, δ-3-carene 0.4–31%, β-caryophyllene 0.7–5.5%, camphene 1.6–3.3%, sabinene 0.2–0.6%, γ-terpinene 0.1–0.5%, trans-ocimene 0.7–1.4%, β-phellandrene 1–2.7%, p-cymene 0–0.2%, terpinolene 0.3–3%
sesquiterpenes longifolene, γ-cadinene 0.5–5.4%, α-copaene 0–0.2%, δ-elemene trace, α-ylangene trace, longifolene 0–0.2%, β-guaiene 0.2–0.7%, β-farnesene trace, γ-muurolene trace–0.4%, α-humulene trace–0.5%, γ-patchoulene 0–0.2%, γ-cadinene trace–0.3%, α-muurolene trace–1%, cubenene trace, calemenene trace

Alcohols
monoterpenols borneol 2%, terpinen-4-ol 1%
sesquiterpenols epi-α-cadinol <1%, epi-α-muurolol <1%, α-cadinol 0–2%

Aldehydes
citronellal 0–0.2%

Esters (1–10%)
bornyl acetate 0–3%

Properties and indications

analgesic	gastralgia, intestinal pains, arthritis, rheumatism
antibacterial	see Table 4.4

antifungal
antiinfectious*   antiseptic (air), respiratory
                         infections, asthma*, bronchitis*,
                         colds, influenza, pneumonia,
                         sinusitis*, tracheitis, tuberculosis,
                         urinary infections (cystitis,
                         prostatitis, pyelitis)
antiinflammatory   inflammatory and allergic
                         conditions, arthritis, gall bladder
                         inflammation, gout, rheumatism
antisudorific   hyperidrosis of the feet
balsamic
cortisonelike   stimulates suprarenal cortex
decongestant   congested lymph, uterine or
                         ovarian congestion, breaks down
                         bronchial secretions
expectorant   respiratory tract
hypertensor*   hypotension*
insulinlike   pancreatic diabetes
litholytic   gallstones
neurotonic*   debility*, fatigue, insufficient
                         semen (nervous origin),
                         multiple sclerosis
rubefacient   arthritis, rheumatism
testosteronelike   impotence

Observations

- no known contraindications
- in patch tests on 21 patients with essential oil dermatoses, positive reactions to full strength or diluted oils including *Pinus sylvestris* oil were attributed to 3-Carene (a major component of pine oil), α-phellandrene and eugenol (Woeber & Krombach 1969)
- no irritation or sensitization at 12% dilution when tested on humans (Opdyke 1976 p. 469)
- no phototoxic effects reported (Opdyke 1976 p. 469)

PIPER NIGRUM fruct. [BLACK PEPPER] PIPERACEAE

Representative constituents

Hydrocarbons
monoterpenes   α-pinene 2–9%, β-pinene 5–14%, α-thujene 0.5–3.5%, sabinene 9–19%, α-terpinene 0.4–2.8%, δ-3-carene 1–15%, myrcene 1.6–2.5%, l-limonene 17%, α-phellandrene 5–9%, δ-elemene 2.6%, *p*-cymene 1–2.8%, γ-terpinene 0.5–3.9%, terpinolene 0.5–1.5%, camphene
sesquiterpenes   β-caryophyllene 9–29%, α-humulene 1–2%, α-guaiene, α- and β-cubebene 0.2–1.6%, α- and β-selinenes 0.5–7.7%, α- and β-elemene 0.3–2.4%, β-bisabolene 2–5%, calamenene, α-copaene 0.5–1.5%, β-farnesene 1–3%, zingiberene trace, bergamotene 0.5%, ar-curcumene 0.5%

Alcohols
monoterpenols   terpinen-4-ol <1%, α-terpineol 0.1%, linalool <1%, trans-pinocarveol, trans-carveol, elemol 0.5%, α-bisabolol 0.1%

Phenolic ethers
p-cymene methyl ether, carvacrol methyl ether trace, myristicin trace, safrole trace

Ketones (1–8%)
di-hydrocarvone 0.05%, piperitone <1%

Aldehydes
piperonal

Oxides
caryophyllene oxide 0.6%

Properties and indications

analgesic*   rheumatic pain, toothache*
antibacterial   see Table 4.4
anticatarrhal   chronic bronchitis, laryngitis,
                        colds
antiseptic   urinary system
eupeptic   sluggish liver, pancreas and
                        digestion
expectorant   bronchitis, coughs
febrifuge   fevers
sexual tonic   frigidity, general

Observations

- no known contraindications
- no irritation or sensitization at 4% dilution when tested on humans (Opdyke 1978 p. 651)
- low-level (insignificant) phototoxic effects (Opdyke 1978 p. 651)
- myristicin and elemicin can be readily modified in the body to amphetamines (Duke 1985)

POGOSTEMON PATCHOULI fol. [PATCHOULI] LABIATAE

Representative constituents

Hydrocarbons
monoterpenes   α-pinene 0.5–1%, β-pinene 0.5–1%, limonene trace
sesquiterpenes (40–50%)   α-bulnesene 10–19.6%, β-bulnesene 14–16%, α-guaiene 6–15%, β-guaiene, α-patchoulene 3–5.3%, β-patchoulene 1.9–6.6%, seychellene 5–12%, cyclo-seychellene <1%, β-caryophyllene 2–4.2%, δ-cadinene 1–2.8%, aromadendrene 10.8–20.9%, 1,5-epoxy-α-guaiene 0.1%, 1,10-epoxy-α-bulnesene 0.2–0.6%

Alcohols
sesquiterpenols (35–45%)   patchoulol 23.6–45.9%, pogostol 1–3%, bulnesol 1%, guaiol, norpatchoulenol <1%

Ketones
patchoulenone trace–2.2%, isopatchoulenone 1%

Oxides
α-guaiene oxide 1%, α-bulnesene oxide 4%, caryophyllene oxide 0.5–1%

Properties and indications

antiinfectious	enteritis
antiinflammatory	acne*, allergies, inflamed skin, seborrhoeic eczema
antifungal	
antiseptic	
decongestant	
cicatrizant	cracked skin, scar tissue, abnormal epidermis
immunostimulant	low natural defences
insect repellent	
phlebotonic*	haemorrhoids*, varicose veins*

Observations

- no known contraindications
- no irritation was produced by the oil on humans at 20% in vaseline or in an ointment, or at 0.1% in a non-irritant cream base in subjects with dermatoses (Fujii et al 1972)
- no irritation or sensitization at 10% dilution when tested on humans (Opdyke & Letizia 1982a)
- no phototoxic effects reported (Opdyke & Letizia 1982a)

RAVENSARA AROMATICA fol.
[AROMATIC RAVENSARA] LAURACEAE

Representative constituents

Hydrocarbons
monoterpenes α-pinene, β-pinene, sabinene 13.5–15%
sesquiterpenes β-caryophyllene

Alcohols
monoterpenols α-terpineol 6–7%, terpinen-4-ol 2%

Esters
terpenyl acetate

Oxides
1,8-cineole 61%

Properties and indications

antibacterial	
antifungal	
antiinfectious*	glandular fever, bronchitis, influenza*, sinusitis, whooping cough
antiinflammatory	rhinopharyngitis
antiviral*	chicken pox, dendritis*, herpes zoster*, viral enteritis, viral hepatitis*
detoxicant	
expectorant*	bronchitis, coughs
nerve tonic	insomnia*, muscle fatigue, neuromuscular problems

Observations

- no contraindications known
- well tolerated on the skin
- relaxing when massaged over the vertebral column

ROSA DAMASCENA, R. CENTIFOLIA flos (dist.) [ROSE OTTO] ROSACEAE

Representative constituents

Hydrocarbons (25%)
monoterpenes stearoptene 16–22%, α-pinene, β-pinene, α-terpinene, limonene, myrcene, ocimene, *p*-cymene, camphene
sesquiterpenes β-caryophyllene 0.3%
other octadecane 0.2%, nonadecane and nonadecene 2–15%

Alcohols
monoterpenols geraniol 15.8–22.2%, citronellol 22.5–60? %, nerol 8.5%, linalool 1.5–2.7%, iso-borneol 0.4%, α-terpineol <1%
sesquiterpenols farnesol 0.2–2%
aromatic phenyl ethyl alcohol 0.9–3%

Aldehydes
neral 0.5%

Esters (2–6%)
citronellyl acetate 0.5%, geranyl and neryl acetate 1.2%

Phenolic ethers
methyl eugenol 1.4%

Oxides
rose oxide 0.3%

Other
damascenone 0.2–1.6%, eicosane 1%, heneicosane, docosane 0.1–0.4%, tricosane 0.04–0.9%, tetracosane 0.2%, pentacosane 0.4%

Properties and indications

antibacterial	see Table 4.4 (pp 61–62)
antiinfectious	acute and chronic bronchitis, asthma, mouth ulcers
antiinflammatory	blotchy skin, gingivitis, conjunctivitis
astringent	
cicatrizant	mouth ulcers, skin problems, sprains, wounds
general tonic	chronic bronchitis
neurotonic*	debility, depression
sexual tonic	frigidity, sexual debility
styptic	wounds

Observations

- no known contraindications
- no irritation or sensitization at 2% dilution when tested on humans (Opdyke 1974 pp. 979–981, 1975 p. 913)
- no phototoxic effects reported (Opdyke 1974 pp. 979–981, 1975 p. 913)
- rose absolute is produced in a different way from rose otto and has a different chemical composition
- French rose absolute produced one sensitization reaction in a test on 25 individuals (Opdyke 1975 p. 911)

ROSMARINUS OFFICINALIS CT. CINEOLE, CT. CAMPHOR fol. [ROSEMARY] LABIATAE

N.B. The cineole and camphor chemotypes have almost the same constituents, properties and indications. They are therefore considered together here

Representative constituents

Hydrocarbons

monoterpenes (30–37%) α-pinene 1.4–12%, β-pinene 3–9%, camphene 3–22%, myrcene 1–2%, α-phellandrene, β-phellandrene, α-terpinene, γ-terpinene, limonene 1.9–2.4%, *p*-cymene 1.1–2%
sesquiterpenes β-caryophyllene 0.9–3%, α-humulene 0.6–1.2%

Alcohols

monoterpenols linalool 0.6–2%, α-terpineol 1–4.5%, borneol 3.4–12%, isoborneol, terpenen-4-ol 0.6–1.5%, cis- and trans-thujanol-4, *p*-cymene-8-ol, verbenol

Esters

iso-bornyl acetate trace–1.2, α-fenchyl acetate

Oxides

1,8-cineole 30–55%, caryophyllene oxide, humulene epoxides

Ketones

monoterpenones α-thujone, β-thujone, camphor 6.4–30%, verbenone trace, carvone 1%
aliphatic 3-hexanone, methyl heptanone

Properties and indications

adrenal cortex stimulant	
analgesic	migraine, painful digestion
antibacterial	see Table 4.4
antifungal	
antiinfectious	chills, diarrhoea, enteritis, influenza
antiinflammatory	cystitis, gout, muscular pains, otitis, rheumatism, inflamed gall bladder
antispasmodic	muscle cramp
antitussive	coughing, whooping cough
antiviral	
cardiotonic	palpitations, weak heart
carminative	flatulence
choleretic*	insufficient bile
cicatrizant	burns, wounds
decongestant (venous)	migraine, headache, poor circulation, arteriosclerosis
detoxicant	hepatitis, jaundice, cirrhosis, enlarged liver, gall bladder malfunction
digestive	indigestion, sluggish digestion, colitis, constipation, painful digestion
diuretic	liver*, gall bladder*
emmenagogic	amenorrhoea, oligomenorrhoea
enuresis	bedwetting
fungicide*	*Candida albicans*
hypertensive (high dose)	hypotension
hypotensive (low dose)	hypertension
litholytic	gall stones
lowers cholesterol	high cholesterol
mucolytic*	chronic bronchitis, sinusitis
neuromuscular action*	multiple sclerosis, painful muscles, epilepsy, neuralgia, rheumatism
neurotonic	fainting, general debility, general fatigue, hysteria, loss of memory, vertigo
sexual tonic	impotence

Observations

- usually regarded as having no contraindications
- there are conflicting opinions regarding the use of rosemary oils in pregnancy and epilepsy:
  —some cite it as an oil to avoid in the first 4 months of pregnancy
  — Roulier (1990) warns against its use in pregnancy but does not give this warning for the verbenone chemotype
  —Franchomme & Pénoël (1990) warn against using the verbenone chemotype on pregnant women, but do not mention the cineole and camphor chemotypes
  —some contraindicate its use on people prone to epilepsy
  — Valnet (1980) recommends its use on epileptics
- bath preparations containing the oil can cause erythema (Duke 1985)
- toiletries containing the oil can cause dermatitis in hypersensitive individuals (Mitchell & Rook 1979)
- the essential oil in wine is said to help cancers (Hartwell 1971)
- no irritation or sensitization at 10% dilution when tested on humans (Opdyke 1974 p. 977)

ROSMARINUS OFFICINALIS CT. VERBENONE fol. [ROSEMARY] LABIATAE

Representative constituents

Hydrocarbons

monoterpenes α-pinene 15–34%, β-pinene, camphene, myrcene, limonene, α-terpinene, terpinolene
sesquiterpenes β-caryophyllene

Alcohols

monoterpenols borneol trace–7%

Esters

bornyl acetate

Ketones

monoterpenones verbenone 15–37%, camphor 1–15%

Oxides

1,8-cineole trace–20%

Properties and indications

antiinfectious	leucorrhoea, vaginitis, candida
anticatarrhal	bronchitis, sinusitis
antispasmodic	
antiviral*	viral colic*, viral hepatitis
antibacterial	
cardiotonic	angina pectoris, arrhythmia, tachycardia
cicatrizant	
detoxicant	liver and bilious affections [but see Observations]
expectorant	bronchitis, coughs
hormone regulator	ovaries and testicles
mucolytic	bronchitis, coughs, sinusitis
nervous system regulator	fatigue, nervous depression, nervous digestive*, sexual problems

Observations

- not normally used on those inclined to liver problems, children, and in pregnancy (except where necessary)
- the oil is neurotoxic and abortive (Franchomme & Pénöel 1990); not to be used in pregnancy (Roulier 1990)

SALVIA OFFICINALIS fol.
[SAGE, DALMATIAN SAGE] LABIATAE

Representative constituents

Hydrocarbons
monoterpenes (3–15%) α-pinene 3.2–6.4%, β-pinene 1.9%, camphene 1–5.4%, myrcene 0.4–1.1%, limonene 0.9–4%, *p*-cymene 1–2%, terpinolene, salvene, α-phellandrene 0.1%, β-phellandrene 0.1%, α-thujene trace, sabinene 0.2%, α-terpinene 0.2%, γ-terpinene 0.3%
sesquiterpenes β-caryophyllene 1–7%, aromadendrene, α-humulene 4–5%, α-cadinene, β-cadinene, β-copaene

Alcohols
monoterpenols (3–38%) linalool 0.4–12%, terpinen-4-ol 0.2–4%, α-terpineol trace–9%, borneol 1.5–14%, salviol, trans-sabinol trace
sesquiterpenols viridiflorol 0–10%

Esters
bornyl acetate 0.1–3%, linalyl acetate 1–2%, sabinyl acetate, linalyl and methyl isovalerates

Phenols
thymol trace

Oxides
1,8-cineole 5–14%, caryophyllene oxide 0.4–2.1%

Ketones
monoterpenones (20–70%) α-thujone 12–35.7%, β-thujone 2–33%, camphor 4.1–26%, fenchone 0.2%

Aldehydes
3-hexanal trace

Coumarins
aesculetine trace

Phenolic ethers
methyl chavicol 0.4%

Other
trans-sabinene hydrate 0.2%, tricyclene 0.3%, cis-2-methyl-3-methylene-5-heptene 0.7%, trans-2-methyl-3-methylene-5-heptene 0.1%, cis-sabinene hydrate trace

Properties and indications

analgesic	angina, rheumatism, toothache
antibacterial	see Table 4.4
anticancer	malignant conditions
anticatarrhal	asthma, bronchitis, coughs
antifungal*	*Candida albicans**
antiinfectious	influenza, gingivitis, insect bites, intermittent fevers, leucorrhoea, sore throat
antipyretic	hot flushes
antispasmodic	dysmenorrhoea
antisudorific	excessive hand and armpit hyperidrosis, night sweating
antiviral	genital herpes, thrush, viral enteritis, viral meningitis, viral neuritis
choleretic	insufficient bile*
cicatrizant	
circulatory regulator	poor circulation, rheumatism, congestion
digestive (low dose)	indigestion, loss of appetite, sluggish digestion
diuretic	oliguria, urinary disorders
drains biliary canal	
emmenagogic	amenorrhoea, irregular periods, scanty periods
expectorant	bronchitis, coughs
hormonal	conducive to conception, facilitates delivery, sterility, menopause, premenopause*
hypertensor	hypotension
hypoglycemiant	prediabetes
insecticidal	
lipolytic*	cellulite
mucolytic	coughs, sinusitis
nerve tonic	alopecia, general debility, nervous debility, tremors, vertigo

Observations

- not normally used for breastfeeding mothers and young children
- antilactogenic: halts lactation in nursing mothers (Roulier 1990, Valnet 1980)
- neurotoxic and abortive (may cause malformed heart in babies if used throughout pregnancy (Franchomme & Pénöel 1990)
- because of its potential toxicity, sage oil, like all essential oils, should be used only in very small quantities (Foster 1993b)

- no irritation or sensitization at 8% dilution when tested on humans (Opdyke 1974 p. 987)
- German authorities recommend an internal dosage level of 1 drop of the essential oil per cup of water in infusion, perhaps taken up to three times per day
- although sage has more thujone than wormwood it seems a far safer plant: but the tea should only be taken for a week or two at a time because of the potentially toxic effects of thujone (Mabey 1988)
- cheilitis and stomatitis follow some cases of sage tea ingestion (Duke 1985)
- the distilled oil is said to be a violent epileptiform convulsant, resembling the essential oils of absinth, nutmeg and wormwood (Duke 1985)

SALVIA SCLAREA flos, fol. [CLARY]
LABIATAE

Representative constituents

Hydrocarbons
monoterpenes (2–3%) α-pinene 0.1–0.25%, β-pinenes 0.3%, sabinene trace, camphene, myrcene 0.1–1.7%, terpinolene, *p*-cymene trace, α-terpinene trace, limonene 0.1–0.8%
sesquiterpenes (5%) β-caryophyllene 0.8–3%, germacrene D 1.6–4%, curcumene, trans calamene, trans-ocimene 0.4–1%, terpinolene 0.1–0.4%, α-cubebene trace, α-copaene 0.1–0.5%, β-bourbonene 0.1%

Alcohols
monoterpenols (15%) linalool 5–26%, α-terpineol 1%, citronellol, nerol trace–1%, geraniol 0.1–3.2%, borneol, isoborneol, thujol, terpinen-4-ol trace–0.1%
sesquiterpenols α-bisabol, junerol
diterpenols (5–7%) sclareol 1–7%
other cis-3-hexanol trace–0.3%, trans-2-hexanol 0.2%, 1-octen-3-ol trace, spathulenol trace

Aldehydes
trans-2-hexanal trace–0.1%, caryophyllenals

Esters
linalyl acetate 49–75%, citronellyl acetate, geranyl acetate 0.3–3.2%, neryl acetate 0.2–1.7%, butyrates, valerates, bornyl acetate 0.2%, α-terpinyl acetate trace–0.1%

Oxides
1,8-cineole, trans-linalool oxide trace, caryophyllene oxide 0.2–0.5%, sclareol oxide, cis-linalool oxide trace

Ketones
α- and β-thujones

Coumarins
coumarin

Properties and indications

antiinfectious	genital infections (connected with hormone deficiency)
antifungal	dermal fungal conditions
antispasmodic	
antisudorific	hyperidrosis
decongestant	dysmenorrhoea
detoxicant	
hormonal (oestrogenlike)	amenorrhoea*, oligomenorrhoea, pre-menopause
neurotonic	epilepsy, nervous fatigue, calming to parasympathetic nervous system, alopecia
phlebotonic	circulatory problems, haemorrhoids, varicose veins, venous aneurism, cholesterol
regenerative	cellular ageing, poor hair growth

Observations

- no known contraindications, but is not normally used on people with cancers or tumours
- no irritation or sensitization at 8% dilution when tested on humans (Opdyke & Letizia 1982b)
- there are in excess of 250 constituents in clary oil
- contains a diterpenol, rare in distilled oils

SANTALUM ALBUM lig. [SANDALWOOD]
SANTALACEAE

Representative constituents

Hydrocarbons
sesquiterpenes α- and β-santalene 10%, epi-β-santalene 6%, α- and β-curcumene, farnesene

Alcohols
sesquiterpenols α-santalol 46–60%, β-santalol 20–30%, epi-β-santalol 4–5%, trans-β-santalol 1–2%, cis-lanceol 1.5%, cis-nuciferol 1%, a monocyclic sesquiterpenol 5%, a tricyclic sesquiterpenol 1%

Aldehydes
sesquiterpenes teresantalal

Properties and indications

antiinfectious	pulmonary: chronic bronchitis, colibacillosis; urinary: cystitis, gonorrhoea, urinary tract infections
astringent	diarrhoea
cardiotonic*	tired heart, haemorrhoids, varicose veins
decongestant*	pelvic congestion*, acne, skin problems
diuretic	
moisturizer	dry skin
nerve relaxant	lumbago, neuralgia, sciatica, meditation
sexual tonic	impotence
tonic	

Observations

- no known contraindications
- regarded as a general and sexual tonic
- does not irritate the mucous linings of the stomach or intestine
- no irritation or sensitization at 10% dilution when tested on humans (Opdyke 1974 p. 987)
- no phototoxic effects reported (Opdyke 1974 p. 987)
- approved for food use (Duke 1985)
- isolated santalol can cause dermatitis in sensitive individuals (Leung 1980)
- the oil has diuretic and urinary antiseptic properties (Leung 1980)

SATUREIA HORTENSIS fol.
[SUMMER OR GARDEN SAVORY] LABIATAE

Representative constituents

Hydrocarbons
monoterpenes (34%) α-thujene <1%, α-pinene <1%, β-pinene trace, myrcene 1–2.8%, α-terpinene 1–3.1%, γ-terpinene 20–24%, *p*-cymene 3.7–15.3%, cymene ?–25%, camphene trace, δ-3-carene, δ-4-carene, α-phellandrene, β-phellandrene trace, limonene trace, sabinene trace
sesquiterpenes (3–4%) β-caryophyllene 2–4%, β-bisabolene 1%, δ-cadinene 3%, calacorene and γ-cadinene 3.6%

Alcohols
monoterpenols linalool, terpinen-4-ol, borneol, α-terpineol, nerol trace, geraniol trace

Phenols (39–40%)
thymol, carvacrol 35–40%, eugenol

Ketones
camphor trace

Aldehydes
piperonal

Oxides
1,8-cineole

Other
damascenone 1%

Properties and indications

antibacterial	see Table 4.4
antifungal	
antiinfectious*	wide range of action
antioxidant	
antiparasitic	
antiviral	
cardiotonic	
choleretic	
digestive tonic	indigestion, facilitates elimination, carminative, sluggish bile
expectorant	
general tonic/stimulant	debility*

nervous system balancer
respiratory antiseptic *
revitalizing
sexual tonic

Observations

- no irritation or sensitization at 6% dilution when tested on humans (Opdyke 1976 p. 859)
- no phototoxic effects reported (Opdyke 1976 p. 859)
- two species of Satureia, *S. hortensis* and *S. montana*, have a pronounced thyme-like odour and flavour, and the oils of the two plants are closely related in chemical composition (Guenther 1949)

SATUREIA MONTANA fol.
[WINTER OR MOUNTAIN SAVORY] LABIATAE

Representative constituents

Hydrocarbons
monoterpenes (40–50%) α- and γ-terpinenes 2–20%, *p*-cymene 10–25%, α-pinene, β-pinene, camphene, sabinene, myrcene, limonene, α-phellandrene
sesquiterpenes β-caryophyllene, α-humulene, aromadendrene, β-bisabolene, α-cadinene, γ-cadinene, calacorene

Alcohols
monoterpenols linalool 9–54%, cis-thujanol-4, trans-thujanol-4, terpinen-4-ol trace–7%, α-terpineol 6–9%, geraniol, borneol

Esters
linalyl acetate, terpinen-4-yl acetate, geranyl acetate, α-terpinyl acetate

Phenols (25–50%)
carvacrol 25–50%, eugenol, thymol 1–5%

Phenolic ethers
carvacrol methyl ether

Oxides
1,8-cineole 1%, caryophyllene oxide

Ketones
camphor

Other
damascenone

Properties and indications

analgesic*	rheumatoid arthritis*
antibacterial	see Table 4.4
anticatarrhal	bronchitis, coughs
antifungal	*Candida albicans*, fungal infections of the mouth
antiinfectious*	wide range of action, colitis, enteritis, tonsillitis, sore throat, tuberculosis, diarrhoea, cystitis, malaria*, skin infections, abscesses, impetigo, lichen

antiparasitic*	oxyures, ascaris, taenia, amoebiasis*
antispasmodic	intestinal spasm, colic, muscle spasms
antiviral	
carminative	flatulence
cicatrizant	insect bites, sores
circulatory tonic	hypotension*
digestive stimulant	painful digestion
expectorant	asthma, bronchitis, catarrh
general tonic*	general debility
immunostimulant	repetitive infections
mental stimulant	mental debility
neurotonic	lymph ganglion inflammation*, debility, nervous fatigue*, depression

Observations

- possible skin irritant and therefore to be used in low concentration
- savory oil is an efficient antidiuretic because of the carvacrol present (Duke 1985)
- winter savory is used for catarrh, colic, otitis, sclerosis and spasms (Duke 1985)

SYZYGIUM AROMATICUM (FORMERLY *EUGENIA CARYOPHYLLATA*) flos
[CLOVE BUD] MYRTACEAE

Representative constituents

Hydrocarbons
monoterpenes   pinene
sesquiterpenes   α- and β-caryophyllene 5–13%, α- and β-humulene 0.5–1.5%, α-cubebene 0.01–0.3%, α-copaene 0.01–0.2%, calamenene 0.2–0.5%

Phenols (60–90%)
eugenol 36–85%, isoeugenol 0.1–0.25%, acetoeugenol 11–21.8%

Esters (20–25%)
eugenyl acetate 0.5–12%, 2-nonanyl acetate trace, α-terpinyl acetate 0.1–0.2%, benzyl acetate trace, methyl benzoate 0.04–0.13%

Oxides
humulene epoxide trace, caryophyllene oxide trace–1.8%

Properties and indications

analgesic	rheumatoid arthritis, toothache, neuralgia*
antibacterial	see Table 4.4
antifungal	
antiinfectious	abscesses, gum infections, infected acne, ulcers, wounds
antiinflammatory	bronchitis, salpingitis

antiseptic	prevention of disease, cystitis, diarrhoea, sinusitis
antispasmodic	diarrhoea, intestinal spasm
antiviral*	enteritis*, influenza, hepatitis, herpes, tuberculosis*
calming	
carminative	flatulence
cicatrizant	infected acne, ulcers, wounds
hormonal	thyroid imbalance
hypertensor	hypotension
immunostimulant	low immunity
insect repellent	mosquitoes, clothes moths
mental stimulant*	memory loss, mental fatigue
neurotonic*	debility, fatigue*
sexual tonic	impotence
unspecified	stimulates secretion of saliva
uterotonic*	difficult labour, long labour

Observations

- should not be applied undiluted to skin because clove oils may cause irritation at high dosage levels
- considered nontoxic at normal usage levels
- 20% dilution of clove bud oil on humans produced erythema in 2 of the 25 tested; no irritation or sensitization occurred at 2%, or at 0.2% on subjects with dermatoses (Fujii et al 1972)
- no irritation or sensitization at 5% dilution when tested on humans (Opdyke 1975 p. 761)
- no phototoxic effects reported for any of the clove oils (Opdyke 1975 p. 761)
- is used as an antiseptic mouthwash
- eugenol sensitizes some people causing contact dermatitis (Duke 1985)
- clove bud oil and savory oil create a synergistic mix (Duraffourd 1982)

THYMUS MASTICHINA flos, fol.
[SPANISH MARJORAM] LABIATAE

Representative constituents

Hydrocarbons
monoterpenes   terpinolene 4%, limonene 2–2.8%, α-pinene 2.6%, β-pinene 2–3%, *p*-cymene 1.3–3.4%, sabinene 0.8–1.1%, α-thujene 0.2–0.5%, myrcene 0.2–1%, camphene 0.2–1.4%, γ-terpinene <1%
sesquiterpenes   β-caryophyllene 0.1%, β-gurjunene 0.3%, allo-aromadendrene 0.2–1%, γ- and δ-cadinene 0.1%, β-bourbonene 0.1%, caryophyllene 1–1.5%

Alcohols
monoterpenols   borneol trace–3.5%, linalool 8.5–43%, α-terpineol 8%, geraniol 0.2%, cis- and trans-thujanol-4 0.2%, trans-pinocarveol 1%, 3-terpinen-1-ol 0.2%, terpinen-4-ol 0.1–0.7%

Phenols
thymol 0–5%

Ketones
camphor trace–4%

Oxides
1,8-cineole 41–75%, caryophyllene oxide trace

Esters
linalyl acetate 1–1.5%, 3-terpinen-1-yl acetate 0.2%,
bornyl acetate 0.2%, trans-pinocarveol acetate 1.5%,
α-terpinyl acetate 3%, geranyl acetate 0.1%

Other
trans-sabinene hydrate 0.2%

Properties and indications

antiinfectious	sinusitis, catarrhal bronchitis*, viral and bacterial infections
antibacterial	see Table 4.4

Observations

- no contraindications known at normal dose
- no irritation or sensitization at 6% dilution when tested on humans (Opdyke 1976 p. 467)
- no phototoxic effects reported (Opdyke 1976 p. 467)

THYMUS VULGARIS herb. population [THYME] LABIATAE

Representative constituents

Hydrocarbons
monoterpenes p-cymene 2.2–42.8%, γ-terpinene 0.3–12.4%,
α-pinene 0.9–3.7%, camphene 0.5–2.4%, myrcene trace–2.6%,
α-terpinene 0.8–1.5%, limonene 0.4–2.1%,
terpinolene trace–2%, α-thujene 0.5%, δ-3-carene 0.1%,
sabinene 0.6%, α-phellandrene 0.1–0.2%, β-pinene trace
sesquiterpenes β-caryophyllene 0.2–2.9%

Phenols
thymol 30–48.2%, carvacrol 0.5–5.5%,
methoxy carvacrol trace

Alcohols
monoterpenols borneol trace–1.8%, linalool 1.3–12.4%,
terpinen-4-ol 0.3–9.5%, α-terpineol 0.4–9.4%,
geraniol 0.1–0.2%, β-terpineol 0.6–0.9%
sesquiterpenols nerolidol 0–0.8%

Ketones
camphor 2.3–16.3%, α-thujone 0.2%

Esters
linalyl acetate 0.9%, α-terpinyl acetate 0.7–1.4%,
geranyl acetate 0–0.5%

Oxides
1,8-cineole 0.4–7.4%, trans-linalool oxide 0.5%,
cis-linalool oxide 1%

Properties and indications

antibacterial	see Table 4.4
antioxidant	
antiseptic	acne, boils, skin problems, etc
antispasmodic	
capillary stimulant	anaemia, circulatory disorders, hair loss
carminative	flatulence
cicatrizant	
digestive tonic	sluggish digestion
diuretic	
expectorant	bronchial secretions, bronchitis, sinusitis, asthma
general tonic	general fatigue
hypertensor	hypotension
mental stimulant	depression, exam nerves
neurotonic	anxiety, debility
parasiticide	
sexual tonic	
stomachic	
sudorific	
vermifuge	intestinal parasites
warming	rheumatism, stiff joints
unspecified	leucorrhoea

Observations

- irritant to the skin
- the volatile oil is toxic in any quantity and internal use should be restricted to professionals (Mabey 1988)
- oil of thyme is largely eliminated through the alveoli of the lung (Weiss 1988)
- the German Bundes Gesundsheitamt (BGA) publishes monographs on acceptable labelling for herb products and permits thyme to be designated for symptoms of bronchitis, whooping cough and catarrh of the upper airways (Foster 1993b)
- it is to be avoided in pregnancy
- thymol is an antiseptic 20 times stronger than phenol, yet, unlike phenol, does not irritate or corrode the skin or mucosa
- thymol can be highly toxic; it is strongly fungicidal, antibacterial, antioxidant and toxic to the hookworm (Foster 1993b)
- thymol is a starting material for synthetic menthone and is used in embalming fluids
- thymol is an effective antifungal agent and anthelmintic: it is poorly absorbed into body fluids, so finds its main use within the gut or on the surface of the body, ideal for toothpastes and mouthwashes (Mills 1991)
- thymol has caused dermatitis in dentists, and (in toothpaste) has caused glossitis (Duke 1985)
- carvacrol stimulates mucosal secretory activity (Mills 1991)
- thyme plants grown from seed (known as population thyme) yield an essential oil with a rich variety of components
- there is wide variation of constituents in oils from *Thymus vulgaris*, hence the broad limits given above
- like many of the herbaceous members of the Labiatae family that have achieved economic importance, there are nomenclatural and botanical authenticity problems associated with thyme (Lawrence 1978); there are about 400 species—or 100 species with 400 names (Foster 1993b). (Phillips 1989, 1991) has attempted to sort out the confusion of species occurring in the USA

- at least nine naturally occurring chemotypes are known
- *T. vulgaris* ct. thymol and *T. vulgaris* ct. carvacrol have thymol and carvacrol respectively as major components
- *T. vulgaris* ct. geraniol has geraniol 60–80%; *T. vulgaris* ct. linalool has linalool 60–80%

THYMUS VULGARIS (ALCOHOL CHEMOTYPES) [SWEET THYME] LABIATAE

Properties and indications

antifungal*	*Candida albicans**
antiinfectious	bronchitis, sinusitis, tuberculosis
antiinflammatory	bronchitis, cystitis, muscular rheumatism, otitis, urethritis, vaginitis, dry eczema, psoriasis, weeping eczema
antiseptic	sore throat, tonsillitis, colitis, infected acne
antispasmodic (ct. linalool)	bronchiole spasm
antiviral*	veruccae, viral enteritis*, people prone to repeated viral attacks*
cardiotonic (ct. geraniol)	tired heart
choleretic	
diuretic (ct. linalool)	
immunostimulant (ct. linalool)	
neurotonic*	fatigue, insomnia
ophthalmic	eye problems (informed use only)
sexual tonic (ct. linalool)	
uterotonic*	facilitates delivery

Observations

- no known contraindications
- sweet thyme oils do not contain the aggressive elements of the red thymes
- preferred for general use, children and the elderly (Price 1993)

THYMUS VULGARIS (PHENOL CHEMOTYPES) [RED THYME] LABIATAE

Properties and indications

anthelmintic*	
antibacterial*	tuberculosis
antidiuretic (ct. carvacrol)	
antifungal* (ct. carvacrol)	
antiinfectious	influenza, general infections*, head colds, infectious diseases, sinusitis
antiparasitic	
mental stimulant	mental strain?
mucolytic*	asthma, emphysema, pulmonary diseases
warming*	rheumatism of joints and muscles, sciatica, lumbago

Observations

- red thymes are powerful antiseptic and antibacterial agents
- to be used with care because of the high phenol content
- no irritation or sensitization at 8% dilution when tested on humans; can be irritating at full strength (Opdyke 1974 p. 1003)
- no phototoxic effects reported (Opdyke 1974 p. 1003)

VETIVERIA ZIZANIOIDES rad. [VETIVER] POACEAE

Representative constituents

Hydrocarbons
sesquiterpenes   vetivene, vetivazulene, tricyclovetivene

Alcohols
sesquiterpenols   vetiverol, bicyclovetiverol 12.1%, tricyclovetiverol 3.3%

Esters (sesquiterpenic)
vetiverol acetate

Ketones (sesquiterpenic)
α-vetiverone 3.9%, β-vetiverone 3%

Acids
vetivenic acid, palmitic acid, benzoic acid

Properties and indications

antiinfectious	general infections, skin infections, acne
circulatory tonic*	inflamed coronary artery
emmenagogic	amenorrhoea, oligomenorrhoea
glandular tonic	insufficient pancreatic secretion, liver congestion
immunostimulant	low immunity
unspecified	arthritis
unspecified	urticaria

Observations

- no known contraindications
- no irritation or sensitization at 8% dilution when tested on humans (Opdyke 1974 p. 1013)
- no phototoxic effects reported (Opdyke 1974 p. 1013)

ZINGIBER OFFICINALE rhiz. [GINGER] ZINGERBERACEAE

Representative constituents

Hydrocarbons
monoterpenes (20%)   α-pinene 0.4–4.2%, β-pinene 0.1–2.3%, camphene 1.1–8%, myrcene 0.1–1%, limonene 1.2–3%, β-phellandrene 1.3–4%
aromatic   p-cymene 0.2–10.8%, toluene decanes
sesquiterpenes (55%)   zingiberene 11.3–50.9%, β-sesquiphellandrene 1.6–9%, ar-curcumene 0.1–32.9%, cis-γ-bisabolene 7%, copaene, sesquithujene, β-ylangene, β-elemene, β-farnesene 19.8%, β-caryophyllene, calamenene, β-bisabolene 0.2%, α-selinene 1.4%

Alcohols

citronellol 6%, linalool 1–5.5%, 2-butanol,
2-nonanol 2.1–7.8%, 2-heptanol trace, nerolidol trace–8.9%,
elemol, β-bisabol, zingiberol, trans-β-sesquiphellandrol,
gingerol, d-borneol 1.3%

Aldehydes

monoterpenes   citronellal, myrtenal, phellandral, neral,
geranial

Ketones

acetone, 2-hexanone, 2-heptanone, methyl-heptanone,
2–nonanone, cryptone, carvotanacetone, gingerone

Oxides

1,8-cineole 1.3%

Properties and indications

analgesic*	angina, painful indigestion, rheumatism, toothache
anticatarrhal	chronic bronchitis
carminative*	flatulence
digestive stimulant	constipation, loss of appetite, sluggish digestion, nausea
expectorant	chronic bronchitis
general tonic	fatigue, impotence
sexual tonic	impotence
stomachic	diarrhoea

Observations

- no known contraindications at normal dose
- gingerols and shagaols do not appear in the distilled essential oil
- no irritation or sensitization at 4% dilution when tested on humans (Opdyke 1974 p. 901)
- low-level insignificant phototoxic effects reported (Opdyke 1974 p. 901)

Appendix B

1. UTEROTONIC OILS WHICH FACILITATE DELIVERY

The percentage figure given for toxic components is the average or a typical range.

Cymbopogon martinii fol. [PALMAROSA]:
  alcohols 80–90% (geraniol).
Foeniculum vulgare var. *dulce* fruct. [SWEET FENNEL]:
  phenolic ether 70%.
Mentha × piperita fol. [PEPPERMINT]:
  ketones 20–30%.
Myristica fragrans sem. [NUTMEG]:
  terpenes 40% , myristicin 2–3%.
Pimenta dioica (= *P. racemosa*) fol. [BAY]:
  phenol 90%. *Difficult deliveries.*
Pimpinella anisum fruct. [ANISEED]:
  phenolic ether 90%.
Szygium aromaticum flos [CLOVE BUD]:
  phenol 70–80%. *Difficult deliveries.*
Thymus vulgaris ct. geraniol, herb. [SWEET THYME]:
  alcohol 60–80%.

2. EMMENAGOGIC ESSENTIAL OILS

The percentage figure given for toxic components is an average. See also Chapter 8.

Achillea millefolium flos [YARROW, MILFOIL]: combined ketone and oxide 30%. Not generally considered to be toxic.
Cinnamomum zeylanicum cort. [CINNAMON]: phenolic ether 60%.
Foeniculum vulgare var. *dulce* fruct. [SWEET FENNEL]:
  phenolic ether 60%. *Also hormonelike, diuretic and lactogenic; facilitates delivery.*
Melaleuca viridiflora fol. [NIAOULI]: oxide 50%. Contains the hormonelike sesquiterpenol viridiflorol.
Myristica fragrans sem. [NUTMEG, MACE]: phenolic ether 6%. Large dose produces narcosis, delirium and death—see also Appendix A. *Also facilitates delivery.*
Petroselinum sativum fruct. [PARSLEY SEED]: phenolic ether 55%.
Pimpinella anisum fruct. [ANISEED]: phenolic ether 83%. *Also hormonelike; facilitates delivery.*
Salvia officinalis fol. [SAGE]: ketone 35%. *Also hormonelike.*

3. DISPUTED EMMENAGOGIC OILS

Essential oils not yet mentioned, which some books suggest are emmenagogic and need care during pregnancy, although there is no research to support or reject these suggestions. See also Chapter 8.

Commiphora molmol (= *C. myrrha*) [MYRRH]: *hormonelike*.
Juniperus communis fruct. [JUNIPER BERRY]: *diuretic*.
Juniperus communis ram. [JUNIPER]: no known toxic component.
Levisticum officinale rad. [LOVAGE]: *diuretic*.
Chamomilla recutita flos [GERMAN CHAMOMILE]: *hormonelike*.
Melaleuca leucadendron fol. [CAJUPUT]: *hormonelike*.
Mentha × piperita fol. [PEPPERMINT]: *hormonelike*.
Ocimum basilicum fol. [BASIL].
Origanum majorana fol. [MARJORAM].
Rosa damascena, R. centifolia flos [ROSE OTTO]: *hormonelike*.
Rosmarinus officinalis ct. camphor [ROSEMARY].
Salvia sclarea [CLARY]: *hormonelike*.
Vetiveria zizanioides rad. [VETIVER].

4. TOXIC, NEUROTOXIC AND ABORTIVE OILS NOT USED IN AROMATHERAPY

This list comprises toxic, neurotoxic and abortive essential oils used by the medical profession in France. Whether or not they are known to aromatherapists, they are not normally used by them. The percentage figure given for toxic components is an average unless otherwise qualified. Common names are given where known.

Acorus calamus [CALAMUS]: phenolic ether 75%.
Agathosma betulina [BUCHU]: ketone 60%.
Artemisia absinthium [WORMWOOD]: ketone 35%.
  Also *emmenagogic*.
Artemisia afra: ketone 40%.
Artemisia annua: ketone 28%. Also *hormonelike*.
Artemisia arborescens: ketone 55%.
Artemisia herba alba: ketone 65%.
Artemisia pallens [DAVANA]: ketone 40%.
Artemisia vulgaris [MUGWORT]. Also *emmenagogic*.
Brassica nigra [MUSTARD]: allylisothiocyanate up to 99%.
Calamintha nepeta [WILD BASIL]: ketone 65%.
Calamintha sylvatica [CALAMINT]: ketone 65%.
Cedrus deodora [HIMALAYAN CEDARWOOD]: ketone 50%.
Chenopodium ambrosioides [WORMSEED]: oxide 60%.
Chrysanthemum balsamita: ketone 75%.
Cinnamomum camphora lig. [BROWN CAMPHOR, BLUE CAMPHOR]: safrole 60%.
Cochlearia armoracia [HORSERADISH]: allylisothiocyanate 90%.
Cupressus arizonica [BLUE CYPRESS]: ketones >50%.
Curcuma longa [TURMERIC]: ketone 60%.
Eucalyptus dives, E. polybractea [eucalyptus]: ketone 45%.
Foeniculum vulgare var *amara* [BITTER FENNEL]: anethole 60%.
Geranium macrorrhizum [BULGARIAN GERANIUM]: ketone 50%.
Gaultheria procumbens [WINTERGREEN]: methyl salicylate 95%.

Illicium verum [STAR ANISE]: phenolic ether 80%—*also hormonelike*.
Juniperus oxycedrus [OIL OF CADE, JUNIPER TAR]. A wood distillate and not an essential oil.
Juniperus sabina [SAVIN]: podophyllotoxine content in the total extract.
Lantana camara [LANTANA]: ketone >50%. Also *emmenagogic*.
Lavandula stoechas [SPANISH LAVENDER]: ketone 75%.
Mentha longifolia [MINT]: oxide 65%. Also *hormonelike*.
Myrica gale [BOG MYRTLE]: ketone >50%.
Ocimum canum ct. camphor [DOG BASIL]: ketone 60%.
Ocotea pretiosa [BRAZILIAN SASSAFRAS]: phenolic ether 85%.
Peumus boldus (= *Boldea fragrans*) [BOLDO]: oxide 30%.
Ruta graveolens [RUE]: ketone 65%.
Santolina chamaecyparissus [LAVENDER COTTON, SANTOLINA]: ketone 35%.
Sassafras officinale [SASSAFRAS]: phenolic ether 85%.
Tanacetum vulgare [TANSY]: ketone 75%.
Thuja occidentalis [THUJA]: ketone 55%.

5. NEUROTOXIC AND/OR ABORTIVE OILS OCCASIONALLY USED IN AROMATHERAPY

The following list comprises essential oils known and used by aromatherapists which are potentially neurotoxic and/or abortive (if used beyond the accepted maximum dosage).

Achillea millefolium [MILFOIL, YARROW]: ketone content variable. (See also Appendix A.)
Anethum graveolens sem. [ANISEED]: ketone 50%.
Artemisia dracunculus [TARRAGON]: phenolic ether 65%. Held to be nontoxic by some.
Carum carvi [CARAWAY]: ketone 50%. Usually held to be nontoxic. Also *diuretic*.
Cedrus atlantica [ATLAS CEDARWOOD]: ketone 20%. Considered toxic in France.
Cinnamomum camphora lig. [CAMPHOR]: ketone and oxide 70%. Camphor from the wood is usually a triple-rectified oil and unsuitable for aromatherapy. The essential oil from the leaves contains mainly alcohols and has no known contraindications.
Hyssopus officinalis [HYSSOP]: ketone 50%. *Not to be used on epileptics*.
Mentha pulegium [PENNYROYAL]: ketone 80%. Also *emmenagogic*.
Mentha spicata [SPEARMINT]: ketone 60%.
Petroselinum sativum fruct. [PARSLEY SEED]: phenol ether (apiole).
Rosmarinus officinalis ct. verbenone [ROSEMARY]: ketone 30%.
Tagetes glandulifera [TAGETTE]: ketone 45%. Also *phototoxic because of coumarin content; also emmenagogic*.

6. POTENTIAL SKIN IRRITANT OILS

These phenolic or aldehydic essential oils generally have no special contraindications in pregnancy. The exceptions are *Cinnamomum cassia* which contains trans-cinnamic aldehyde and *Cinnamomum zeylanicum* cort. which is also emmenagogic.

Cinnamomum cassia [CASSIA]: aldehyde 78–88%;
    phenol 5–6% typically. *Very caustic on the skin.*
Cinnamomum zeylanicum cort. [CINNAMON BARK]:
    aldehyde 40–76%. *Neurotoxic.*
Cinnamomum zeylanicum fol. [CINNAMON LEAF]:
    phenol 70–96%.
Cuminum cyminum fruct. [CUMIN]: aldehyde 20–50%.
Cymbopogon citratus fol. [LEMONGRASS]: aldehyde 60–86%.
Origanum heracleoticum fol. [OREGANO]: phenol 51–63%.
Origanum vulgare fol. [OREGANO]: phenol 22–83%.
Syzygium aromaticum caul. [CLOVE STEM]: aldehyde 90–95%.
Syzygium aromaticum flos [CLOVE BUD]: aldehyde 60–90%.
Syzygium aromaticum fol. [CLOVE LEAF]: aldehyde 82–88%.
Thymus serpyllum herb. [WILD or CREEPING THYME]:
    phenol 20–30%.
Thymus vulgaris ct. phenol herb. [RED THYME]:
    phenol 50–60%.

7. PHOTOTOXIC OILS

Some essential oils may render the skin hypersensitive to ultraviolet rays, producing the protective tanning reaction. Photosensitizing essential oils may contain up to approximately 2% furocoumarins, generally found in the expressed citrus oils.

Angelica archangelica fruct., rad. [ANGELICA ROOT, SEED].
Carum carvi fruct. [CARAWAY]: low level phototoxicity.
Cinnamomum cassia fol. [CASSIA]: low level phototoxicity.
Cinnamomum zeylanicum cort. [CINNAMON BARK]:
    low level phototoxicity.
Citrus aurantifolia per. [LIME].
Citrus aurantium var. *amara* per. [BITTER ORANGE].
Citrus bergamia per. [BERGAMOT].
Citrus limon per. [LEMON].
Cuminum cyminum fruct. [CUMIN].
Levisticum officinale fol. [LOVAGE].
Lippia citriodora [LEMON VERBENA]: low level phototoxicity.
Melissa officinalis fol. [MELISSA]: low level phototoxicity.
Ruta graveolens herb. [RUE]. See also Appendix B.4.
Zingiber officinale rhiz. [GINGER]: low level phototoxicity.

Generally speaking the maximum concentration of essential oils in a carrier should not exceed 5% (equivalent to 10 drops of essential oils in 10 ml of carrier). Regarding phototoxicity and sensitization, even this quantity can be too much for a few oils, as the following information (extracted from the Code of Practice of the International Fragrance Association) shows. [p] = phototoxic, [s] = sensitizer. See also Appendix B.8.

Angelica Root Oil [p]	3.9% max
Bergamot Oil [p+s]	2.0% max
Orange Oil [p]	7.0% max
Cassia Oil [s]	1.0% max
Cinnamon Bark Oil [s]	0.1% max
Costus Root Oil [s]	0.1% max
Cumin Oil [p]	0.1% max
Fig Leaf Oil [p+s]	0.0%
Lemon Oil [p]	10.0% max
Lime Oil [p]	3.5% max
Rue Oil [p]	3.5% max
Savin Oil	0.0%
Verbena Oil [p+s]	0.0%

8. CONTACT-SENSITIZING OILS

Sensitization is a type of allergic reaction which can occur when a substance comes into contact with the body. A few essential oils applied to the skin may cause sensitization, perhaps only after repeated application (the amount used is not significant). The skin reaction appears as redness, irritation and perhaps vesiculation.

Cananga odorata flos [YLANG YLANG].
Cinnamomum cassia fol. [CASSIA].
Cinnamomum zeylanicum cort. [CINNAMON BARK OIL].
Costus speciosus rad. [COSTUS ROOT].
Citrus bergamia per. [BERGAMOT].
Ficus carica fol. [FIG LEAF].
Inula helenium rhiz. [ELECAMPANE].
Lippia citriodora [VERBENA].
Pimpinella anisum fruct. [ANISEED].
Szygium aromaticum caul. [CLOVE STEM].
Szygium aromaticum flos [CLOVE BUD].

Cross-sensitization

With some essential oils an allergic reaction to one oil may lead to sensitivity to other material(s). Little is known of cross-sensitization reactions, but the risk is slight. Two examples are:

- benzoin resinoid cross colophony (a resin) cross *Mentha × piperita* cross Peru balsam (not distilled cross turpentine (a rectified oil)
- *Laurus nobilis* ram. et fol. cross *Costus speciosus* rad. cross *Cinnamomum zeylanicum* cort.

Some individuals show patch test reactions to *Achillea millefolium* [YARROW] and cross-sensitivity between this oil and other Asteraceae has been demonstrated (Duke 1985).

9. GENERAL PROPERTIES OF ESSENTIAL OILS

This table shows general properties attributed to essential oils. Refer to relevant chapters in the text and to Appendix A for details.

	Analgesic	Antianaemic	Antibacterial	Antidiabetic	Antifungal	Antihistaminic, antiallergic	Antinfectious	Antiinflammatory	Antiirritant	Antimigraine	Antioxidant	Antiparasitic	Antiseborrhoeic	Antispasmodic	Antistress/anxiety	Antisudorific	Antitumoral
Achillea millefolium [YARROW]								X									
Boswellia carteri (res. dist.) [FRANKINCENSE]	X						X	X				X					
Cananga odorata [YLANG YLANG]				X										X			
Carum carvi (fruct.) [CARAWAY]			X		X									X			
Cedrus atlantica (lig.) [ATLAS CEDARWOOD]			X														
Chamaemelum nobile (flos) [ROMAN CHAMOMILE]		X						X		X		X		X			
Chamomilla recutita (flos) [GERMAN CHAMOMILE]						X		X						X			
Citrus aurantium var. amara (flos) [NEROLI BIGARADE]			X				X					X					X
Citrus aurantium var. amara (fol.) [PETITGRAIN BIGARADE]			X				X	X						X			
Citrus aurantium var. amara (per.) [ORANGE BIGARADE]								X							X		
Citrus bergamia (per.) [BERGAMOT]			X				X							X			
Citrus limon (per.) [LEMON]		X	X				X	X						X			
Citrus reticulata (per.) [MANDARIN]					X									X			
Coriandrum sativum (fruct.) [CORIANDER]	X		X				X							X			
Cupressus sempervirens (fol.) [CYPRESS]			X				X							X		X	
Eucalyptus globulus (fol.) [TASMANIAN BLUE GUM]			X		X		X	X				X					
Eucalyptus smithii (fol.) [GULLY GUM]	X						X										
Eucalyptus staigeriana (fol.) [LEMON SCENTED IRON TREE]							X	X						X	X		
Foeniculum vulgare var. dulce (fruct.) [FENNEL]	X		X				X							X			
Hyssopus officinalis [HYSSOP]			X				X	X									
Juniperus communis (fruct.) [JUNIPER BERRY]	X			X													
Juniperus communis (ram.) [JUNIPER TWIG]	X							X					X				
Lavandula angustifolia [LAVENDER]	X		X		X			X		X				X	X		
Lavandula × intermedia 'Super' [LAVANDIN]					X					X							
Melaleuca alternifolia (fol.) [TEA TREE]	X		X		X		X					X			X		
Melaleuca leucadendron (fol.) [CAJUPUT]	X		X				X							X			
Melaleuca viridiflora (fol.) [NIAOULI]	X		X				X	X				X					X
Melissa officinalis (fol.) [MELISSA]								X						X			
Mentha × piperita (fol.) [PEPPERMINT]	X		X		X		X	X	X	X				X			
Myristica fragrans (sem.) [NUTMEG]	X		X														
Nardostachys jatamansi (rad.) [SPIKENARD]														X			
Nepeta cataria var. citriodora (fol.) [CATNEP]							X	X									
Ocimum basilicum (fol.) [BASIL]	X		X		X		X			X				X	X		
Origanum majorana (fol.) [MARJORAM]	X		X				X			X				X			
Ormenis mixta (flos) [MOROCCAN CHAMOMILE]			X				X	X	X								
Pelargonium graveolens (fol.) [GERANIUM]	X		X	X	X		X	X						X	X		
Pimpinella anisum (fruct.) [ANISEED]	X									X				X			
Pinus sylvestris (fol.) [PINE]	X		X		X		X	X								X	
Piper nigrum (fruct.) [BLACK PEPPER]	X		X														
Pogostemon patchouli (fol.) [PATCHOULI]					X		X	X									
Ravensara aromatica (fol.) [RAVENSARA]			X				X	X									
Rosa centifolia (flos), R. damascena [ROSE OTTO]			X				X	X									
Rosmarinus officinalis [ROSEMARY]	X		X		X		X	X		X				X			
Rosmarinus officinalis ct. verbenone [ROSEMARY]			X											X			
Salvia officinalis (fol.) [SAGE]	X		X		X		X							X		X	
Salvia sclarea [CLARY]					X		X							X		X	
Santalum album (lig.) [SANDALWOOD]							X										
Satureia hortensis (fol.) [SUMMER SAVORY]			X		X		X					X	X				
Satureia montana (fol.) [WINTER SAVORY]	X		X		X		X						X	X			
Styrax benzoin, S. tonkinensis [BENZOIN]																	
Syzygium aromaticum (flos) [CLOVE BUD]	X		X		X		X							X			
Tagetes glandulifera (flos) [TAGETES]					X							X					
Thymus mastichina [SPANISH MARJORAM]			X				X										
Thymus satureioides [THYME]			X				X	X									
Thymus vulgaris (population) [THYME]			X								X			X	X		
Thymus vulgaris ct. alcohol [SWEET THYME]					X		X	X						X			
Thymus vulgaris ct. phenol [RED THYME]			X				X							X			
Vetiveria zizanioides (rad.) [VETIVER]							X										
Zingiber officinale (rhiz.) [GINGER]	X																

General properties of essential oils *(cont'd)*

	Antitussive	Antiviral	Appetite stimulating	Balancing	Balsamic	Cardiotonic	Carminative	Cholagogic, choleretic	Circulation stimulant	Decongestant	Detoxicant, depurative	Stomachic, digestive, stimulant	Diuretic	Emmenagogic	Eupeptic	Expectorant	Febrifuge
Achillea millefolium [YARROW]								x		x		x	x	x		x	x
Boswellia carteri (res. dist.) [FRANKINCENSE]																	
Cananga odorata [YLANG YLANG]				x													
Carum carvi (fruct.) [CARAWAY]			x				x	x					x	x			
Cedrus atlantica (lig.) [ATLAS CEDARWOOD]									x								
Chamaemelum nobile (flos) [ROMAN CHAMOMILE]								x				x		x			
Chamomilla recutita (flos) [GERMAN CHAMOMILE]										x		x					
Citrus aurantium var. *amara* (flos) [NEROLI BIGARADE]												x					
Citrus aurantium var. *amara* (fol.) [PETITGRAIN BIGARADE]				x													
Citrus aurantium var. *amara* (per.) [ORANGE BIGARADE]								x				x					
Citrus bergamia (per.) [BERGAMOT]		x	x									x					
Citrus limon (per.) [LEMON]		x					x					x	x				
Citrus reticulata (per.) [MANDARIN]								x				x			x		
Coriandrum sativum (fruct.) [CORIANDER]							x					x					
Cupressus sempervirens (fol.) [CYPRESS]	x												x				
Eucalyptus globulus (fol.) [TASMANIAN BLUE GUM]		x			x					x						x	
Eucalyptus smithii (fol.) [GULLY GUM]		x	x							x		x				x	
Eucalyptus staigeriana (fol.) [LEMON SCENTED IRON TREE]																	
Foeniculum vulgare var. *dulce* (fruct.) [FENNEL]							x	x	x	x		x	x	x			
Hyssopus officinalis [HYSSOP]	x									x		x	x			x	
Juniperus communis (fruct.) [JUNIPER BERRY]											x	x	x				
Juniperus communis (ram.) [JUNIPER TWIG]											x		x			x	
Lavandula angustifolia [LAVENDER]							x										
Lavandula × *intermedia* 'Super' [LAVANDIN]		x														x	
Melaleuca alternifolia (fol.) [TEA TREE]		x															
Melaleuca leucadendron (fol.) [CAJUPUT]										x						x	
Melaleuca viridiflora (fol.) [NIAOULI]		x										x				x	x
Melissa officinalis (fol.) [MELISSA]								x				x					
Mentha × *piperita* (fol.) [PEPPERMINT]		x					x					x				x	x
Myristica fragrans (sem.) [NUTMEG]							x		x			x		x			
Nardostachys jatamansi (rad.) [SPIKENARD]						x											
Nepeta cataria var. *citriodora* (fol.) [CATNEP]		x															
Ocimum basilicum (fol.) [BASIL]		x					x	x							x		
Origanum majorana (fol.) [MARJORAM]												x	x			x	
Ormenis mixta (flos) [MOROCCAN CHAMOMILE]																	
Pelargonium graveolens (fol.) [GERANIUM]										x		x					
Pimpinella anisum (fruct.) [ANISEED]			x				x	x		x			x	x		x	
Pinus sylvestris (fol.) [PINE]					x					x						x	
Piper nigrum (fruct.) [BLACK PEPPER]															x	x	x
Pogostemon patchouli (fol.) [PATCHOULI]										x							
Ravensara aromatica (fol.) [RAVENSARA]		x									x					x	
Rosa centifolia (flos), *R. damascena* [ROSE OTTO]																	
Rosmarinus officinalis [ROSEMARY]	x	x					x	x	x	x		x	x	x			
Rosmarinus officinalis ct. verbenone [ROSEMARY]		x					x					x				x	
Salvia officinalis (fol.) [SAGE]		x					x	x				x	x	x		x	x
Salvia sclarea [CLARY]												x	x				
Santalum album (lig.) [SANDALWOOD]						x						x		x			
Satureia hortensis (fol.) [SUMMER SAVORY]		x					x	x				x				x	
Satureia montana (fol.) [WINTER SAVORY]		x						x	x			x				x	
Styrax benzoin, S. tonkinensis [BENZOIN]																	
Syzygium aromaticum (flos) [CLOVE BUD]		x					x										
Tagetes glandulifera (flos) [TAGETES]														x			
Thymus mastichina [SPANISH MARJORAM]																	
Thymus satureioides [THYME]																	
Thymus vulgaris (population) [THYME]							x		x			x	x			x	
Thymus vulgaris ct. alcohol [SWEET THYME]		x					x	x									
Thymus vulgaris ct. phenol [RED THYME]												x	x	x		x	
Vetiveria zizanioides (rad.) [VETIVER]									x					x			
Zingiber officinale (rhiz.) [GINGER]							x					x				x	

General properties of essential oils *(cont'd)*

	Hepatic stimulant	Hormonelike	Hypertensor	Hypotensor	Immunostimulant	Insecticidal, parasiticidal	Insect repellent	Lactogenic	Larvicidal	Lipolytic	Litholytic	Mental stimulant	Mucolytic, anticatarrhal	Neurotonic, antidepressive	Oestrogenic	Ophthalmic
Achillea millefolium [YARROW]				x								x	x			
Boswellia carteri (res. dist.) [FRANKINCENSE]					x								x	x		
Cananga odorata [YLANG YLANG]				x												
Carum carvi (fruct.) [CARAWAY]									x				x			
Cedrus atlantica (lig.) [ATLAS CEDARWOOD]										x			x			
Chamaemelum nobile (flos) [ROMAN CHAMOMILE]																x
Chamomilla recutita (flos) [GERMAN CHAMOMILE]		x														
Citrus aurantium var. *amara* (flos) [NEROLI BIGARADE]														x		
Citrus aurantium var. *amara* (fol.) [PETITGRAIN BIGARADE]																
Citrus aurantium var. *amara* (per.) [ORANGE BIGARADE]																
Citrus bergamia (per.) [BERGAMOT]														x		
Citrus limon (per.) [LEMON]					x	x					x					
Citrus reticulata (per.) [MANDARIN]	x															
Coriandrum sativum (fruct.) [CORIANDER]								x						x		
Cupressus sempervirens (fol.) [CYPRESS]														x		
Eucalyptus globulus (fol.) [TASMANIAN BLUE GUM]							x						x			
Eucalyptus smithii (fol.) [GULLY GUM]													x			
Eucalyptus staigeriana (fol.) [LEMON SCENTED IRON TREE]																
Foeniculum vulgare var. *dulce* (fruct.) [FENNEL]		x						x		x					x	
Hyssopus officinalis [HYSSOP]			x							x	x		x			
Juniperus communis (fruct.) [JUNIPER BERRY]																
Juniperus communis (ram.) [JUNIPER TWIG]													x	x		
Lavandula angustifolia [LAVENDER]				x										x		
Lavandula × *intermedia* 'Super' [LAVANDIN]													x	x		
Melaleuca alternifolia (fol.) [TEA TREE]					x									x		
Melaleuca leucadendron (fol.) [CAJUPUT]		x					x									
Melaleuca viridiflora (fol.) [NIAOULI]	x	x		x	x						x		x			
Melissa officinalis (fol.) [MELISSA]				x												
Mentha × *piperita* (fol.) [PEPPERMINT]	x	x	x				x						x	x		
Myristica fragrans (sem.) [NUTMEG]														x		
Nardostachys jatamansi (rad.) [SPIKENARD]																
Nepeta cataria var. *citriodora* (fol.) [CATNEP]												x				
Ocimum basilicum (fol.) [BASIL]	x			x			x							x		
Origanum majorana (fol.) [MARJORAM]		x		x										x		
Ormenis mixta (flos) [MOROCCAN CHAMOMILE]														x		
Pelargonium graveolens (fol.) [GERANIUM]							x									
Pimpinella anisum (fruct.) [ANISEED]								x							x	
Pinus sylvestris (fol.) [PINE]		x	x									x		x		
Piper nigrum (fruct.) [BLACK PEPPER]													x			
Pogostemon patchouli (fol.) [PATCHOULI]					x		x									
Ravensara aromatica (fol.) [RAVENSARA]														x		
Rosa centifolia (flos), *R. damascena* [ROSE OTTO]														x		
Rosmarinus officinalis [ROSEMARY]			x	x								x	x	x		
Rosmarinus officinalis ct. verbenone [ROSEMARY]	x												x			
Salvia officinalis (fol.) [SAGE]	x	x					x		x				x	x		
Salvia sclarea [CLARY]	x													x		
Santalum album (lig.) [SANDALWOOD]																
Satureia hortensis (fol.) [SUMMER SAVORY]														x		
Satureia montana (fol.) [WINTER SAVORY]					x							x	x	x		
Styrax benzoin, S. tonkinensis [BENZOIN]																
Syzygium aromaticum (flos) [CLOVE BUD]			x		x	x						x		x		
Tagetes glandulifera (flos) [TAGETES]													x			
Thymus mastichina [SPANISH MARJORAM]																
Thymus satureioides [THYME]					x									x		
Thymus vulgaris (population) [THYME]			x			x						x		x		
Thymus vulgaris ct. alcohol [SWEET THYME]														x		x
Thymus vulgaris ct. phenol [RED THYME]			x											x		
Vetiveria zizanioides (rad.) [VETIVER]					x											
Zingiber officinale (rhiz.) [GINGER]													x			

General properties of essential oils *(cont'd)*

	Phlebotonic	Photosensitizer	Psychoactive	Radioprotective	Reproductive stimulant	Respiratory tonic	Rubefacient	Scalp tonic	Sedative, calming, soporific	Styptic, haemostatic, astringent	Sudorific	Tonic (general), energizing	Uterotonic	Vasodilator	Vermifuge, anthelmintic	Vulnerary, cicatrizant
Achillea millefolium [YARROW]																x
Boswellia carteri (res. dist.) [FRANKINCENSE]												x				x
Cananga odorata [YLANG YLANG]					x			x	x							
Carum carvi (fruct.) [CARAWAY]								x	x							
Cedrus atlantica (lig.) [ATLAS CEDARWOOD]								x								x
Chamaemelum nobile (flos) [ROMAN CHAMOMILE]									x		x	x				x
Chamomilla recutita (flos) [GERMAN CHAMOMILE]									x							x
Citrus aurantium var. *amara* (flos) [NEROLI BIGARADE]	x								x							
Citrus aurantium var. *amara* (fol.) [PETITGRAIN BIGARADE]									x				x			
Citrus aurantium var. *amara* (per.) [ORANGE BIGARADE]		x							x				x			
Citrus bergamia (per.) [BERGAMOT]		x							x							x
Citrus limon (per.) [LEMON]	x								x	x						
Citrus reticulata (per.) [MANDARIN]									x							
Coriandrum sativum (fruct.) [CORIANDER]			x													
Cupressus sempervirens (fol.) [CYPRESS]	x								x	x						
Eucalyptus globulus (fol.) [TASMANIAN BLUE GUM]							x									
Eucalyptus smithii (fol.) [GULLY GUM]									x							
Eucalyptus staigeriana (fol.) [LEMON SCENTED IRON TREE]									x							
Foeniculum vulgare var. *dulce* (fruct.) [FENNEL]						x										
Hyssopus officinalis [HYSSOP]									x	x		x			x	x
Juniperus communis (fruct.) [JUNIPER BERRY]									x							
Juniperus communis (ram.) [JUNIPER TWIG]																
Lavandula angustifolia [LAVENDER]									x			x				x
Lavandula × *intermedia* 'Super' [LAVANDIN]									x			x				
Melaleuca alternifolia (fol.) [TEA TREE]	x			x												
Melaleuca leucadendron (fol.) [CAJUPUT]	x			x							x					
Melaleuca viridiflora (fol.) [NIAOULI]	x			x								x				
Melissa officinalis (fol.) [MELISSA]									x					x		
Mentha × *piperita* (fol.) [PEPPERMINT]					x								x			
Myristica fragrans (sem.) [NUTMEG]			x									x	x			
Nardostachys jatamansi (rad.) [SPIKENARD]	x								x							
Nepeta cataria var. *citriodora* (fol.) [CATNEP]									x							
Ocimum basilicum (fol.) [BASIL]															x	
Origanum majorana (fol.) [MARJORAM]					x				x					x		
Ormenis mixta (flos) [MOROCCAN CHAMOMILE]					x								x			
Pelargonium graveolens (fol.) [GERANIUM]	x									x						x
Pimpinella anisum (fruct.) [ANISEED]			x	x	x				x				x			
Pinus sylvestris (fol.) [PINE]						x										
Piper nigrum (fruct.) [BLACK PEPPER]					x											
Pogostemon patchouli (fol.) [PATCHOULI]	x															x
Ravensara aromatica (fol.) [RAVENSARA]																
Rosa centifolia (flos), *R. damascena* [ROSE OTTO]					x					x		x				x
Rosmarinus officinalis [ROSEMARY]					x											x
Rosmarinus officinalis ct. verbenone [ROSEMARY]												x				x
Salvia officinalis (fol.) [SAGE]																x
Salvia sclarea [CLARY]	x								x							
Santalum album (lig.) [SANDALWOOD]					x				x			x				
Satureia hortensis (fol.) [SUMMER SAVORY]					x											
Satureia montana (fol.) [WINTER SAVORY]												x				x
Styrax benzoin, S. tonkinensis [BENZOIN]																
Syzygium aromaticum (flos) [CLOVE BUD]					x				x				x			x
Tagetes glandulifera (flos) [TAGETES]															x	
Thymus mastichina [SPANISH MARJORAM]																
Thymus satureioides [THYME]					x							x	x			
Thymus vulgaris (population) [THYME]					x						x				x	x
Thymus vulgaris ct. alcohol [SWEET THYME]					x								x			
Thymus vulgaris ct. phenol [RED THYME]		?										x				x
Vetiveria zizanioides (rad.) [VETIVER]																
Zingiber officinale (rhiz.) [GINGER]												x				

REFERENCES TO APPENDICES

Achterrath-Tuckerman U, Kunde R, Flaskamp O, Theimer I, Theimer K 1980 Pharmacological investigations with compounds of chamomile. V. Investigations on the spasmolytic effect of compounds of chamomile. Planta Medica, Stuttgart 39: 38–50

Åkesson H O, Wälinder J 1965 Nutmeg intoxication. Lancet i: 1271

Bassett I B, Pannowitz D L, Barmetson R St C 1990 A comparative study of tea tree oil versus benzoyl peroxide in the treatment of acne. Medical Journal of Australia 153: 455–458

Belaiche P 1979 Traité de phytothérapie et d'aromathérapie. Maloine, Paris

Buckle J 1993 Does it matter which lavender essential oil is used? Nursing Times 89(20): 32–35

Bunny S (ed.) 1984 Illustrated book of herbs. Octopus, London

Burkhill J H 1966 A dictionary of the economic products of the Malay Peninsula. Art Printing Works, Kuala Lumpur

Corbier B, Teisseire P 1974 Contribution to the knowledge of neroli oil from Grasse. Recherches 19: 289–290

Dale H H 1909 Nutmeg. Society of experimental biology. New York 23: 69

Draize J H 1959 Dermal toxicity. In: Appraisal of the safety of chemicals in foods, drugs and cosmetics. Association of Food and Drug Officials of the United States, Austin, p. 52

Duke J A 1985 Handbook of medicinal herbs. CRC Press, Boca Raton

Duraffourd P 1982 En forme tous les jours. La Vie Claire, Périgny

Duthie H L 1981 The effect of peppermint oil on colonic motility in man. British Journal of Surgery 68: 820

Emboden W A Jr 1972 Narcotic plants. Macmillan, New York

Forbes P D, Urbach F, Davies R E 1977 Phototoxicity testing of fragrance raw materials. Food and Cosmetics Toxicology 15: 55–60

Ford R A, Letizia C S, Api A M 1988 Tea tree oil. Food and Chemical Toxicology 26(4): 407

Ford R A, Api A M, Letizia C S 1992a Petitgrain bigarade oil. Food and Chemical Toxicology 30 (supplement): 101S

Ford R A, Api A M, Letizia C S 1992b Mandarin oil. Food and Chemical Toxicology 30 (supplement): 69S

Foster S 1991 *Chamomile, Matricaria recutita* and *Chamaemelum nobile*. Botanical Series no. 307, American Botanical Council, Austin

Foster S 1993a Chamomile. The Herb Companion December /January: 64–68

Foster S 1993b Herbal renaissance. Gibbs Smith, Layton

Franchomme P, Pénoël D 1990 L'aromathérapie exactement. Jollois, Limoges

Fujii T, Furukawa S, Suzuki S 1972 Studies on compounded perfumes for toilet goods: On the non-irritative compounded perfumes for soaps. Yukugaku 21(12): 904–908

Garg S C 1974 Antifungal effects of *Boswellia serrata* leaf oil. Indian Journal of Pharmacy 36: 46

Goodman L, Golman A 1942 The pharmacological basis of therapeutics. Macmillan, New York

Habersang S, Leuschner O, Theimer I, Theimer K 1979 Pharmacological studies of chamomile constituents. IV. Studies on the toxicity of (-)-α-bisabolol. Planta Medica 35: 118–124

Harry R G 1948 Cosmetic materials. vol. 2. Hill, London

Hartwell J L 1971 Plants used against cancer: a survey. Lloydia 30

Hausen B M, Busker E, Carle R 1984 The sensitizing capacity of Compositae plants. VII. Experimental investigations with extracts and compounds of *Chamomilla recutita* (L.) Rauschert and *Anthemis cotula* (L.). Planta medica 229–234

Isaac O 1979 Pharmakologische Untersuchungen von Kamillen-Inhaltsstoffen I. Zur Pharmakologie des (-)-α-bisabolols und der Bisabololoxide (Übersicht). Planta Medica 35: 118–124

Jakovlev V et al 1979 Pharmacological investigations with compounds of chamomile. II. New investigations on the antiphlogistic effects of (-)-α-bisabolol and bisabolol oxides. Planta Medica 35: 125–140

Lawrence B M 1977 Progress in essential oils. Perfumer & Flavorist February/March 2(1): 3

Lawrence B M 1984 Progress in essential oils. Perfumer & Flavorist August/September 9(4): 37

Lawrence B M 1989a Essential oils 1981–1987. Allured, Wheaton

Lawrence B M 1989b Progress in essential oils. Perfumer & Flavorist 14(3): 71

Leung A Y 1980 Encyclopedia of common natural ingredients used in foods, drugs and cosmetics. Wiley, New York

List P H, Horhammer L 1969–1979 Hagers Handbuch der pharmazeutischen Praxis. Springer-Verlag, Berlin

Loveman A B 1938 Stomatitis venenata: report of a case of sensitivity of the mucous membranes and the skin to oil of anise. Archiva Dermatologica 38: 906

Löwenfeld W 1932 Ekzematose Überempfindlichkeit gegen Eukalyptusöl. Dermatologie Wochenschrift 95: 1281

Mabey R (ed.) 1988 The complete new herbal. Elm Tree Books, London

Maruzella J C, Sicurella N A 1960 Antibacterial acivity of essential oil vapours. Journal of American Pharmaceutical Association 49: 692

Marzulli F N, Maibach H I 1970 Perfume phototoxicity. Journal of the Society of Cosmetic Chemists 21: 695

Mills S Y 1991 The essential book of herbal medicine. Penguin Arkana, Harmondsworth

Mitchell J C, Rook A 1979 Botanical dermatology. Greenglass, Vancouver

Morton J F 1981 Atlas of medicinal plants of Middle America. Thomas, Springfield

Murray F A 1921 Dermatitis caused by bitter orange. British Medical Journal 1: 739

Musajo L, Rodighiero G, Caporale G 1953 The photodynamic activity of the natural coumarins. Chimica Industria Milan 35: 13–15

Musajo L, Rodighiero G, Caporale G 1954 The photodynamic activity of the natural coumarins. Bulletin Société de Chimie et Biologie 36: 1213–1224

Nano G M, Sacco T, Frattini C 1974 Botanical and chemical research on *Anthemis nobilis* L. and some of its cultivars. Paper no. 114, Sixth International Essential Oil Congress, San Francisco

Ognyanov I 1984 Bulgarian lavender and Bulgarian lavender oil. Perfumer & Flavorist 8(6): 29–41

Opdyke D L J 1973 In: Food and Cosmetics Toxicology 11

Opdyke D L J 1974 In: Food and Cosmetics Toxicology 12. Special issue I: Monographs on fragrance raw materials

Opdyke D L J 1975 In: Food and Cosmetics Toxicology 13. Special issue II: Monographs on fragrance raw materials

Opdyke D L J 1976 In: Food and Cosmetics Toxicology 14. Special issue III: Monographs on fragrance raw materials

Opdyke D L J 1978 In: Food and Cosmetics Toxicology 16. Special issue IV: Monographs on fragrance raw materials

Opdyke D L J, Letizia C 1982a Patchouly oil. Food and Chemical Toxicology 20 (supplement): 791

Opdyke D L J, Letizia C 1982 Clary oil. In: Food and Chemical Toxicology 20 (supplement): 823

Pathak M A, Fitzpatrick T B 1959 Relation of molecular configuration to the furocoumarins which increase the cutaneous responses following long wave ultraviolet radiation. Journal of Investigative Dermatology 32: 255–262

Pénoël D 1993 A special eucalyptus (*E. smithii*). The Aromatherapist 1(2): insert

Pénoël D 1994 A staple essential oil: presentation of a new eucalyptus oil—*Eucalyptus staigeriana*—for aromatherapists. The Aromatherapist 1(3): 22–27

Perry L M 1980 Medicinal plants of East and Southeast Asia. MIT Press, Cambridge, Mass., p. 620

Peterson H R, Hall A 1946 Dermal irritating properties of perfume materials. Drug and Cosmetic Industry, January 58: 113

Phillips H F 1989 What thyme is it? A guide to the thyme taxa cultivated in the United States. In: Simon J E (ed.) Proceedings of the fourth national herb growing and marketing conference. International Herb Growers and Marketers Association, Silver Spring

Phillips H F 1991 The best of thymes. The Herb Companion April /May: 22–29

Prager M J, Miskiewicz M A 1979 Gas chromatographic-mass spectrometric analysis, identification and detection of adulteration of lavender, lavandin and spike lavender oils. J A O A C 62: 1231–1238

Prakash V 1990 Leafy spices. CRC Press, Boca Raton

Price S 1993 The aromatherapy workbook. Thorsons, London

Rao B G V N, Joseph P L 1971 Die Wirksamt einiger ätherischer Öle gegenüber phytopathogenen Fungi. Riechstoffe Aromatische 21: 405

Reichling J, Becker H, Drager P-D 1978 Herbicides in chamomile cultivation. Acta Horticultiva 73: 331–338

Roulier G 1990 Les huiles essentielles pour votre santé. Dangles, St-Jean-de-Braye

Schwarz L 1934 Skin hazards in American industry. Part 1. US Publication Health Bulletin no. 215

Schwarz L, Peck S M 1946 Cosmetics and dermatitis. Hoeber, New York

Schwarz L, Tulipan L, Peck S M 1947 Occupational diseases of the skin. Lea and Febiger, Philadelphia

Secondini O 1990 Handbook of perfumes and flavors. Chemical Publishing, New York

Shu C K, Waradt J P, Taylor W I 1975 Improved methods for bergapten determination by high performance liquid chromatography. Journal of Chromatography 106: 271–282

Sigmund C J, MacNally E F 1969 The action of a carminative on the lower oesophageal sphincter. Gastroenterology 56: 13–18

Stevenson C J 1994 The psychophysiological effects of aromatherapy massage following cardiac surgery. Complementary Therapies in Medicine 2: 27–35

Szelenyi I et al 1979 Pharmacological investigations with compounds of chamomile. III. Experimental studies of the ulcerprotective effect of chamomile. Planta Medica 35: 218–227

Taylor B D, Luscombe D K, Duthie H L 1983 Inhibitory effect of peppermint oil on gastrointestinal smooth muscle. Gut 24: 992

Tester-Dalderup C B M 1980 Drugs used in bronchial asthma and cough. In: Dukes M N G (ed.) Meyler's side effects of drugs, 9th edn. Excerpta Medica, Amsterdam

Trease G E, Evans W C 1983 Pharmacognosy, 13th edn. Baillière Tindall, Eastbourne

Tulipan L 1938 Cosmetic irritants. Archiva Dermatologica 38: 906

Tyler V E 1982 The honest herbal: a sensible guide to the use of herbs and related remedies. Stickley, Philadelphia

Tyler V E 1992 Phytomedicines in Western Europe: their potential impact on herbal medicine in the United States. Lecture delivered at the annual meeting of the American Chemical Society, San Francisco, April

Valnet J 1980 The practice of aromatherapy. Daniel, Saffron Walden

Vömel A, Reichling J, Becker H, Dräger P D 1977 Herbicides in the cultivation of *Matricaria chamomilla*. 1st Communication: Influence of herbicides on flower and weed production. Planta Medica 31: 378–379

Wagner H, Bladt S, Zgainski E M 1984 Plant drug analysis. Springer-Verlag, Berlin p. 13

Weiss R F 1988 Herbal medicine. Beaconsfield Publishers, Beaconsfield

Winter R 1984 A consumer's dictionary of cosmetic ingredients. Crown, New York

Woeber K, Krombach M 1969 Zur Frage der Sensibilisierung durch Ätherische Öle (Vorläufige Mitteilung). Berufsdermatosen 17: 320

Wren R C (ed.) 1988 Potter's new cyclopedia of botanical drugs and preparations, 8th ed. Daniel, Saffron Walden

Zheng G Q, Kenney P M, Lam K K T 1992 Anethofuran, carvone and limonene: potential cancer chemopreventative agents from dill weed oil and caraway oil. Planta Medica 58: 338–341

SOURCES

Agnel R, Teisseire P 1984 Essential oil of French lavender: its composition and its adulteration. Perfumer & Flavorist 9(2) 53–56

Alberto-Puleo M 1980 Fennel and anise as estrogenic agents. Journal of Ethnopharmacology 2(4): 337–344

Arctander S 1960 Perfume and flavor materials of natural origin. Published by the author, Elizabeth, NJ

Bardeau F 1976 La médecine aromatique. Robert Laffont, Paris

Becker H, Förster W 1984 Biologie, Chemie und Pharmakologie pflanzlicher Sedativa. Zeitschrift für Phytotherapie, Stuttgart 5: 817–823

Benigni R, Capra C, Cattorini P E 1962 Piante medicinali: chimica farmacologia e terapia. Inverni & Della Beffa, Milan

Bernadet M 1983 La phyto-aromathérapie pratique. Dangles, St-Jean-de-Braye

British Herbal Pharmacopoeia 1983 British Herbal Medicine Association, Cowling

Chandler R F, Hooper S N, Harvey M J 1982 Ethnobotany and phytochemistry of yarrow, *Achillea millefolium*, Compositae. Economic Botany 36(2): 203–223

Council of Scientific and Industrial Research 1948–1976 The Wealth of India, 11 vols. New Delhi

Denny E F K 1981 The history of lavender oil: disturbing inferences for the future of essential oils. Perfumer & Flavorist 6: 23–25

De Vincenzi M, Dessi M R 1991 Botanical flavouring substances used in foods: proposal of classification. Fitoterapia 62(1): 39–63

Duraffourd P 1987 Les huiles essentielles et la santé. La Maison de Bien-Etre, Montreuil-sous-Bois

Forster H B, Niklas H, Lutz S 1980 Planta Medica 40(4): 309

Franchomme P, Pénoël D 1985 Aromatherapy: advanced therapy for infectious illnesses (1). Phytoguide no. 1, International Phytomedical Foundation, La Courtête

Gattefossé R-M 1937 Aromathérapie. Girardot, Paris. (English trans. 1993 Daniel, Saffron Walden)

Guenther E 1949 The essential oils, 6 Vols. Van Nostrand, New York

Gümbel D 1986 Principles of holistic skin therapy with herbal essences. Haug, Heidelberg

Harkiss K J 1993 Eight peak index of essential oils, version 2.2. Published by the author, Bingley

Herrmann E C, Kucera L S 1967 Proceedings of the Society of Experimental Biology and Medicine 124: 865

Hoffman W 1979 Lavendel-Inhaltsstoffe und ausgewählte Synthesen. Seifen-Öle-Fette-Wachse 105: 287–291

Huang T C, Liu P K, Chang C F, Chou, Tseng H L 1981 Study of antiasthmatic constituents in *Ocimum basilicum* Benth. Yao Hsueh T'ung Pao 16(4): 56

International Fragrance Association 1992 Code of practice. IFA, Geneva

Lautié R, Passebecq A 1979 Aromatherapy. Thorsons, Wellingborough

Law D 1982 The concise herbal encyclopedia. Bartholomew, Edinburgh

Lawrence B M 1979 Essential oils 1976-1978. Allured, Wheaton

Lawrence B M 1981 Essential oils 1979-1980. Allured, Wheaton

Lawrence B M 1987/1988 Progress in Essential Oils. Perfumer & Flavorist 12 (6): 59

Lawrence B M 1993 Essential oils 1988–1991. Allured, Wheaton

Mailhebiau P 1989 La nouvelle aromathérapie. Vie Nouvelle, Toulouse

Melegari M et al 1988 Chemical characteristics and pharmacological properties of the essential oils of *Anthemis nobilis*. Fitoterapia, Milan 59(6): 449–455

Opdyke D L J (ed.) 1979 Monographs on fragrance raw materials. Pergamon Press, Oxford

Pénoël D, Pénoël R-M 1992 Pratique aromatique familiale. Osmobiose, Aoûste

Perry L M 1980 Medicinal plants of East and Southeast Asia. MIT Press, Cambridge

Price S 1993 The aromatherapy workbook. Thorsons, London

Renz-Rathfelder S 1986 Vom Duft der Pflanzen. Palmengarten, Frankfurt

Reynolds J E F (ed.) 1993 Martindale: the extra pharmacopoeia, 30th edn. The Pharmaceutical Press, London

Salamon I 1992 Chamomile production in Czecho-Slovakia. Focus on Herbs 10: 1–8

San Martin R, Granger R, Adzet T, Passer J, Tevlade-Arbousset M G 1973 Chemical polymorphism in two Mediterranean labiates, *Satureia montana* L. and *Satureia obovata* Lag. Plantes Médicinales et Phytothérapie 7: 95

Stewart M 1987 The encyclopedia of herbs and herbalism. Black Cat, London

Tucker A O, Tucker S S 1988 Catnip and the catnip response. Economic Botany 42(2): 214–231

Viaud H 1983 Huiles essentielles: hydrolats. Présence, Sisteron

Glossary

abortifacient: inducing an abortion; causing expulsion of the foetus

adaptogenic: having a positive general effect on the body irrespective of disease condition, especially under stress

alcohols: group of hydrocarbon compounds frequently found in volatile oils

aldehydes: class of organic compounds standing between alcohols and acids

allopathy: system of medicine which uses drugs with effects opposite to the symptoms produced by the disease (in contrast to homoeopathy)

amenorrhoea: absence of menstruation outside pregnancy in premenopausal women

anaphrodisiac: of a drug, diminishing sexual drive

anodyne: relieving pain; analgesic

anthelmintic: destructive of intestinal worms

antiphlogistic: counteracting inflammation or fever; antipyretic

antithermic: cooling; antipyretic

antitussive: relieving or preventing coughing

anxiolytic: relieving anxiety and tension

aperient: mildly laxative

aperitive: stimulating the appetite

aromatic: organic chemical compound derived from benzene; also called aromatic compound

astringent: causing contraction of living tissues (often mucous membranes), reducing haemorrhages, secretions, diarrhoea etc.

balneotherapy: treatment by medicinal baths

bitters: botanical drugs with bitter-tasting constituents used to stimulate the gastrointestinal tract; also used as antiinflammatory agents and as relaxants

calmative: mildly sedative

cardiotonic: having a tonic effect on the heart

carminative: relieving flatulence

cathartic: strongly laxative

chemotype: visually identical plants with significantly different chemical components, resulting in different therapeutic properties; abbreviated to ct. as in *Thymus vulgaris* ct. alcohol

cholagogic: stimulating gallbladder contraction to promote the flow of bile

choleretic: stimulating the production of bile in the liver

cicatrizant: promoting formation of scar tissue and healing

coumarin: a chemical compound, $C_9H_6O_2$, with a high boiling point (290ºC) found within the lactones; hardly volatile with steam thus found mainly in expressed oils and sparingly in some distilled essential oils; characteristic smell of new-mown hay

cultivar: *culti*vated *variety*: a plant produced by horticulture or agriculture not normally occurring naturally; labelled by adding a 'name' to the species as in *Lavandula angustifolia* 'Maillette'

depurative: purifying or cleansing

diaphoretic: causing or increasing perspiration; sudorific

digestive: aiding digestion

dysmenorrhoea: painful or difficult menstruation

dyspepsia: disturbed digestion

emmenagogic: inducing or regularizing menstruation; euphemism for abortifacient

erethism: abnormal irritability or sensitivity

essential oil: plant volatile oil obtained by distillation

eubiotic: brings about conditions favourable to life and healing

eupeptic: aiding digestion

febrifuge: agent which reduces temperature; antipyretic

fixed oil: nonvolatile oil; plant oils consist of esters of fatty acids, usually triglycerides

forma: lowest botanical rank in general use, denoting trivial differences within a species

fruit: the ripe seeds and their surrounding structures, which can be fleshy or dry

galactagogic: promoting the secretion of milk; lactogenic

genus: important botanical classification of related but distinct species given a common name; genera (pl.) are in turn grouped into families; the first word of the binomial botanical name denotes the genus

glycoside: sugar-derivative found in certain plants (e.g. digoxin, used to treat heart failure)

haemostatic: checking blood flow

hallucinogen: agent affecting any or all of the senses, producing a wide range of distorted perceptions and reactions

herb: non-woody soft leafy plant; plant used in medicine and cooking

homoeopathy: system of medicine using tiny amounts of drugs which would produce in a healthy body symptoms similar to those of the disease (as distinct from allopathy)

hybrid: natural or manmade plant produced by the fertilization of one species by another; indicated by × as in *Mentha × piperita*

hypermenorrhoea: profuse or prolonged menses

hypertensor: increasing blood pressure; pressor

hypotensor: reducing blood pressure; antihypertensive

immunostimulant: stimulating the immune system

lactogenic: promoting the secretion of milk

laxative: loosening the bowel contents, promoting evacuation

lipid: a fat or fat-like substance insoluble in water and soluble in fat solvents

lipolytic: breaking down fat

lipophilic: having strong affinity for lipids

maceration: the extraction of substances from a plant by steeping in a fixed oil

menorrhagia: excessive periods

metrorrhagia: uterine haemorrhage occurring outside menstrual periods

narcotic: inducing insensibility (sleep) and relieving pain in small dose, toxic in high dose

oestrogenic: simulating the action of female hormones

officinalis: used in medicine; recognized in the pharmacopoeia

organic: grown without the use of chemical fertilizers, pesticides, etc.

organoleptic: concerned with testing the effects of a substance on the senses, particularly taste and smell

percutaneous: applied through the skin

pharmacokinetics: study of absorption, distribution, metabolism and elimination of drugs

photosensitization: abnormally increased sensitivity of the skin to ultraviolet radiation or natural sunlight; can follow ingestion of or contact with various substances

phytotherapy: treatment of disease by the use of plants and plant extracts; herbalism

polymenorrhea: unusually short menstrual cycles

probiotic: favouring the beneficial bacteria in the body, while inhibiting harmful microbes; literally 'for life' as distinct from antibiotic, 'against life'

prophylactic: preventing disease

psychopharmaceutical: pertaining to drugs affecting the mind or mood

psychotropic: of a drug, affecting the brain and influencing behaviour

purgative: strongly laxative

rhizome: underground stem bearing roots, scales and nodes

rubefacient: increasing local blood circulation causing redness of the skin

spasmolytic: relieving convulsions, spasmodic pains and cramp

stomachic: agent which stimulates the secretory activity of the stomach

styptic: arresting haemorrhage by means of an astringent quality; haemostatic

subspecies: subdivision of a species, often denoting a geographic variation; structure or colour are peculiar to subspecies and are more definite than characteristics identifying varieties; subspecies can interbreed; abbreviated to subsp.

sudorific: inducing sweating

synergy: increased effect of two or more medicinal substances working together

taxonomy: scientific classification of living things

thymoleptic: antiseptic

tonic: producing or restoring normal vigour or tension (tone)

trichome: hairlike structure on the epidermis of a plant

variety: indicates a botanical rank between subspecies and forma; abbreviated to var. as in *Citrus aurantium* var. *amara*

vermifugal: expelling intestinal worms

vesicant: producing blisters (therapeutically, to induce counter-irritant serosity)

vulnerary: agent promoting healing of wounds

Useful addresses

GREAT BRITAIN

Supplies

For list of suppliers of aromatherapy products (essential oils, diffusers, cream and lotion bases etc.):

Aromatherapy Trades Council
PO Box 38
Romford
Essex RM1 2DN
Tel: 01702 390625

Members include:

Shirley Price Aromatherapy Ltd
Essentia House
Upper Bond Street
Hinckley
Leics LE10 1RS
Tel: 01455 615466
Fax: 01455 615054

Also:

Herbal Garden
20 Eldon Gardens
Percy Street
Newcastle upon Tyne
Tyne & Wear NE1 7RA
Tel: 0191-230-3126

Preston Health Food Stores
Guildhall Street
Preston
Lancs

Aromatology/Aromatherapy Associations

For lists of accredited training organisations and registered therapists, send an A5 s.a.e. to:

Aromatherapy Organizations Council
3 Latymer Close
Braybrooke
Market Harborough
Leicestershire
LE16 8LN
Tel: 01858 434242

Members include:

Shirley Price Aromatherapy Ltd.
Essential House
Upper Bond Street
Hinckley
Leics.
LE10 1RS
Tel: 01455 615466

Aromatology Association
23 Magdalen Road
Tetbury
Gloucestershire
GL8 8LG

WORLDWIDE

Aromatherapy training and essential oils

Australia

Margaret Tozer
PO Box 187
Montrose 3765
Victoria
Australia
Tel: 03 9 723 2531
       03 9 723 2509

Germany

Forum Essenzia
Panoramastr 17
87477 Sulzberg-Moosbach
Germany
Tel: (49) 8376 8591

Northern Ireland

Mary Thompson
European College of Natural Therapies
16 North Parade
Belfast
Northern Ireland BT7 2GG
Tel: 01232 641454

Republic of Ireland

Mary Cavanagh
Chamomile
Three Mile Water
Wicklow
Eire
Tel: (353) 404 47319

South Africa

Lucile Bischoff
PO Box 743
Gallo Manor
South Africa 2052
Tel: (27) 11 804 2365

Switzerland

VEROMA
Alte Gasse 19
C11-6390 Engelberg
Switzerland
Tel: (41) 94 2040

Sara Gelzer
Eigentalstr 552, No. 14
8425 Oberembrach
Switzerland
Tel: (41) 1865 4996

USA

Bonne Santé
462 62nd Street
Brooklyn
NY 1120
USA
Tel: (1) 718 492 9514

Margot Latimer
PO Box 65
Pineville
PA 18946
USA
Tel: (1) 215 598 3802

Index